New Developments in Medical Research

nova
Medicine & Health
New York

New Developments in Medical Research

Leptin and its Role in Health and Disease
Stephen E. Bradley (Editor)
2023. ISBN: 979-8-89113-274-0 (Softcover)
2023. ISBN: 979-8-89113-334-1 (eBook)

Inflammation and Chronic Disorders: The Secret Connection
Ashwani K. Dhingra, PhD (Editor)
Priyanka Kriplani, PhD (Editor)
Bhawna Chopra, PhD (Editor)
Ajmer Singh Grewal, PhD (Editor)
Geeta Deswal, PhD (Editor)
Peeyush Kaushik, M. Pharm (Editor)
2023. ISBN: 979-8-88697-980-0 (eBook)

Antidiabetic Plants: Properties and Applications
Arpita Roy, PhD (Editor)
2023. ISBN: 979-8-88697-957-2 (Hardcover)
2023. ISBN: 979-8-88697-982-4 (eBook)

The Dangers of Psychoactive Substances
Denise J. Burton (Editor)
2023. ISBN: 979-8-88697-705-9 (Softcover)
2023. ISBN: 979-8-88697-712-7 (eBook)

An Innovative Program at Alfaisal Medicine: A Brief History and Guide to Success
Paul Ganguly, MBBS, MD, FACA (Editor)
2023. ISBN: 979-8-88697-638-0 (Softcover)
2023. ISBN: 979-8-88697-703-5 (eBook)

More information about this series can be found at
https://novapublishers.com/product-category/series/new-developments-in-medical-research/

Nazan Yurtcu
Emel Güler
Editors

Current Clinical Recommendations and Applications for the Uses of Platelet Rich Plasma

nova
Medicine & Health
New York

DOI: https://doi.org/10.52305/DCWZ2342

Library of Congress Cataloging-in-Publication Data

ISBN: 979-8-89113-723-3 (hardcover)
ISBN: 979-8-89113-726-4 (e-book)

Published by Nova Science Publishers, Inc. † New York

Contents

Preface

This first edition of Current Clinical Recommendations and Application for Use of Platelet Rich Plasma is written by many of the leading scientists and clinicians who have been responsible for the dramatic progress in platelet rich plasma use. The purpose of the book is to deal with all aspects of its usage areas. The authors have met the expectation that practice guidelines be based either on convincing available evidence or on consensus statements of authoritative organizations. The book will be useful for dermatologists, obstetricians, urologists, orthopedics, physical therapy, and rehabilitation specialists.

Chapter 1 - In this section of the book, the definition of Platelet Rich Plasma (PRP) and its subtypes of platelet concentrates (PC) are discussed, along with the preparation stages of these subtypes and PRP. Towards the end of the section, a summary of the preparation stages of PRP and its subtypes described in some articles is provided in a table. There have been various approaches to the preparation of PRP and its subtypes. These procedures differ in terms of centrifuge speed and duration, the use of anticoagulants and activators, and other factors.

Chapter 2 - In recent years, there has been a significant increase in the use of platelet-rich plasma (PRP) in all medical branches, especially in the Orthopedics and Traumatology departments. Due to its compatibility with the biological structure of the body, low adverse reactions have made PRP attractive in musculoskeletal pathologies. PRP is promising as an alternative to surgical treatment by stimulating curative-enhancing pathways and suppressing inflammation. Although its use in the future is exciting, consistent results have not been achieved in studies so far, and it is not possible to talk about a common treatment algorithm. When the results of the current literature are evaluated, it cannot be said that the use of PRP in surgical and non-surgical shoulder pathologies can be supported or rejected. Although poorly reported, cost-benefit analyses of the use of PRP in rotator cuff repairs show that it does not cover the cost. For this reason, studies with a large standardized patient group are required to better understand the effectiveness and negative consequences of PRP use in shoulder pathologies.

Chapter 3 - Platelet-rich plasma (PRP) is one of the treatment options in the field of regenerative medicine. It aims to enhance the tissue repair process through the local administration of autologous bioactive agents to influence critical physiological mechanisms such as inflammation, angiogenesis, or extracellular matrix synthesis. The use of PRP and its derivatives in the treatment of musculoskeletal system injuries is increasing rapidly. Although promising results are observed especially in preclinical studies, there are highly controversial results in clinical trials. The content of platelet-rich plasma and differences in the techniques of its application make it difficult to report homogeneous results in clinical trials. In addition, changing both the time and content of PRP application according to the stage of the specific disease whose treatment is targeted is a candidate to be the subject of study in the near future. In the current review, findings on the efficacy of PRP and its derivatives in various musculoskeletal system diseases are presented under the guidance of current literature information presented with strong evidence.

Chapter 4 - Platelet-rich plasma (PRP) has gained recognition as a valuable treatment option in orthopedic medicine for accelerating tissue repair. This chapter focuses on the use of PRP in the treatment of hip disorders, including hip osteoarthritis, avascular necrosis of the femoral head, hamstring tendinopathy, adductor tendinopathy, and muscle strains around the hip. PRP is derived from the patient's own blood and contains various growth factors and bioactive molecules that promote tissue regeneration. In hip osteoarthritis, PRP injections have shown promising results in improving functional scores compared to traditional treatments, although no significant structural changes have been observed. In avascular necrosis of the femoral head, PRP has been used both as a nonsurgical injection and as an adjuvant in surgical procedures, demonstrating positive outcomes in select cases. For hamstring and adductor tendinopathies, PRP injections have yielded positive outcomes, reducing pain intensity and facilitating a faster return to activity. Additionally, PRP has shown promise in the treatment of adductor and hamstring tendinopathy, exhibiting a reduction in the size of the lesion and improved functional outcomes. Moreover, PRP has been used in the treatment of muscle strains around the hip. While PRP offers advantages such as simplicity and safety, image-guided methods are often required for accurate administration. Although the use of PRP in other hip-related conditions is limited to case reports and small studies, it presents a promising avenue for future research and clinical applications.

Chapter 5 - Avascular necrosis is the necrosis of bone tissue that can be due to many reasons. Today, a clear treatment algorithm has not been established yet. Platelet-rich plasma therapy is a method that has been widely used in regenerative medicine. Considering the mechanisms of action, it emerges as a method that can affect the histopathological changes due to avascular necrosis and ensure the appropriate differentiation of mesenchymal cells in the environment. Although the information in our literature is limited, the results are quite promising.

Chapter 6 - Lateral epicondylitis (LE), also termed tennis elbow, is a tendonitis of the extensor carpi radialis brevis (ECRB) muscle. Involvement of the extensor carpi radialis longus and the extensor carpi ulnaris may also be observed. Its incidence in society is between 1% and 3%. Medial epicondylitis (ME), also known as golfer's elbow, occurs as a result of microtrauma and degeneration of the forearm flexor muscles at the common insertion point in the medial epicondyle of the elbow, which is similar to LE. It occurs between the fourth and sixth decades of life and affects both males and females equally.

Elbow epicondylitis is associated with excessive use combined with repetitive wrist flexion, extension, supination, and pronation movements. There are many treatment options for lateral and medial epicondylitis. The first choice is usually conservative treatment, and success is often achieved. Commonly used treatments include rest, activity modification, nonsteroidal anti-inflammatory drugs (NSAIDs), physiotherapy, injections (corticosteroids, platelet-rich plasma, prolotherapy), and orthotics. Surgical treatment can also be implemented in resistant cases.

Chapter 7 - Achilles Tendinopathy is a common foot and ankle condition that cannot be easily treated. More than one treatment modality for the cure has been tried, such as physiotherapy, immobilization, injections, shockwave therapy, and surgical intervention. Among these treatments, injections, especially Platelet-Rich Plasma (PRP) treatment, are frequently used. It is obtained after centrifugation of blood and has a highly concentrated platelet content compared to plasma. Platelets are a natural human body product and have an important role in the clotting cascade, promoting the healing process of inflammatory tissue. Because PRP contains recovery speed-up autologous materials such as some cytokines and growth factors, it has recently become more popular in orthopedic practice, especially in the treatment of tendon injuries. Platelet-rich plasma (PRP) injections have been studied since the

1970s and are widely used for tendinopathies. More than a dozen studies have been conducted in recent years to assess the effectiveness of the Platelet-rich plasma injection method for Achilles tendon problems. However, there was still controversy about whether PRP injection had a beneficial effect on Achilles tendinopathy and other tendinopathies. On the other hand, many articles in the literature support the success of the treatment and the positive impact of PRP on Achilles tendinopathy.

Chapter 8 - Achilles Tendinopathy is a common foot and ankle condition that cannot be easily treated. More than one treatment modality for the cure has been tried, such as physiotherapy, immobilization, injections, shockwave therapy, and surgical intervention. Among these treatments, injections, especially Platelet-Rich Plasma (PRP) treatment, are frequently used. It is obtained after centrifugation of blood and has a highly concentrated platelet content compared to plasma. Platelets are a natural human body product and have an important role in the clotting cascade, promoting the healing process of inflammatory tissue. Because PRP contains recovery speed-up autologous materials such as some cytokines and growth factors, it has recently become more popular in orthopedic practice, especially in the treatment of tendon injuries. Platelet-rich plasma (PRP) injections have been studied since the 1970s and are widely used for tendinopathies. More than a dozen studies have been conducted in recent years to assess the effectiveness of the Platelet-rich plasma injection method for Achilles tendon problems. However, there was still controversy about whether PRP injection had a beneficial effect on Achilles tendinopathy and other tendinopathies. On the other hand, many articles in the literature support the success of the treatment and the positive impact of PRP on Achilles tendinopathy.

Chapter 9 - Platelet-rich plasma (PRP) has been actively practiced in treatment for the last 30 years because of the indication of its effect on the healing process of tissue and nerve damage. PRP has shown an effective role in the healing process of nerve damage by accelerating axonal regeneration. The mechanism of action occurs through the effect of regulating inflammation and increasing the angiogenesis and growth factors released from alpha granulations of platelets, especially axonal regeneration, such as platelet-derived growth factor (PDGF), vascular endothelial growth factor (VEGF), transforming growth factor-beta (TGF-β), epidermal growth factor (EGF), and insulin-like growth factor (IGF). Platelets and growth factors physiologically released from platelets have an important role in the healing processes of nerve damage. Therefore, it has been considered that it might be useful to apply PRP to the area of nerve damage. Hence, PRP has been practiced in cases where neuronal damage is observed, such as nerve injuries, nerve damage as the reason for crushing, carpal tunnel syndrome, and polyneuropathy in treatment. While there are studies indicating that PRP is effective in these diseases, there are also in vitro, animal, and clinical testing indicating that it has no effect. Therefore, there is a need for more studies evaluating the efficiency of PRP in nerve damage.

Chapter 10 - Diabetes mellitus is a metabolic and chronic disease caused by the combination of a sedentary lifestyle and genetic factors. Increasing life expectancy, the increase in the elderly population, and the fight against diabetes and its complications are becoming important social problems. Despite known debridement, antibiotherapy, and surgical approaches, amputations due to diabetic foot threaten human health and cause an increase in the resources allocated by the states to health. Therefore, there is a need for new treatment approaches besides known and established treatments. Platelet-rich plasma (PRP) treatments, which are encouraging right now, have given satisfactory results in the treatment of patients with diabetic foot. The isolated and combined development of ischemic and neurological processes on different grounds from patient to patient in the formation of diabetic ulcer complicates a single treatment approach. With the understanding that there is no disease, there is a patient, a detailed examination of each patient, and a detailed examination of the formation of the diabetic foot appear to be effective in the wound healing of PRP, which is started on an appropriate basis, and in preventing the loss of limb of the patient. For this treatment to become widespread, it needs to be tested in larger populations and a timeline of proven literature.

Chapter 11 - Diabetes mellitus is a metabolic and chronic disease caused by the combination of a sedentary lifestyle and genetic factors. Increasing life expectancy, the increase in the elderly population, and the fight against diabetes and its complications are becoming important social problems. Despite known debridement, antibiotherapy, and surgical approaches, amputations due to diabetic foot threaten human health and cause an increase in the resources allocated by the states to health. Therefore, there is a need for new treatment approaches besides known and established treatments. Platelet-rich plasma (PRP) treatments, which are encouraging right now, have given satisfactory results in the treatment of patients with diabetic foot. The isolated and combined development of ischemic and neurological processes on different grounds from patient to patient in the formation of diabetic ulcer complicates a single treatment approach. With the understanding that there is no disease, there is a patient, a detailed examination of each patient, and a detailed examination of the formation of the diabetic foot appear to be effective in the wound healing of PRP, which is started on an appropriate basis, and in preventing the loss of limb of the patient. For this treatment to become widespread, it needs to be tested in larger populations and a timeline of proven literature.

Chapter 12 - Platelet concentrates collected from the patient's blood were first presented over 20 years ago. The aim of this technique was to collect the maximum number of platelets and growth factors and implement them during surgery. This relatively "new" regenerative method could surely be applied to various clinical procedures in dentistry with favorable results and low risks. The PRF membrane helps in the wound healing process, protecting the surgical area and stimulating soft tissue repair. When PRF is mixed with bone graft, it may attract stem cells and provide neo-angiogenesis. The following chapter attempts to summarize the significant literature regarding the technique of PRF application, focusing on its preparation, advantages, and disadvantages of using it in dental procedures.

Chapter 13 - The World Health Organization currently defines infertility as 'a disease of the male or female reproductive system defined by the failure to achieve a pregnancy after 12 months or more of regular unprotected sexual intercourse.' A male factor is solely responsible for about 20% of infertile couples and contributes to another 30-40%. Azoospermia, defined as the complete absence of sperm from the ejaculate, is present in about 1% of all men and in approximately 10-15% of infertile men. Azoospermia is classified into two categories in clinical practice: Obstructive azoospermia (OA) and non-obstructive azoospermia (NOA). Platelets are known for their therapeutic effects, containing many active proteins that are involved in mitogenic, chemotactic, adhesion, angiogenic, antiangiogenic, and neurotrophic processes. In recent years, the successful use of PRP in many clinical fields has led to research on its use in male infertility. Despite the limited availability of data in the literature, the use of PRP therapy is a promising new experimental method in the field of male infertility. However, further investigation with randomized controlled trials is needed to refine the technique and determine the effectiveness of this therapy.

Chapter 14 - Genital aesthetics (cosmetic) is all of the procedures for the correction of genital organs that are defective or are believed to be defective. The genital aesthetic applications are as follows; labiaplasty, vaginoplasty, perineoplasty, hymenoplasty, G shot, O shot applications, genital laser applications, and PRP applications. Aesthetic concerns have been in women for centuries. With the widespread use of the Internet, access to information has become easier, so the perception of beauty has changed, and people have been searching for it. Socially, the growing importance given to appearance has increased the interest in aesthetic applications. While aesthetic applications are increasing rapidly, new alternative applications to surgical treatment have emerged. PRP is obtained by centrifuging one's blood. Genital PRP is a non-surgical, functional injection applied in the genital area. The advantages of PRP are that it can be taken from the person and injected in the same session without anesthesia, and it is not allergic. PRP is extremely effective in wound and tissue healing with its high amount of growth factors in platelets.

Chapter 15 - Erectile dysfunction is a health problem that is believed to affect millions of men around the world. It is considered a precursor of cardiovascular diseases. Due to its organic and psychological reasons, it required multidisciplinary treatment. Various protocols are applied in their treatment that range from patient education and lifestyle changes to penile prosthesis surgery. Platelet-rich plasma has been the focus of attention in recent years because it reduces the need for medical treatment and provides spontaneous erection. It provides tissue regeneration due to the growth factors, cytokines, and chemokines it contains. In preclinical studies, it has been observed to increase intracavernosal pressure and reverse the pathological process. In recent clinical studies, it has provided a noticeable change in the IIEF-5 scores of patients. However, no controlled studies have been conducted with large participation homogenized groups for PRP treatment in erectile dysfunction and no standard treatment protocol has been established. With large-scale studies and standardized treatment protocols, PRP is likely to take its place in the future in the treatment of erectile dysfunction.

Chapter 16 - Sexual dysfunction occurs in men and women, and the prevalence increases with age. Dysfunction can occur in one or more areas of the normal sexual response cycle: desire, arousal, or orgasm. It can also be due to pain. In addition to medical and surgical treatments, PRP has recently been tested in patients with sexual dysfunction. Platelet-rich plasma (PRP) found its use in the treatment of different conditions and diseases because concentrated plasma PRP consists of many growth factors. Their interaction with surrounding cells, intracellular matrix, and mediators at the site of injection leads to tissue regeneration. Due to the angiogenic, vasculogenic, and regenerative effects of PRP, it has recently been widely used in the treatment of male and female sexual dysfunctions. Platelet-rich plasma (PRP) treatments, which seem to offer hope here, have given satisfactory results in the treatment of patients with this dysfunction. PRP is an innovative therapeutic modality, as it is affordable, simple, easily performed, and effective. It is also a non-invasive modality with promising results and no side effects. For this treatment to become widespread, it needs trials in larger populations and a timeline of proven literature.

Chapter 17 - An anal fistula is one of the common benign illnesses of the anorectum seen by coloproctologists. The main goal of surgery is to eradicate the fistula and preserve anal continence. However, anal fistula treatment, especially in complex fistulas, still had a high risk of recurrences ranging to %50 despite these surgical techniques. Local application of platelet-rich plasma PRP can be a new era in the treatment of anal fistula, both alone and in order to increase surgical success. Having been defined as a treatment in selected complex cryptogenic fistula –in-ano, autologous PRP is regarded safe and equivalent to commercial fibrin glue, which is less expensive. The combined the Lift-Prp technique in a high perianal fistula increases healing results from 59% to 77% compared to the alone LIFT technique. The combined use of PRP with other surgical techniques accelerates the range of cure rate to 83%. Another difficult problem to overcome is the anal fistulas that develop due to inflammatory bowel diseases. Combining the mucosal advancement flap with platelet-rich plasma in patients suffering from Crohn's disease–related high perianal fistulas enables moderate consequences such as the healing rate accounting for 70% of the total figure. In conclusion, the use of PRP for the closure of the perianal fistula is a novel alternative method that may offer significant benefits. Platelet-rich plasma can be considered a safe, effective, alternative, and additional treatment to surgery in the anal fistula.

Chapter 18 - Platelets are involved in different stages of wound healing through the growth factors and cytokines they contain. Different platelet-rich plasma products containing higher platelets than normal blood have been applied in experimental and clinical studies in different areas of regenerative medicine to use these effects of platelets. Wound healing is one of these areas, and these products show their effects by increasing angiogenesis and re-epithelialization, stimulating migration, proliferation, and differentiation of cells involved in wound healing. These effects are variable due to the variety of platelet-derived products, preparation, and application methods. Factors such as wound location, wound type, and comorbidities of the patient also contribute to this variability. With the development of more effective products with innovative methods and comprehensive studies to ensure the standardization of application doses and routes, platelet-rich plasma applications, which have been observed to have positive effects, have the potential to be used frequently in the healing process of different wounds in the future.

Chapter 19 - Although bone tissue has the potential to heal after trauma, the healing capacity of bone tissue depends on many factors, such as fracture type, age, and genetic bone disorders. The risk of non-union or delayed union varies worldwide but ranges from 1.9% to 4.9%. In elderly patients with lower extremity fractures, long-term immobilization after non-union, thromboembolism, pulmonary infection, and bed sores may increase the risk of death. Today, the basic treatment principle for fractures is surgery for a stable fixation or a plaster or splint. Platelet-rich plasma (PRP) can be used alone or in combination to increase bone regeneration. PRP is produced by the centrifugation of peripheral blood. Containing high levels of bioactive substances, PRP plays a role in neovascularization, tissue remodeling, and the regulation of inflammation. In recent years, the use of PRP has gained popularity for accelerating fracture healing and treating non-union fractures.

Chapter 20 - Platelet-rich plasma therapy is an autologous blood product that is obtained by centrifugation of blood and contains high concentrations of platelets. Platelets contain many growth factors with regenerative properties that are involved in cell proliferation and differentiation, angiogenesis, and extracellular matrix production. Because of these unique properties, PRP has been used in many different fields such as dermatology, plastic surgery, orthopedics, urology, and obstetrics. Recently, PRP applications in skin diseases have become more and more prevalent. PRP will be used in dermatology for skin diseases, mainly alopecia, acne scars, skin rejuvenation, striae, and vitiligo. The results obtained from the studies are promising and point to a new indication every day. Although promising results have been obtained with the use of PRP, larger studies are needed to prove its effectiveness.

Chapter 21 - Although the etiology of in vitro fertilization (IVF) failures has not been fully elucidated, the quality of transferred embryos and endometrial receptivity are the main factors that determine the success of implantation. The condition of the uterine cavity is known to be effective in the implantation process. The quality and number of ovum also increase the number of pregnancies obtained. Various methods have been tried to increase endometrial thickness and impact the ovary. Platelet-rich plasma (PRP) is one of them.

The PRP method can be defined in detail as administering plasma rich in platelets and growth factors to organs and/or tissues for treatment purposes.

It has been used for a long time to help tissue and organ repair in the treatment of various injuries, particularly in branches such as orthopedics, plastic reconstructive and aesthetic surgery, and medical aesthetics.

In the PRP method, plasma is acquired by separating the blood taken from the patient by a special procedure. The obtained plasma is rich in platelets, whose main function in the body is blood coagulation. This plasma is given back to the patient through injection. Platelets help cell regeneration with the growth factors in their content. Administering PRP in the case of a thin endometrium is still an experimental intervention, there is no convincing scientific evidence that PRP applications are beneficial due to early menopause and deficiency of the ovarian reserve, and it is an experimental practice.

As an experimental intervention, PRP can only be administered under controlled research conditions, with the approval of the ethical committee and the permission for the experimental intervention acquired from the relevant units of the Ministry of Health, by explaining the possible risks.

Chapter 22 - The use of Platelet-Rich Plasma (PRP) in the treatment of tendon injuries has gained significant attention. Tendons, which connect muscles to bones, frequently experience injuries. PRP is a plasma solution derived from the patient's own blood and contains a high concentration of platelets. Platelets release growth factors that are essential for blood clotting and initiate the healing process. PRP is used to expedite the natural healing of tendon injuries. Research studies have demonstrated that PRP promotes tendon healing and reduces pain. It is believed that PRP stimulates tendon cells, increases collagen production, and facilitates tissue remodeling. However, debates regarding the efficacy of PRP persist, necessitating further research. In summary, PRP is considered a potential treatment option for tendon injuries due to its potential to accelerate the healing process. Nonetheless, additional studies are required to evaluate its full effectiveness and long-term outcomes.

Chapter 23 - Plantar fasciitis (PF) is very common in the community and is one of the most common causes of heel pain. It is especially seen in those with foot anomalies, those who stand for a long time, runners, and obese people. PF is a degenerative disease that occurs in the calcaneal tubercle, which is the origin of the plantar fascia. Platelet-rich plasma (PRP) therapy is used as a safe treatment option for tendon, muscle, bone, and cartilage injuries. PRP therapy can be a good alternative, especially in resistant cases, due to the high amount of growth factors and cytokines it contains. With

PRP treatment, both good functional and pain-reducing results can be obtained.

Chapter 1

PRP Preparation Protocol-PRP and Subgroup Type

Yasemin Savranlar*, MD
Department of Histology and Embryology, Nuh Naci Yazgan University, Kayseri, Turkiye

Abstract

In this section of the book, the definition of Platelet Rich Plasma (PRP) and its subtypes of platelet concentrates (PC) are discussed, along with the preparation stages of these subtypes and PRP. Towards the end of the section, a summary of the preparation stages of PRP and its subtypes described in some articles is provided in a table. There have been various approaches to the preparation of PRP and its subtypes. These procedures differ in terms of centrifuge speed and duration, the use of anticoagulants and activators, and other factors.

Keywords: PRP, PRF, PRP subgroup type

Introduction

Platelets, which are also known as thrombocytes, are small, disc-shaped bodies found in the blood. They are formed by the fragmentation of the cytoplasm of large cells called megacaryocytes, which are located in the bone marrow. There are normally 150-450 x 10^9/L platelets of blood.

* Corresponding Author's Email: ysavranlar@nny.edu.tr.

In: Current Clinical Recommendations ...
Editors: Nazan Yurtcu and Emel Güler
ISBN: 979-8-89113-723-3

Platelets have oval or round biconvex discoid structures about 2 - 3 μm in diameter (Ross & Pawlina, 2016; Bos-Mikich et al., 2019).

PRP

Platelet-rich plasma (PRP) is a plasma component obtained by centrifuging whole blood, which contains a higher concentration of platelets than whole blood (Yilmaz & Kesikburun, 2013) (Figure 1). For the treatment of different dermatological conditions using PRP, it is suggested to use a platelet concentration of 1–1.5 million platelets per microliter (μL) (An et al., 2017). High platelet concentrations are preferred for most treatments. PRP is considered natural and safe because it comes from an autologous source, is prepared with minimal manipulation, has fewer risk of infection and has no immune reactivity (Kawase et al., 2020; Nabavizadeh et al., 2022). The granules found in platelets contain numerous cytokines, various growth factors, and proteins (Table 1) (Tey et al., 2022; Atkinson et al., 2021; Hauseuer & Jones, 2019; Cognasse et al., 2021). When a cut or injury occurs in the body, platelets are activated and secrete these molecules that act synergistically on regional cells to promote wound healing, turning the biological environment into a suitable regenerative environment. Platelets are anucleated cells. Anucleated platelets in circulation do not synthesize new proteins. All cytokines and growth factors present in the granules of platelets and transmitted by platelets are produced by megakaryocytes, their source cell (Bos-Mikich et al., 2019).

There are various factors that determine the therapeutic effect of PRP. These are (compared to whole blood/plasma measurements) platelet count/folds of platelet concentration, levels of cytokines, anti-inflammatory and proinflammatory factors, adhesion molecules, growth factors, lysosomal enzymes, chemokines and extracellular vesicles (Table 1) (Cognasse et al., 2021).

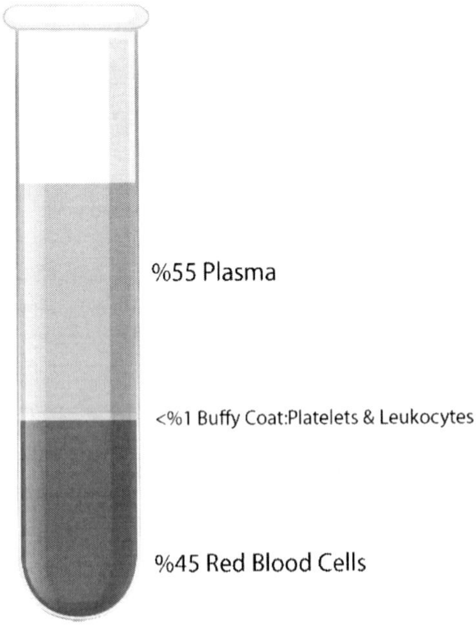

Figure 1. The image was formed after the whole blood in the tube was centrifuged.

Table 1. Cytokines and growth factors in platelet granules

Cytokines and growth factors in platelet granules:	
Cytokines/Chemokines/Immunologic molecules:	Anti-Angiogenic mediators:
IL-1β, IL-1α, IL-6, IL-8, IL-13, IL-27 HMGB1, BMP2-6, CCL1-2-3-4-5-7-17 CXCL-5-7-8-12-17, OX40L, mtDNA, CD154, CD62P, TNF- α, LIF: leukemia inhibitory factor	Thrombospondin-1, Angiostatin, Endostatin, CXCL-4, TGF-β, PAI-1, TIMP-4, TIM-1-4, PF-4
Growth Factors:	Adhesion molecules:
FGF- β: Fibroblast growth factor β VEGF: Vascular endothelial growth factor PDGF: Platelet-derived growth factor ILGF1-2: Insulin-like growth factor 1-2 CTGF: Connective tissue growth factor HGF: Hepatocyte growth factor EGF: Epidermal growth factor EGF: Endothelial growth factor CCN2: Connective tissue growth factor CSF-1: Colony stimulating factor 1 AGF, PD-ECGF, TGF- β, VEGFC, GM-CSF	Fibronectin, Osteonectin, PECAM, GPIba, Multimerin, P-selectin, vWF, Vitronectin, aV β 3, CD9

Table 1. (Continued)

Cytokines and growth factors in platelet granules:	
Pro-Angiogenic Mediators:	Coagulation Factors:
VEGF, β FGF, IGF1-2, HGF, S1P, LPA, EGF, Deoxyribose-1-phosphate, PDGF, Angiopoietin-1, PDEGF, SDF-1α, BFGF, Heparanase, MMP2-9	TFPI, Factor V-VIII-XI-XIII, α2-antiplasmin, α2-antityripsin, α2-macroglobulin, Antithrombin, Fibrinogen, Plasmin, Protease, PAI-1 Nexin-2, Protein-S, Prothrombin
Lipid mediator:	
S1P, sphingosine-1-phosphate	
Lysosomal Enzymes:	
Acid proteases, Acid phosphatases, Arylsulphatases, Carboxypeptidase A-B, CathepsinD-E, Collagenase, Proline, Elastase, Acid hydrolases, β glucoronidase, α-annosidase, β-N-acetyl-hexosaminidase, α-β fucosidase, α-β galactosidase, α-β glucosidase, α-arabinosidase, Arabinofuranosidase	
Membrane proteins:	Hormones:
LAMP-1-2, CD63	Seratonin

PRP Subgroup Types

During the preparation of this chapter, the term *"Platelet Concentrate-PC"* was encountered while conducting research. Platelet concentrates (PCs) are autologous origin and contain high concentrations of platelets, leukocytes, and growth factors (Shirbhate & Bajaj, 2022). The platelet concentrate can be examined in four generations from 1 to 4 (Kawase et al., 2020). The main contents of platelet concentrate can be summarized as follows:

1. *First generation platelet concentrates:* Concentrated platelet count and growth factors have been validated and devices are being developed for automated PRP preparation.
2. *Second generation platelet concentrates:* Development of new platelet-rich plasma derivatives, such as platelet-rich fibrin (PRF), with modifications to previous preparation techniques. PRF is a breakthrough at this stage, and freeze-dried PRP can also be included in this group. Freeze-dried platelets were developed primarily for military use (Horimizu et al., 2013). Because freeze-dried PRP was prepared from allogeneic blood, this technique was never considered worthy of further clinical study due to economic and safety concerns (Kawase et al., 2020). Therefore, allogeneic PRP would be more viable when PRP could be regenerated by

combining platelets derived from iPSC (induced Pluripotent Stem Cell), including clotting factors, with major plasma components. PRP will be a "game changer" in the development of PC therapy when derived from iPSC (Kawase et al., 2020).

3. *Third generation platelet concentrates:* In the third generation, more attention was paid to comparisons between PRP derivatives. Here, in particular, the ability of PRP to uptake and release growth factors and the distribution of leukocytes and platelets have been further investigated. However, comprehensive and fair comparisons between the major derivatives listed are insufficient (Saini et al., 2020; Kawase et al., 2020; Dohan Ehrenfest et al., 2009 Nadra et al., 2022; Melnikov et al., 2020). The main PRP derivatives are:
   - P-PRP; Pure plateler rich plasma,
   - PRP lysate
   - CGF; Concentrated growth factors,
   - L-PRP; Leukocyte and platelet-rich plasma,
   - PRGF; Plasma rich in growth factors,
   - A-PRF+; Advanced Platelet-rich fibrin plus,
   - I-PRF; Injectable Platelet-rich fibrin,
   - T-PRF; Titanium Platelet-rich fibrin,
   - L-PRF; Leukocyte and platelet-rich fibrin,
   - A-PRF; Advanced platelet-rich fibrin, etc.
4. *Fourth generation platelet concentrates:* Includes research on tissue engineering. Conventional PCs do not contain sufficient amounts of mesenchymal and hematopoietic stem cells. If we think of it as three important parts, the first is a scaffold, the second is growth factors, and the third is stem cells. However, we can think of it as a triple leg, while the PCs contain scaffold materials (fibrin) and growth factors, the third piece can be regenerated by adding appropriate stem cells (Kawase et al., 2020). This generation looks like it will be popular in the future.

A good and simple summary would be to classify and present platelet-rich forms as follows (Pietruszka et al., 2021; Mariani et al., 2014; Varshney et al., 2019):

1-PRP: Platelet Rich Plasma (Figure 2);

a-L-PRP: Leukocyte- and platelet-rich plasma

b-P-PRP: Pure platelet-rich plasma
2-PRF: Platelet-rich fibrin (Figure 3);
a-L-PRF: Leukocyte- and platelet-rich fibrin
b-P-PRF: Pure platelet-rich fibrin
c-I-PRF: Injectable PRF (I-PRF).

Apart from these four generations, it is also desirable to mention the production of PRP from a slightly different source and a different product of PRP. These are hUC-PRP and PRP-EVs.

Human umbilical cord (hUC) PRP: The use of hUC-PRP in clinical settings is still considered experimental (Rodríguez-Eguren et al., 2022). Studies have found that human umbilical cord platelet-rich plasma (hUC-PRP) contains a higher concentration of growth factors, cytokines, and chemokines compared to adult peripheral blood PRP. This can contribute to tissue regeneration by enhancing platelet-derived growth factor (PDGF) and vascular endothelial growth factor (VEGF) (Castellano et al., 2017; Lehallier et al., 2019). hUC-PRP contains minimal pro-inflammatory cytokines (Romanov et al., 2019). Interestingly, hUC-PRP has demonstrated promising preclinical results for conditions such as oral mucositis (Piccin et al., 2017), epidermolysis bullosa (Gelmetti et al., 2018), reversing chemotherapy-induced ovarian damage (Buigues et al., 2021), and foot ulcers associated with diabetes (Volpe et al., 2017). The cord blood required for the procedure is taken and processed according to the cellular treatments guidelines of the centers. The cord blood collection set is used.

Towards the end of this chapter, *Platelet-rich plasma-derived extracellular vesicles* will be briefly discussed. In 1967, Wolf was the first to describe the platelet-derived extracellular vesicle (EV), which is a combination of exosomes and micro-vesicles (Wolf, 1967). In the 1980s and 1990s, the terms "microvesicle" and "exosome" were introduced by scanning the web and PubMed. An article from that period specifically referred to microvesicles and exosomes derived from platelets. Microvesicles (1nm-1μ) could be detected by flow cytometry, but not exosomes (40 nm-100nm), probably because of the small size of the latter (Heijnen et al., 1999). One of the most ground-breaking developments in the field of cell biology over the last few decades has been the discovery of extracellular vesicles (EVs) (Raposo & Stoorvogel, 2013). Extracellular vesicles (EVs) are exosomes and microvesicles that carry cytoplasmic constituents of intracellular origin and membrane, and they can transfer microRNAs, long-coding RNA, messenger RNAs, circular RNA, bioactive lipids, proteins, and growth factors (bFGF,

VEGF, PDGF-BB, TGF-β1) to target cells to affect their function and phenotype. These target cells have specific surface receptors. EVs are examined under the heading of acellular therapies in publications (Rodríguez-Eguren et al., 2022; Kawase et al., 2020) Table 2 contains an example of the preparation of PRP-EVs.

Obtaining PRP-EVs can be summarized under 3 headings (Wu et al., 2021):

1. Obtaining PRP
2. PRP activation
3. Differential centrifugation

Preparation Methods for PRP and PRP-Subgroup Type

The known methods for the preparation of PRP are as follows;

1. Manual preparation,
2. Using commercial kits,
3. Automated system.

The preparation of the PC types mentioned above is summarized in Table 2. The prepared PRP solutions are usually divided into small pieces of 5 mL each and stored. One of these pieces is sent to the laboratory for platelet count and bacteriological examination. Frequently, anticoagulants such as heparin, EDTA, Acid citrate dextrose-A (ACD-A), Trisodium citrate (TSC), Citrate phosphate dextrose adenine (CPDA), or others are often required in the process of preparing PRP. Acid citrate dextrose-A (ACD-A) was found to be more effective than heparin, CPDA, and TSC. However, TSC and ACD-A are considered acceptable anticoagulants (An et al., 2017).

The number of thrombocytes in PRP can increase up to *eight times* more than in the initial blood, depending on the preparation method employed. Double centrifugation can produce a higher concentration of thrombocytes and leukocytes compared to single centrifugation (Pietruszka et al., 2021).

Venous blood is collected in a tube with anticoagulant

↓

Soft Spin centrifugation: low RPM (Round Per Minute)

↓

Supernatant is transferred to another tube (No anticoagulant added)

↓

Hard Spin: higher RPM

↓

Platelets confirm a pellet at the bottom of the tube

↓

2/3 upper part of supernatant-PPP (Platelet Pure Plasma) is removed

↓

PRP: 1/3 lower part is resuspended gently

Figure 2. PRP preparation with the *double-spin open method* (Revised from An et al., 2017).

There are two primary manual methods for preparing PRP: the *"PRP production"* method and the *"buffy coat"* method. With the "PRP production" method, whole blood is subjected to an initial slow centrifugation, referred to as a "soft spin," which produces an upper layer containing platelets and leukocytes, a middle layer called the buffy coat (rich in white blood cells), and a bottom layer containing mostly red blood cells (Figure 3). After extracting the upper layer and superficial buffy coat, they undergo a second round of centrifugation at a higher speed, known as a "hard spin," resulting in the formation of soft pellets primarily composed of platelets, as well as platelet-poor plasma (PPP). The PPP is removed, leaving PRP. The "buffy coat" method begins by subjecting whole blood to a heavy spin, which separates it into a top layer of platelet-poor plasma (PPP), a middle layer consisting of the buffy coat (containing PRP), and a bottom layer of red blood cells (RBC) (Figure 3). The supernatant plasma is removed, and the buffy coat undergoes a soft spin, resulting in the extraction of pure PRP and leukocytes, which are then disposed of (Hauseuer & Jones, 2019). The *buffy coat* and *PRP production* methods mentioned here can be called the *double spin method* (Figure 2). The *plasma method* is mentioned as the *single spin method*. PRP is prepared by swing-rotor centrifugation (Figure 5). The suggested centrifuge settings for preparing PRP involve a first spin at 100-300 g for 5-10 minutes, followed by a second spin at 400-700 g for 10-17 minutes. For the treatment of dermatologic conditions, a recommended platelet concentration in PRP is 1-1.5 million platelets/μL. Activation of PRP is not necessary when administered by injection into soft tissue. Thrombin, collagen type 1, and calcium chloride can be used as an activator for PRP.

Although there are many studies, there is no standardization in the preparation of PRP (An et al., 2017). However, the double spin method has been confirmed as the standard method for the preparation of PRP in both the American Association of Blood Banks Technical Manual and some articles (An et al., 2017; Harrison et al., 2020).

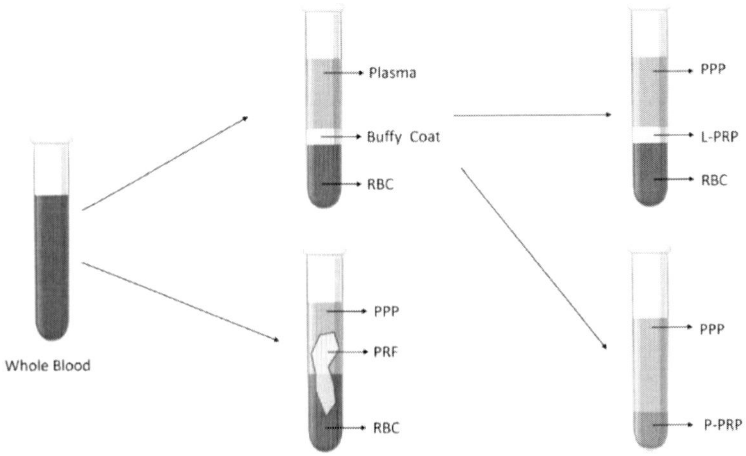

Figure 3. Preparation of PRF, L-PRF, and P-PRF. (PPP: platelet poor plasma, RBC: red blood cell).

Choukroun et al. have recently created a technique for producing fibrin gels (PRF), which does not need the use of external additives. Therefore, another feature of Choukroun's PRF is that the fibrin gel obtained is softer than that prepared with the addition of thrombin. When the fibrin clot formed during the preparation of PRF is divided horizontally into three parts and examined, it has been determined that the section closest to the RBC (part I) has four times more platelets than the upper (part III) and middle (part II) sections, especially in the part close to the bottom of the tube (Kobayashi et al., 2012) (Figure 4). PRF is prepared by angle-rotor centrifugation (Figure 5).

At the end of this section, where preparation techniques are mentioned, a small amount of tubes and needles used can be mentioned. It has been determined that plastic vacutainers contain endotoxin and pyrogen. Its diagnostic use is recommended. For this reason, a glass vacutainer should be preferred instead of a plastic vacutainer in the preparation of PRP to be used in treatment. Tunali et al. (2015) mentioned titanium tubes in their publications. They found that titanium-induced platelet aggregation is similar to that in glass tubes. The clot formed in titanium tubes exhibited clinical characteristics indistinguishable from those formed in glass tubes. Furthermore, they revealed that the fibrin carpet formed with titanium exhibited a more compact mesh structure, and its absorption within the tissue persisted for an extended period (Tunali et al., 2015). Harrison et al. (2020) and Gupta et al. (2020) emphasized that platelet counts are 2.5 and 4.8 times higher in PRP prepared with commercial kits. These commercial kits have a closed system of narrow neck tube construction. The commercial kits use three methods separately: gel separation method, automated cell separation, and narrow neck tube method. And finally, the needle thickness should be 21G and above when taking blood (An et al., 2017).

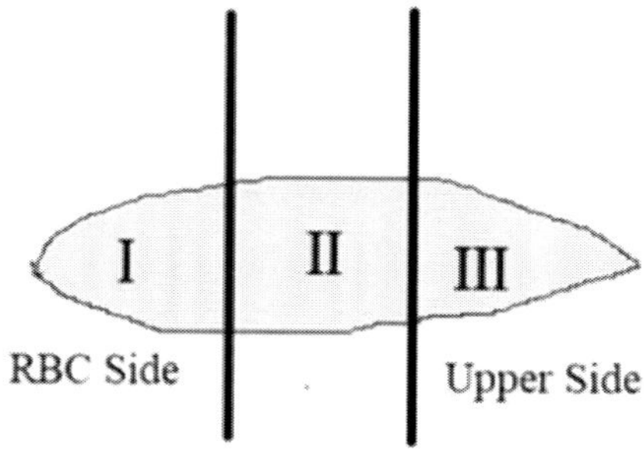

Figure 4. The shape of the PRF (Platelet Rich Fibrin) transversely divided into 3 parts (I, II, III).

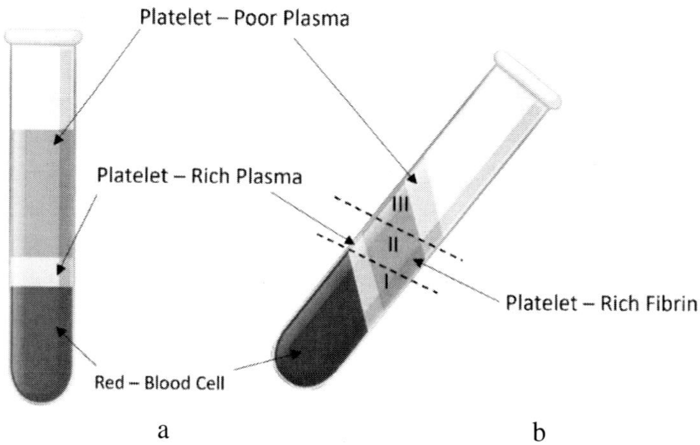

Figure 5. Swing-rotor (A) and angle-rotor (B) centrifugation.

Table 2. Some Examples of Preparation PRP and PRP subgroup types

PC Type	*Processing time*	*Blood Volume/ Weight*	*Stages*	*The rate of the centrifuge (rpm or G)*	*Time-minute*	*Anticoagulant*	*Platelet concentration*	*For activation of PRP*	*References*
A-PRF+	Immediately		1- Blood samples are collected in vacuum plain glass tubes 2- Centrifugated by an A-PRF centrifugation system 3- Eliminate the RBC fraction 4- CGF clots are placed on a dry gauze-10 s-for eliminate excess serum	Angle rotor, 1300 rpm/ 198 g	8 min	No			(Masuki et al., 2016)
P-PRP and PPP		55 mL (11 mL per 1 tube-separated 5 tubes)	1- Centrifugation 2- 1 mL of the upper plasma is harvested as PPP and after about that 1 mL of P-PRP is harvested from the upper part of remained plasma	460g	8 min	1 mL Tri-sodium citrate per tube	P-PRP: 290 X 10^3/µL (<200/ µL WBC) PPP: 6 X 10^3/µL (undetectable WBC)		(Mariani et al., 2014)
PRF	Immediately	10 mL		3000 rpm or 800 g	10 min	-			(Kobayashi et al., 2012)
I-PRF		9 mL	- Plastic blood tube is used. - After centrifugation, 5 mL of supernatant is collected with an 18G hypodermic needle in a 20 cc syringe	3300 RPM Horizontal centrifuge	2 min				(Almeida Barros Mourão et al., 2015)

Table 2. (Continued)

PC Type	*Processing time*	*Blood Volume/ Weight*	*Stages*	*The rate of the centrifuge (rpm or G)*	*Time-minute*	*Anticoagulant*	*Platelet concentration*	*For activation of PRP*	*References*
T-PRF	Immediately	10 mL	- Titanium tube is used - The cloth is removed with tweezers - The cloth is separated from the base of red blood cells (RBC) and pressed between two pieces of gauze	3500 RPM	15 min				(Tunali et al., 2015)
hUC-PRP	In 48 hours	300-410 g	1- Cord Blood pool centrifugation 2- The obtained PRP is passed through the automatic separator- it retains the leukocytes 3- Centrifugation of the PRP obtained 4- PRP was divided into 5 mL aliquots in small bags and frozen at −80°C	799×g 3845×g	4 min 6 min	20 mL of CPD- current in Cord blood collection set	1000×10^9/L ± 20% (4-5 times)	%10 calcium gluconate added before usage of PRP	(Mazzotta et al., 2022)
PRGF		9.6 mL	1- Blood samples were collected with an 18 G needle in a PRGF-Endoret tube (containing sodium citrate) 2- The fraction above the buffy coat was collected and stored at -80°C	Swing rotor, 1850 rpm/ 580 g	8 min	0.2 mL sodium citrate			(Masuki et al., 2016)

PC Type	*Processing time*	*Blood Volume/ Weight*	*Stages*	*The rate of the centrifuge (rpm or G)*	*Time-minute*	*Anticoagulant*	*Platelet concentration*	*For activation of PRP*	*References*
PRP		150 mL	1- Centrifugation 2- Plasma and buffy coat are transferred to a second bag in a closed circuit, centrifuged, and the supernatant is removed. 3- PRP is divided into 5 mL aliquots in small bags and frozen at −30°C	1800 rpm 3800 rpm	15 min 10 min		1000×10^9/L ± 20% (4-5 times)	10% calcium gluconate added before usage of PRP	(Mazzotta et al., 2022)
PRP		150 mL	1- Blood sample collection and centrifugation 2- Centrifugation 3- PRP is divided into 5 mL small units, one is used in 2 hours, and others are stored at −30°C	1500 rpm 3500 rpm	6 min 12 min	21 mL of Sodium citrate			(Görmeli et al., 2017)
PRP		12 mL	1- Centrifugation 2- PRP fractions (buffy coat) were collected with long needles	Swing rotor, 3200 rpm/ 1800 g	4 min x2				(Masuki et al., 2016)
PRP		54 mL	1- Blood is collected with an 18 G syringe 2- PPP is removed	3200 rpm/ 1600 g	15 min	6 mL Citrate			(Yilmaz & Kesikburun, 2013)
L-PRP		9 mL	1- Centrifugation 2- The Plasma+buffy coat is collected 3- CaCl2 is added and stayed at 37°C for 1 hour 4- Supernatant is collected	580 g	8 min	04 mL of 3.8% Sodium citrate		10% CaCl2	(Anitua et al., 2022)

Table 2. (Continued)

PC Type	*Processing time*	*Blood Volume/ Weight*	*Stages*	*The rate of the centrifuge (rpm or G)*	*Time-minute*	*Anticoagulant*	*Platelet concentration*	*For activation of PRP*	*References*
CGF	Immediately		1- Blood samples are collected in vacuum plain glass tubes 2- Centrifugated by a Medifuge centrifugation system in order 3- Eliminate the RBC fraction 4- CGF clots are placed on a dry gauze -10 s- to eliminate excess serum	Angle rotor, -2700 rpm/ 692 g -2400 rpm/ 547 -2700 rpm/ 692 g -3000 rpm/ 855 g	2 min 4 min 4 min 3 min	No			(Masuki et al., 2016)
PRP lysate		8 mL	1- The whole blood is centrifugated: PPP+PRP–plasma1 is collected 2- Remaining blood is centrifugated PPP+PRP=plasma2 is collected 3- Plasma1+Plasma2 are added together and centrifuged 4- The activation protocol: 250 µL of 10% CaCl2 into 10 mL PRP 5- Incubation at 37°C for 1 h	1200 RCF 1200 RCF 1200 RCF	2 min 2 min 5 min	1/4: ACD/ blood (2/8 mL)		CaCl2	(Nadra et al., 2022)

PC Type	*Processing time*	*Blood Volume/ Weight*	*Stages*	*The rate of the centrifuge (rpm or G)*	*Time-minute*	*Anticoagulant*	*Platelet concentration*	*For activation of PRP*	*References*
PRP-EVs			Platelet isolation: 1- PRP diluted, washed-twice and resuspended with Krebs Ringer buffer 2- EDTA and amino ethyl-benzene sulfonyl fluoride (AEBSF) are added to the suspension	180 g	10 min at 22°C	1/10 vol of 0.13 mol/L Sodium citrate			(Heijnen et al., 1999)
			Isolation of vesicles: 1- 5 mL releases of 4 to 12 / 10^6/µL washed platelets	10.000 g	30 min at 4°C	EDTA (5 mmol/L)			
			2- Platelet suspension is stimulated with 15 µmol/L TRAP:10 min at 37°C 3- Supernatant platelet release is centrifugated	65.000 g	16 hours at 4°C				
			4- Supernatant is resuspended with sucrose, HEPES, and EDTA 5- The suspension in the 4th stage is staged in the bottom and different sucrose gradient is layered on top of this suspension and centrifugated 6- 500 µL fractions were collected from the top of the gradient	20.000 g	60 min				

Table 2. (Continued)

PC Type	*Processing time*	*Blood Volume/ Weight*	*Stages*	*The rate of the centrifuge (rpm or G)*	*Time-minute*	*Anticoagulant*	*Platelet concentration*	*For activation of PRP*	*References*
			7- The fraction is diluted with PBS+EDTA and ultracentrifugated. 8- Samples of the pellets are incubated at 95°C for 5 minutes in SDS buffer.						

In summary:

- The PRP preparation technique should be chosen, open or closed method.
- The double spin method has been confirmed as the standard method for the preparation of PRP.
- The blood tube should be glass vacutainer for therapeutic purposes.
- In an open procedure, PRP must be prepared under laminar airflow for aseptic conditions. Sterile gowns, face masks, and sterile disposable gloves should be used.
- The thickness of the needle should be 21G and above when taking blood.
- The automated system has a much higher platelet count but is an expensive method.

Conclusion

The number of factors, such as chemokines and cytokines, detected in PRP appears to increase with studies to be conducted in the coming years.

To summarize, over the past two to three decades, pre-clinical and clinical studies on PC therapy have consistently taken precedence over basic PC studies and have evaluated their effectiveness in various clinical scenarios. Nonetheless, a significant breakthrough in the field of PCs remains elusive and will require compelling evidence from primary studies to be achieved.

The diversity in the preparation of PRP is an indication that there will still be many articles on this subject in the future, and micro-nano-level applications will develop in cell-derived therapies.

More studies are needed to obtain the ideal PRP solution. To advance PC therapy in the future, researchers and clinicians can focus on standardizing the protocols, quality, and diagnosis. This will help ensure consistency in the treatment approach and allow for a better comparison of results across different studies.

References

Almeida Barros Mourão, C. F. De, Valiense, H., Melo, E. R., Freitas Mourão, N. B. M., & Maia, M. D. C. (2015). Obtention of injectable platelets rich-fibrin (i-PRF) and its polymerization with bone graft: technical note. *Revista Do Colegio Brasileiro de Cirurgioes*, *42*(6), 421–423. https://doi.org/10.1590/0100-69912015006013.

An, I., Harman, M., & Ibiloglu, I. (2017). Topical Ciclopirox Olamine 1%: Revisiting a Unique Antifungal. *Indian Dermatology Online Journal*, *10*(4), 481–485. https://doi.org/10.4103/idoj.IDOJ.

Anitua, E., Pino, A., Azkargorta, M., Elortza, F., & Prado, R. (2022). High-Throughput Proteomic Analysis of Human Dermal Fibroblast Response to Different Blood Derivatives: Autologous Topical Serum Derived from Plasma Rich in Growth Factors (PRGF) versus Leukocyte- and Platelet-Rich Plasma (L-PRP). *Biomolecules*, *12*(7). https://doi.org/10.3390/biom12071002.

Atkinson, L., Martin, F., & Sturmey, R. G. (2021). Intraovarian injection of platelet-rich plasma in assisted reproduction: Too much too soon? *Human Reproduction*, *36*(7), 1737–1750. https://doi.org/10.1093/humrep/deab106.

Bos-Mikich, A., Ferreira, M. O., de Oliveira, R., & Frantz, N. (2019). Platelet-rich plasma or blood-derived products to improve endometrial receptivity? *Journal of Assisted Reproduction and Genetics*, *36*(4), 613–620. https://doi.org/10.1007/s10815-018-1386-z.

Castellano, J. M., Mosher, K. I., Abbey, R. J., McBride, A. A., James, M. L., Berdnik, D., Shen, J. C., Zou, B., Xie, X. S., Tingle, M., Hinkson, I. V., Angst, M. S., & Wyss-Coray, T. (2017). Human umbilical cord plasma proteins revitalize hippocampal function in aged mice. *Nature*, *544*(7651), 488–492. https://doi.org/10.1038/nature22067.

Cognasse, F., Hamzeh-Cognasse, H., Mismetti, P., Thomas, T., Eglin, D., & Marotte, H. (2021). The Non-Haemostatic Response of Platelets to Stress: An Actor of the Inflammatory Environment on Regenerative Medicine? *Frontiers in Immunology*, *12*(September), 10–12. https://doi.org/10.3389/fimmu.2021.741988.

Dohan Ehrenfest, D. M., Rasmusson, L., & Albrektsson, T. (2009). Classification of platelet concentrates: from pure platelet-rich plasma (P-PRP) to leucocyte- and platelet-rich fibrin (L-PRF). *Trends in Biotechnology*, *27*(3), 158–167. https://doi.org/10.1016/j.tibtech.2008.11.009.

Görmeli, G., Görmeli, C. A., Ataoglu, B., Çolak, C., Aslantürk, O., & Ertem, K. (2017). Multiple PRP injections are more effective than single injections and hyaluronic acid in knees with early osteoarthritis: a randomized, double-blind, placebo-controlled trial. *Knee Surgery, Sports Traumatology, Arthroscopy*, *25*(3), 958–965. https://doi.org/10.1007/s00167-015-3705-6.

Gupta, V., Parihar, A. S., Pathak, M., & Sharma, V. K. (2020). Comparison of Platelet-Rich Plasma Prepared Using Two Methods: Manual Double Spin Method versus a Commercially Available Automated Device. Indian dermatology online journal, 11(4), 575–579. https://doi.org/10.4103/idoj.IDOJ_653_19.

Harrison, T. E., Bowler, J., Levins, T. N., Cheng, A. L., & Reeves, K. D. (2020). Platelet yield and yield consistency for six single-spin methods of platelet rich plasma preparation. *Platelets*, *31*(5), 661–666. https://doi.org/10.1080/09537104.2019.1663808.

Hauseuer, A. M., & Jones, D. H. (2019). *PRP and Microneedling in Aesthetic Medicine.* Thieme.

Heijnen, H. F. G., Schiel, A. E., Fijnheer, R., Geuze, H. J., & Sixma, J. J. (1999). Activated platelets release two types of membrane vesicles: Microvesicles by surface shedding and exosomes derived from exocytosis of multivesicular bodies and α-granules. *Blood*, *94*(11), 3791–3799. https://doi.org/10.1182/blood.v94.11.3791.

Horimizu, M., Kawase, T., Nakajima, Y., Okuda, K., Nagata, M., Wolff, L. F., & Yoshie, H. (2013). An improved freeze-dried PRP-coated biodegradable material suitable for connective tissue regenerative therapy. *Cryobiology*, *66*(3), 223–232. https://doi.org/10.1016/j.cryobiol.2013.01.006.

Kawase, T., Mubarak, S., & Mourão, C. F. (2020). The platelet concentrates therapy: From the biased past to the anticipated future. *Bioengineering*, *7*(3), 1–20. https://doi.org/10.3390/bioengineering7030082

Kobayashi, M., Kawase, T., Horimizu, M., Okuda, K., Wolff, L. F., & Yoshie, H. (2012). A proposed protocol for the standardized preparation of PRF membranes for clinical use. *Biologicals*, *40*(5), 323–329. https://doi.org/10.1016/j.biologicals.2012.07.004.

Lehallier, B., Gate, D., Schaum, N., Nanasi, T., Lee, S. E., Yousef, H., Moran Losada, P., Berdnik, D., Keller, A., Verghese, J., Sathyan, S., Franceschi, C., Milman, S., Barzilai, N., & Wyss-Coray, T. (2019). Undulating changes in human plasma proteome profiles across the lifespan. *Nature Medicine*, *25*(12), 1843–1850. https://doi.org/10.1038/s41591-019-0673-2.

Mariani, E., Filardo, G., Canella, V., Berlingeri, A., Bielli, A., Cattini, L., Landini, M. P., Kon, E., Marcacci, M., & Facchini, A. (2014). Platelet-rich plasma affects bacterial growth in vitro. *Cytotherapy*, *16*(9), 1294–1304. https://doi.org/10.1016/j.jcyt.2014.06.003.

Masuki, H., Okudera, T., Watanebe, T., Suzuki, M., Nishiyama, K., Okudera, H., Nakata, K., Uematsu, K., Su, C.-Y., & Kawase, T. (2016). Growth factor and pro-inflammatory cytokine contents in platelet-rich plasma (PRP), plasma rich in growth factors (PRGF), advanced platelet-rich fibrin (A-PRF), and concentrated growth factors (CGF). *International Journal of Implant Dentistry*, *2*(1). https://doi.org/10.1186/s40729-016-0052-4.

Mazzotta, A., Pennello, E., Stagni, C., Del Piccolo, N., Boffa, A., Cenacchi, A., Buzzi, M., Filardo, G., & Dallari, D. (2022). Umbilical Cord PRP vs. Autologous PRP for the Treatment of Hip Osteoarthritis. *Journal of Clinical Medicine*, *11*(15). https://doi.org/10.3390/jcm11154505.

Melnikov, D. V., Kirillova, K. A., Zakharenko, A. S., Sinelnikov, M. Y., Ragimov, A. A., Istranov, A. L., & Startseva, O. I. (2020). Effect of cryo-processing on platelet-rich autoplasma preparations. *Sovremennye Tehnologii v Medicine*, *12*(6), 54–60. https://doi.org/10.17691/stm2020.12.6.07.

Nabavizadeh, S. S., Talaei-Khozani, T., Zarei, M., Zare, S., Hosseinabadi, O. K., Tanideh, N., & Daneshi, S. (2022). Attenuation of osteoarthritis progression through intra-articular injection of a combination of synovial membrane-derived MSCs (SMMSCs), platelet-rich plasma (PRP) and conditioned medium (secretome).

Journal of Orthopaedic Surgery and Research, *17*(1), 1–12. https://doi.org/10.1186/s13018-021-02851-2.

Nadra, M., Niu, W., Kurisawa, M., Rousson, D., & Spector, M. (2022). Platelet-Rich Plasma Lysate-Incorporating Gelatin Hydrogel as a Scaffold for Bone Reconstruction. *Bioengineering*, *9*(10). https://doi.org/10.3390/bioengineering 9100513.

Pietruszka, P., Chruścicka, I., Duś-Ilnicka, I., & Paradowska-Stolarz, A. (2021). Prp and prf—subgroups and divisions when used in dentistry. *Journal of Personalized Medicine*, *11*(10). https://doi.org/10.3390/jpm11100944.

Raposo, G., & Stoorvogel, W. (2013). Extracellular vesicles: Exosomes, microvesicles, and friends. *Journal of Cell Biology*, *200*(4), 373–383. https://doi.org/ 10.1083/jcb.201211138.

Rodríguez-Eguren, A., Gómez-Álvarez, M., Francés-Herrero, E., Romeu, M., Ferrero, H., Seli, E., & Cervelló, I. (2022). Human Umbilical Cord-Based Therapeutics: Stem Cells and Blood Derivatives for Female Reproductive Medicine. *International Journal of Molecular Sciences*, *23*(24). https://doi.org/10.3390/ijms232415942.

Romanov, Y. A., Vtorushina, V. V., Dugina, T. N., Romanov, A. Y., & Petrova, N. V. (2019). Human Umbilical Cord Blood Serum/Plasma: Cytokine Profile and Prospective Application in Regenerative Medicine. *Bulletin of Experimental Biology and Medicine*, *168*(1), 173–177. https://doi.org/10.1007/s10517-019-04670-2.

Ross, M. H., & Pawlina, W. (2016). *Histology: A Text and Atlas* (Seventh Edition). Lippincott Williams & Wilkins.

Saini, K., Chopra, P., & Sheokand, V. (2020). Journey of platelet concentrates: A review. *Biomedical and Pharmacology Journal*, *13*(1), 185–191. https://doi.org/ 10.13005/bpj/1875.

Shirbhate, U., & Bajaj, P. (2022). Third-Generation Platelet Concentrates in Periodontal Regeneration: Gaining Ground in the Field of Regeneration. *Cureus*, *14*(8), 4–10. https://doi.org/10.7759/cureus.28072.

Tey, R. V., Haldankar, P., Joshi, V. R., Raj, R., & Maradi, R. (2022). Variability in Platelet-Rich Plasma Preparations Used in Regenerative Medicine: A Comparative Analysis. *Stem Cells International*, *2022*. https://doi.org/10.1155/2022/3852898.

Tunali, M., Özdemir, H., Küçükodaci, Z., Ezirganli, Ş., Bariş, E., Akman, S., Atay, A., & Firatli, E. (2015). A novel platelet concentrate for guided bone regeneration: Titanium prepared platelet-rich fibrin (T-PRF). *Gulhane Medical Journal*, *57*(2), 102–106. https://doi.org/10.5455/gulhane.173504.

Varshney, S., Dwivedi, A., & Pandey, V. (2019). Antimicrobial effects of various platelet rich concentrates-vibes from in-vitro studies-a systematic review. *Journal of Oral Biology and Craniofacial Research*, *9*(4), 299–305. https://doi.org/10.1016/ j.jobcr.2019.06.013.

Wolf, P. (1967). The nature and significance of platelet products in human plasma. *British Journal of Haematology*, *13*(3), 269–288. https://doi.org/10.1111/j.1365-2141.1967.tb08741.x.

Wu, J., Piao, Y., Liu, Q., & Yang, X. (2021). Platelet-rich plasma-derived extracellular vesicles: A superior alternative in regenerative medicine? *Cell Proliferation*, *54*(12), 1–13. https://doi.org/10.1111/cpr.13123.

Yilmaz, B., & Kesikburun, S. (2013). Plateletten Zengin Plazma Uygulamaları [Platelet-Rich Plasma Applications]. *Turkiye Fiziksel Tip ve Rehabilitasyon Dergisi*, *59*(4), 338–344. https://doi.org/10.4274/tftr.78700.

Chapter 2

PRP Treatment for Shoulder

M. Fatih Serttaş*, MD
Department of Orthopedics and Traumatology, Sakarya University, Sakarya, Turkiye

Abstract

In recent years, there has been a significant increase in the use of platelet-rich plasma (PRP) in all medical branches, especially in the Orthopedics and Traumatology departments. Due to its compatibility with the biological structure of the body, low adverse reactions have made PRP attractive in musculoskeletal pathologies. PRP is promising as an alternative to surgical treatment by stimulating curative-enhancing pathways and suppressing inflammation. Although its use in the future is exciting, consistent results have not been achieved in studies so far, and it is not possible to talk about a common treatment algorithm. When the results of the current literature are evaluated, it cannot be said that the use of PRP in surgical and non-surgical shoulder pathologies can be supported or rejected. Although poorly reported, cost-benefit analyses of the use of PRP in rotator cuff repairs show that it does not cover the cost. For this reason, studies with a large standardized patient group are required to better understand the effectiveness and negative consequences of PRP use in shoulder pathologies.

Keywords: platelet-rich plasma, PRP, shoulder, rotator cuff tear

* Corresponding Author's Email: mfserttas@gmail.com.

In: Current Clinical Recommendations ...
Editors: Nazan Yurtcu and Emel Güler
ISBN: 979-8-89113-723-3

Introduction

In recent years, there has been a significant increase in the use of platelet-rich plasma (PRP) in all medical branches, especially in the Orthopedics and Traumatology departments (Hussain et al., 2017; Charles et al., 2018). There are theories that PRP, which is an autologous derivative of whole blood taken from the patient, has positive effects on healing in inflammatory pathways and is rich in growth factors that influence recovery in the musculoskeletal system (Charles et al., 2018; Andia et al., 2018; Klatte-Schulz et al., 2018; Kim et al., 2018). The low incidence of adverse reactions due to its compatibility with the biological structure of the body has made PRP attractive in musculoskeletal pathologies (Garbis et al., 2011). However, studies on the efficacy of PRP on these pathologies are unclear and contradictory. In this article, our objective is to review the results of using PRP in combination with conservative treatment or surgical treatment in common pathologies of the shoulder such as biceps tendinopathy, labral tears, calcific tendinitis, and rotator cuff tendinopathy.

Non-Surgical Indications and Outcomes of PRP in the Shoulder

It is seen that interest in the literature review on the use of PRP shoulder pathologies in the conservative treatment and follow-up process is increasing day by day; It is very difficult to evaluate the collective results of these studies due to differences in the way of preparation and application (Hussain et al., 2017; Miranda et al., 2017; Zhang et al., 2016). It has been shown that physical therapy, non-steroidal anti-inflammatory, and corticosteroid injection treatments are effective in the regression and improvement of complaints in patients with rotator cuff tears (Shams et al., 2016). PRP is the conservative treatment of partial rotator cuff tears; it is promising in terms of being an alternative to surgical treatment by stimulating the curative enhancement pathways and suppressing inflammation. Generally, studies have focused on the comparison of PRP and corticosteroid injections. Shams et al. conducted a prospective randomized control study in 40 symptomatic patients with partial rotator cuff tears (Shams et al., 2016). He divided the patients into two groups, administered subacromial corticosteroids to one group and subacromial PRP to the other group, and evaluated the functional results of both groups at the end of the 6th, 12th, and 24th weeks. As a result of the study, he reported that there was no significant difference between functional results in the 24th week in terms of functional results. As a result of this study, we present evidence that PRP is a good alternative in patients with rotator cuff tears who fear corticosteroid injections. Apart from this, some studies compare PRP with placebo. Kesikburun et al. prospectively evaluated the results of PRP and placebo injection in 40 patients with partial rotator cuff tear or tendinopathy who had a symptomatic course (Kesikburun et al., 2013). They included patients in the rehabilitation program following the injection and evaluated their pain and functional outcomes in a double-blind randomized manner in the 3rd week, 6th week, 12th week, 24th week, and 1st year time periods. They reported no significant difference between the groups at any time in the study.

Apart from these, there are very few studies on the use of PRP in subacromial bursitis, biceps tendinitis, calcific tendinitis, and labral tears. It is concluded that the thoughts on the use of PRP in these pathologies are generally based on the experience and transfer of the surgeons who are interested in shoulder surgery. Moon et al. divided 100 patients who had pain for 1 year and proximal biceps tendinitis on magnetic resonance imaging into two groups and applied PRP to the first group and prolotherapy to the second group (Moon et al., 2011). When they evaluated the functional results of the patients at the 1st, 3rd, 6th, and 12th months, they reported that there were no functionally significant differences between the 1st-month results and that the results of the PRP group were better in the 3rd, 6th, and 12th-month evaluations. In conclusion, he reported that PRP was effective in the non-surgical treatment of biceps tendinopathy. Say et al. compared 50 patients with calcific tendinitis by dividing them into 2 groups (Say et al., 2016). The PRP injection in one of the groups and the corticosteroid injection in the other were administered subacromially once. Constant-Murley and VAS scores increased significantly at 6 months in both groups. No difference was reported in terms of the joint range of motion between the two groups. Nejati et al. divided the patient group diagnosed with subacromial impingement into two and applied PRP injection to one group and physical therapy to the other group for 3 months (Nejati et al., 2017). They reported that there was an improvement from baseline in both groups and that the group that received physical therapy was superior in terms of functional outcomes.

These studies have shown that PRP alone is effective in pathologies such as partial rotator cuff tears, subacromial impingement, calcific tendinitis, and biceps tendinopathy. However, some studies use physical therapy with PRP.

And since there is no difference between corticosteroid injection applications, there is no consensus in the literature. Since very few publications have been reported on the negative effects of PRP, it should be considered a more valid treatment method in cases where the corticosteroid injection has refrained, and it is safer than corticosteroids.

Surgical Indications and Outcomes of PRP in the Shoulder

In recent years, the number of studies on the use of PRP to increase healing after surgical treatment of rotator cuff tears has increased rapidly (Hussain et al., 2017; Meadows et al., 2017; Fu et al., 2017). In addition, differences such as the size of the lesion, and the way and time of PRP application make it difficult to evaluate the overall results in this regard.

There are many studies that examine the clinical results of the use of PRP after surgical treatment. Randelli et al. evaluated the effect of PRP in patients with full-thickness rotator cuff tears for whom arthroscopic repair was performed (Nejati et al., 2017). During the postoperative period, the PRP group had lower pain scores in the first month than the non-PRP group and higher functional scores in the 3rd month. However, they reported that there was no significant difference between the groups in terms of functional outcomes after 24 months of postoperative follow-up. Hurley et al. reported a meta-analysis in which they examined the efficacy of PRP in 18 randomized controlled trials in which arthroscopic rotator cuff repair was performed (Hurley et al., 2018). As a result of the analysis, it was found that the PRP group had an increase in tendon healing compared to the control group. In addition, a positive result was found in favor of the group applied to PRP in pain scores. Saltzman et al. evaluated the systematic review of meta-analyses in 2015 (Saltzman et al., 2016). They compared patients who underwent PRP during rotator cuff repair with those who did not. In the study, in which seven meta-analyses were included, they observed that there was no significant difference between clinical results when the mean follow-up of 3193 patients was examined for 12-31 months.

There are studies evaluating structural results in patients who used PRP after surgical treatment of rotator cuff tears. Jo et al. examined the structural results of patients who underwent arthroscopic rotator cuff repair and PRP (Jo et al., 2013). Patients who did not undergo PRP were used as the control group. Structural improvement was demonstrated in patients who underwent PRP, and 20% recurrence was observed in the control group, while only 3%

recurrence was observed in the PRP group. However, when they evaluated the cross-sectional area of the supraspinatus tendon in early postoperative and postoperative 1-year MRI images, they reported that there was a significant increase in the PRP group. He reported that there was no significant difference in the rate of recovery and functional outcome evaluations.

There are not many studies reported on the use of PRP in combination with the surgical treatment of other pathologies in the shoulder. Carr et al. evaluated patients who underwent arthroscopic acromioplasty alone and PRP together in their study on 60 patients with rotator cuff tendinopathy (Carr et al., 2015). They evaluated functional outcomes and tissue biopsies. Although there was no significant difference in terms of functional results in the 2-year follow-up period, they reported a decrease in vascularity and an increase in apoptosis levels in the tissue biopsy of the PRP group.

Conclusion

The use of PRP in orthopedics continues to increase day by day in surgical and non-surgical treatments (Hussain et al., 2017; Zhang et al., 2016; Jo et al., 2015). In experimental animal studies, it is thought that PRP increases platelets to high concentrations and secretes healing and growth-enhancing factors (Warth et al., 2015; Jo et al., 2013; Vayken et al., 2015; Carr et al., 2015). Although it is exciting for its use in the future, consistent results have not been achieved in studies so far, and it is not possible to talk about a common treatment algorithm.

When the current literature results are evaluated, it cannot be said that the use of PRP in surgical and non-surgical shoulder pathologies can be supported or rejected. Although its adverse effects have been under-reported, cost-benefit analysis of the use of PRP in rotator cuff repairs show that it does not cover the cost (Vayken et al., 2015). More double-blind, randomized controlled trials with large sample sizes and optimized PRP preparations are needed to better assess the efficacy and cost-effectiveness of PRP in shoulder pathologies.

References

Andia, I., Martin, J. I., & Maffulli, N. (2018). Advances with platelet rich plasma therapies for tendon regeneration. *Expert Opinion on Biological Therapy*, *18*(4), 389-398. https://doi.org/10.1080/14712598.2018.1424626.

Carr, A. J., Murphy, R., Dakin, S. G., Rombach, I. N. E. S., Wheway, K. I. M., Watkins, B., & Franklin, S. L. (2015). Platelet-rich plasma injection with arthroscopic acromioplasty for chronic rotator cuff tendinopathy: a randomized controlled trial. *The American journal of sports medicine*, *43*(12), 2891-2897. https://doi.org/10.1177/0363546515608485.

Charles, M. D., Christian, D. R., & Cole, B. J. (2018). The role of biologic therapy in rotator cuff tears and repairs. *Current Reviews in Musculoskeletal Medicine*, *11*, 150-161. https://doi.org/10.1007/s12178-018-9469-0.

Fu, C. J., Sun, J. B., Bi, Z. G., Wang, X. M., & Yang, C. L. (2017). Evaluation of platelet-rich plasma and fibrin matrix to assist in healing and repair of rotator cuff injuries: a systematic review and meta-analysis. *Clinical Rehabilitation*, *31*(2), 158-172. https://doi.org/10.1177/0269215516634815.

Garbis, N., Romeo, A. A., Van Thiel, G., Ghodadra, N., Provencher, M. T., Cole, B. J., & Verma, N. (2011). Clinical indications and techniques for the use of platelet-rich plasma in the shoulder. *Operative Techniques in Sports Medicine*, *19*(3), 165-169. https://doi.org/10.1053/j.otsm.2011.03.002.

Hurley, E. T., Lim Fat, D., Moran, C. J., & Mullett, H. (2019). The efficacy of platelet-rich plasma and platelet-rich fibrin in arthroscopic rotator cuff repair: a meta-analysis of randomized controlled trials. *The American Journal of Sports Medicine*, *47*(3), 753-761. https://doi.org/10.1177/0363546517751397.

Hussain, N., Johal, H., & Bhandari, M. (2017). An evidence-based evaluation on the use of platelet rich plasma in orthopedics–a review of the literature. *SICOT-J*, *3*. https://doi.org/10.1051/sicotj/2017036.

Jo, C. H., Shin, J. S., Lee, Y. G., Shin, W. H., Kim, H., Lee, S. Y., Yoon, K. S., & Shin, S. (2013). Platelet-rich plasma for arthroscopic repair of large to massive rotator cuff tears: a randomized, single-blind, parallel-group trial. *The American journal of sports medicine*, *41*(10), 2240-2248. https://doi.org/10.1177/0363546513497925.

Jo, C. H., Shin, J. S., Shin, W. H., Lee, S. Y., Yoon, K. S., & Shin, S. (2015). Platelet-rich plasma for arthroscopic repair of medium to large rotator cuff tears: a randomized controlled trial. *The American journal of sports medicine*, *43*(9), 2102-2110. https://doi.org/10.1177/0363546515587081.

Kesikburun, S., Tan, A. K., Yılmaz, B., Yaşar, E., & Yazıcıoğlu, K. (2013). Platelet-rich plasma injections in the treatment of chronic rotator cuff tendinopathy: a randomized controlled trial with 1-year follow-up. *The American journal of sports medicine*, *41*(11), 2609-2616. https://doi.org/10.1177/0363546513496542.

Kim, S. J., Kim, E. K., Kim, S. J., & Song, D. H. (2018). Effects of bone marrow aspirate concentrate and platelet-rich plasma on patients with partial tear of the rotator cuff tendon. *Journal of orthopaedic surgery and research*, *13*, 1-7. https://doi.org/10.1186/s13018-017-0693-x.

Klatte-Schulz, F., Schmidt, T., Uckert, M., Scheffler, S., Kalus, U., Rojewski, M., Schrezenmeier, H., Pruss, A., & Wildemann, B. (2018). Comparative analysis of different platelet lysates and platelet rich preparations to stimulate tendon cell biology: an in vitro study. *International journal of molecular sciences*, *19*(1), 212. https://doi.org/10.3390/ijms19010212.

Meadows, M. C., Levy, D. M., Ferry, C. M., Gardner, T. R., Teratani, M. T., & Ahmad, C. S. (2017). Effects of platelet-rich plasma and indomethacin on biomechanics of rotator cuff repair. *Am J Orthop*, *46*(5), E336-E343.

Miranda, I., Sánchez-Alepuz, E., Lucas, F. J., Carratalá, V., GonzálezJofre, C. A. (2017). Use of platelet-rich plasma in the treatment of rotator cuff pathology. What has been scientifically proven? *Rev Esp Cir Ortop Traumatol, 61*(4):249–58. https://doi.org/10.1016/j.recot.2017.03.001.

Moon, Y. L., Ha, S. H., Lee, Y. K., & Park, Y. K. (2011). Comparative studies of platelet-rich plasma (PRP) and prolotherapy for proximal biceps tendinitis. *Clinics in Shoulder and Elbow*, *14*(2), 153-158. https://doi.org/10.5397/CiSE.2011.14.2.153.

Nejati, P., Ghahremaninia, A., Naderi, F., Gharibzadeh, S., & Mazaherinezhad, A. (2017). Treatment of subacromial impingement syndrome: platelet-rich plasma or exercise therapy? A randomized controlled trial. *Orthopaedic journal of sports medicine*, *5*(5), 2325967117702366. https://doi.org/10.1177/2325967117702366.

Saltzman, B. M., Jain, A., Campbell, K. A., Mascarenhas, R., Romeo, A. A., Verma, N. N., & Cole, B. J. (2016). Does the use of platelet-rich plasma at the time of surgery improve clinical outcomes in arthroscopic rotator cuff repair when compared with control cohorts? A systematic review of meta-analyses. *Arthroscopy: The Journal of Arthroscopic & Related Surgery*, *32*(5), 906-918. https://doi.org/10.1016/j.arthro.2015.10.007.

Say, F., Gürler, D., & Bülbül, M. (2016). Platelet-rich plasma versus steroid injection for subacromial impingement syndrome. *Journal of Orthopaedic Surgery*, *24*(1), 62-66. https://doi.org/10.1177/230949901602400115.

Shams, A., El-Sayed, M., Gamal, O., & Ewes, W. (2016). Subacromial injection of autologous platelet-rich plasma versus corticosteroid for the treatment of symptomatic partial rotator cuff tears. *European Journal of Orthopaedic Surgery & Traumatology*, *26*, 837-842.

Vavken, P., Sadoghi, P., Palmer, M., Rosso, C., Mueller, A. M., Szoelloesy, G., & Valderrabano, V. (2015). Platelet-rich plasma reduces retear rates after arthroscopic repair of small-and medium-sized rotator cuff tears but is not cost-effective. *The American journal of sports medicine*, *43*(12), 3071-3076. https://doi.org/10.1177/0363546515572777.

Warth, R. J., Dornan, G. J., James, E. W., Horan, M. P., & Millett, P. J. (2015). Clinical and structural outcomes after arthroscopic repair of full-thickness rotator cuff tears with and without platelet-rich product supplementation: a meta-analysis and meta-regression. *Arthroscopy: The Journal of Arthroscopic & Related Surgery*, *31*(2), 306-320.

Zhang, J. Y., Fabricant, P. D., Ishmael, C. R., Wang, J. C., Petrigliano, F. A., & Jones, K. J. (2016). Utilization of platelet-rich plasma for musculoskeletal injuries: an analysis of current treatment trends in the United States. *Orthopaedic journal of sports medicine*, *4*(12), 2325967116676241. https://doi.org/10.1177/2325967116676241.

Chapter 3

PRP Treatment for Knee

M. Cemil Gün[1,*], MD and Uğur Özdemir[2], MD

[1]Department of Orthopaedics and Traumatology, Sakarya University Faculty of Medicine, Sakarya, Turkiye
[2]Department of Orthopaedics and Traumatology, Bandırma Onyedi Eylül University Faculty of Medicine, Balıkesir, Turkiye

Abstract

Platelet-rich plasma (PRP) is one of the treatment options in the field of regenerative medicine. It aims to enhance the tissue repair process through the local administration of autologous bioactive agents to influence critical physiological mechanisms such as inflammation, angiogenesis, or extracellular matrix synthesis. The use of PRP and its derivatives in the treatment of musculoskeletal system injuries is increasing rapidly. Although promising results are observed especially in preclinical studies, there are highly controversial results in clinical trials. The content of platelet-rich plasma and differences in the techniques of its application make it difficult to report homogeneous results in clinical trials. In addition, changing both the time and content of PRP application according to the stage of the specific disease whose treatment is targeted is a candidate to be the subject of study in the near future. In the current review, findings on the efficacy of PRP and its derivatives in various musculoskeletal system diseases are presented under the guidance of current literature information presented with strong evidence.

[*] Corresponding Author's Email: mcemil23@gmail.com.

In: Current Clinical Recommendations ...
Editors: Nazan Yurtcu and Emel Güler
ISBN: 979-8-89113-723-3

Keywords: platelet-rich plasma (PRP), growth factors, knee diseases

Introduction

Platelet-rich plasma (PRP) was first used for medical treatment for regeneration in the 1980s and 1990s, and it was first recorded for use in heart disease, dental diseases, and maxillofacial operations (Wu et al., 2016). Developments in the field of cell science and molecular biology and their development in tissue regeneration have been used in orthopedics and traumatology as well as in many branches of medicine. Plasma products (autologous fibrin glue) have been used to accelerate regeneration during the treatment of complex skin fistulas and have recently become popular in musculoskeletal diseases as well as in many areas of medicine due to their high content of growth factors (Abel et al., 1993). Platelet-rich plasma (PRP), platelet-rich growth factor (PRGF), and platelet-rich fibrin (PRF) are the leading biological agents. Platelet-rich plasma is an autologous blood product prepared by centrifugation of whole blood, and it contains a higher concentration of platelets and growth factors than normal levels (Paoloni et al., 2011). The growth factors it contains by injection into the damaged area provide an accelerating effect of regeneration in damaged chondral, tendinous, and osseous structures. In recent years, it has been seen that many scientific studies on PRP application in orthopedics and traumatology patient groups have been published with increasing frequency. In this review article, basic principles and different confusing nomenclatures will be tried to be explained in a clear way and relevant articles in the literature will be examined, especially in the common areas of use in knee pathologies.

PRP Application Areas

Concentrated plasma products (thrombin and fibrinogen) have been widely used in many areas of medicine since the 1990s. In the early 2000s, their use in maxillofacial surgery became widespread and started to be used in many musculoskeletal problems after the approval of the United States Food and Drug Administration (FDA) in 2012. In the field of orthopedics and traumatology, it is used in different pathologies, especially in osteoarthritis, tendinopathies, sports injuries, delays in wound healing, and fracture fusion.

Complications and Contraindications

In the early period of platelet-rich plasma administration, there may be an increase in the inflammatory response, which may cause an increase in the level of pain in patients. Reducing this effect with the addition of local anesthetics may be a recommendation. Studies show that the effectiveness of PRP decreases since there may be changes in ambient pH in the use of local anesthetics (Sampson et al., 2008). Relatively common complications include local sensitivity at the injection site and infection, while calcification and scar formation are rarer complications. It is not suitable for use in the case of possible tumor presence, metastatic diseases, active infections, and during pregnancy or lactation periods in the area to be applied in the patient. In addition, the presence of thrombocytopenia and anemia, as well as very rare bovine thrombin allergy, are contraindications (Sampson et al. 2008).

Clinical Studies

When the literature is evaluated, it is seen that studies in the field of orthopedics and traumatology related to PRP are frequently focused on knee osteoarthritis, meniscus pathologies, effect on healing after anterior cruciate ligament reconstruction, rotator cuff tendinopathies, delayed fracture union, lateral epicondylitis, Achilles tendinopathy, and patellar tendinopathy. Due to its non-liquid structure, platelet-rich fibrin is applied directly to the damaged area during orthopedic surgery, and studies on rotator cuff and meniscus pathologies are common in the literature.

PRP Applications in Knee Osteoarthritis

The mechanism of action of PRP in osteoarthritis (OA) has been supported by in vitro studies. Some of these studies show that PRP significantly increases chondrogenic and osteogenic markers in synovial tissue. Because of these properties, it is believed that PRP causes mesenchymal stem cells (MSCs) to transform into chondrocytes and osteocytes in vitro (Mishra et al., 2018).

Belk et al. reported in their meta-analysis of involving a total of 811 patients that intra-articular PRP therapy in patients with knee osteoarthritis had a higher curative effect on pain scores than hyaluronic acid (HA) applications (Belk et al., 2021). In addition, it has been reported that better results are obtained with leukocyte-poor P-PRP than with leukocyte-rich L-PRP (Belk et al., 2021). In another meta-analysis that examined seven randomized controlled trials, PRP, HA, and placebo treatments were compared in patients with knee osteoarthritis. It was reported that there was no certain difference between the platelet-rich plasma-injected patients and the HA-injected group and the placebo group in terms of the Western Ontario and McMaster Universities Osteoarthritis Index (WOMAC) score, Lequesne scores, and side effects (Kanchanatawan et al., 2016). Joshi Jubert et al. compared PRP with local anesthetic and corticosteroid injections in a prospective randomized controlled trial of 75 patients in 2017. While both groups showed an improvement in post-injection pain scores, they could not find a significant difference between the groups (Joshi Jubert et al., 2017).

In another study (Marmotti et al., 2015), 808 patients with symptomatic knee OA for three months or more were injected intraarticularly with P-PRP three times at two-week intervals. At month six, when they evaluated the subject, improvement was shown in scores on the 36-item short-form health questionnaire (SF-36), the visual analogue pain scale (VAS), and WOMAC, as well as the Lequesne Algofunctional Index, an index that analyzes the severity of pain. This index is based on pain/discomfort, maximum walking distance, and performance for daily living activities. But the results, although improved at baseline, were only not permanent, with a decrease that occurred approximately 12 and 24 months after injection. The fact that no effect of different PRP concentrations was reported in this study confirms the previous findings (Association et al., 2017). The positive effects of PRP on OA appear to be influenced by personal factors and injection frequencies; additionally, better results were seen in the earliest age, male gender, patients with milder cartilage degeneration, a lower BMI, and an increased injection frequency (Mangone et al., 2018).

A retrospective comparison study of HA versus PRP in stage I/II Kellgren-Lawrence scale gonarthrosis in the early stages of arthritis showed certain improvements in VAS and CSR scores in both these groups 2 months and 6 months after injection. However, the improvement of the PRP group was better, in general (Guler et al., 2015). Because of this, PRP can be a more effective treatment choice in patients who were in the early stage of OA. In fact, current clinical practice guidelines put forward by the American Academy of Orthopedic Surgery (AAOS) do not suggest the use of HA in symptomatic knee OA in their "strong" recommendations (Treatment of osteoarthritis of the knee, 2018).

Corticosteroid (CS) injections have been used in the practice of knee OA for more than 50 years. Also, CS injections are suggested by the latest American College of Rheumatology (ACR) (Hochberg et al., 2012) guidelines (updated in 2012) for the symptomatic treatment of knee OA. To understand the comparison of PRP and CS effects in the context of knee OA, Forogh et al. conducted a randomized controlled trial of one-time PRP and CS injections in patients with moderate knee OA (CL grade II/III). Four of the pain intensity (over VAS scores), the 20 m walk (20 MW) test and five KOOS outcome scores (excluding the sport parameter) were found to improve significantly 2 and 6 months after the intervention in the PRP group compared to the CS group (Forogh et al., 2015). Additionally, a pilot study that estimates the benefit of combining PRP and CS showed a synergistic effect with significantly lower scores of WOMAC (at 1 and 3 months) and VAS (at 1, 3, and 6 months) compared to PRP in the combined group. However, 12 months after the injection, the benefits were no longer apparent (Camurcu et al., 2018).

According to these outcomes, PRP could be a more effective treatment choice than CS in terms of pain relief and life quality in patients with moderate knee OA, and although we need more research, the two modalities may have a synergistic effect in reducing disability and pain.

PRP Applications in High Tibial Osteotomy

HTO is a general treatment for OA of the medial compartment and varus sequencing disorder [a36]. The number of studies that consider the use of PRP in HTO is very limited to two studies. In a dog model, PRP and saline injections following an HTO for precall ligament rupture were compared (Franklin et al., 2017). In this study, they found that there was no difference in MRI or ultrasonographic healing on the 28th, 49th, and 70th days following the procedure.

In addition, PRP has not been found to reduce bone fusion in these studies. In fact, a study shows that patients who underwent HTO with PRP mixed into the allograft bone had an increased risk of non-fusion compared to those who underwent allograft alone (Giuseffi et al., 2015).

PRP Applications in Total Knee Arthroplasty

PRP injections during surgery or immediately after total knee arthroplasty (TKA) were examined according to various clinical results, including pain scores, some studies (Muchedzi et al., 2017; Guerreiro et al., 2015). PRP has been documented to have a positive effect on postoperative time, between zero and two months after surgery (Morishita et al., 2014). Despite being statistically significant, studies demonstrating improvement in pain scores in the postoperative 2-6 months could not reach clinical significance (Muchedzi et al., 2017; Guerreiro et al., 2015). In the group using double-centrifugal L-PRP, which had platelet concentrations between two and four times that of the physiological group, compared to the group using PRP, postop showed improvement in the verbal pain score from 24 hours to two months. On the contrary, Morishita et al., in the study in which each of the 20 patients was divided into control and PRP groups, shows us that intraoperative PRP gel applications did not certainly improve the quality of life in the short term (0-28 days) measured by CSR and KOOS (Morishita et al., 2014). In addition, there was no significant difference between the two groups in terms of swelling, pain, bleeding, and range of motion muscle strength recovery.

In a review of 17 studies and 2328 patients (Muchedzi et al., 2017), statistically significant differences in pain after PRP treatment after TKA were found in five of these studies (although there was a significant heterogeneous difference between the data).

There was also progress in knee function in patients with OA that were performed with PRP injections. On the other hand, there was no improvement in knee function and life quality after TKA, as well as secondary results such as length of hospital stay and wound scores.

Additionally, a meta-analysis of six studies also measured postoperative complications such as a decrease in hemoglobin, blood loss, and length of hospital stay (Ma et al., 2017). Intraoperative PRP has been shown to not increase postoperative complications and may be effective in reducing TKA-related blood loss and hemoglobin decrease. Because of these, inhibition of these inflammatory pathways must be a potential mechanism by which PRP can help heal and repair the meniscus. Interestingly, milder OA, which was also found to be the best response to PRP, has been shown to be a positive factor for PRP efficacy following arthrosis (Muchedzi et al., 2017). It can be concluded that any positive effect of PRP after TKA is limited to progressions in pain scores in the early postoperative period and may not reflect improved function.

PRP Applications in Meniscus Pathologies

Belk et al., who compared 309 patients who underwent PRP simultaneously with meniscus repair and 445 patients who did not undergo it, found no significant differences between the groups (Belk et al., 2020). However, in another meta-analysis, it was stated that recovery rates were higher after PRP administration simultaneously with meniscus repair (Sochacki et al., 2020). Alessio-Mazzola et al. administered PRP injections to 69 patients with degenerative meniscopathy and stated that the 12-month results were successful, but more accurate results could be obtained with large studies involving control groups (Alessio-Mazzola et al., 2022).

Pujol et al. evaluated the effect of injected PRP in open meniscus surgery in grade II and III horizontal cleavage tears extending to the avascular region in young patients. In this study, no difference was observed in return to work, postoperative range of motion, level of basic activity or participation in sports, or International Knee Documentation Committee (IKDC) scores among patients who underwent fibrin matrix and sutured meniscus. However, this study had several limitations, including the inability to distinguish between the type of meniscus tear in the PRP and control groups (small sample sizes such as 15 and 20), and significant heterogeneity in key features (including age and BMI) between the groups (Griffin et al., 2015). Following this, Kaminski et al. conducted a prospective, double-blind, randomized, controlled study in which they supported arthroscopically repaired vertical red-white region meniscus tears with saline L-PRP (Kaminski et al., 2018). After 2-3 years of follow-up, they found a significant improvement in the mean COOS score in sports categories and the pain in the PRP group. Additionally, the MRI evaluation performed in year 1 showed that meniscus hyperintension was completely recovered in 75% of the patients in the PRP group compared to 40% in the control group (Pujol et al., 2014).

PRP Applications in Anterior Cruciate Ligament Reconstruction

Zhang et al. revealed that the PRP application stimulated bone marrow mesenchymal stem cells in rabbit model studies and stated that in vitro anterior cruciate ligament (ACL) reconstruction accelerated early healing at bone tendon junctions (Zhang et al., 2018). However, in a meta-analysis published in 2019 that included seven randomized controlled trials and a total of 765 patients, it was observed that the use of PRP in ACL reconstruction did not make an absolute difference in graft healing, donor site morbidity, and postoperative pain and function scores (Davey et al., 2020).

Clinical trials using human subjects have shown conflicting results in terms of the effect of PRP on ACL reconstructions. PRP applied through collagen scaffolding has been shown to be useful in some studies (Steiner et al., 2008) in terms of maximal load, linear hardness, and efficiency following ACL repair, but not in others (Murray et al., 2013). In a meta-analysis of eight studies, PRP was shown to improve ACL graft healing by an average of 20-30% compared to the control group (Vavken et al., 2011).

PRP Applications in Patellar Tendinopathies

The PRP application for patellar tendinopathy is quite common, and there are various results in the literature. In patients who underwent PRP injection due to patellar tendinopathy, the return rate to the pre-symptom sports level was reported to be between 22-81% (Liddle et al., 2015; Gosens et al., 2012). Cervellin et al. stated that PRP application reduced donor field morbidities and anterior knee pain in patients who received patellar bone-tendon grafts for ACL reconstruction (Cervellin et al., 2012). However, there are different conclusions about this in the literature. Walters et al. could not find a significant difference in terms of pain in the donor field in the groups with and without PRP in patients who used patellar bone-tendon grafts for ACL reconstruction (Walters et al., 2018).

PRP Applications in Osteochondritis Dissection

Osteochondritis dissection (OCD) is a common disease in the knee and can be treated with different methods depending on the stability of the chondral fragment and the age of the patient. Osteochondritis dissection has been observed in previous studies when treated with ICRS type III lesion, i.e., absence but the absence of dislocation, variable rate of boiling and high non-fusion, arthroscopic or open reduction, and fixation. In this study, it is aimed to extend the benefit of PRP with osteochondritis dissection lesion. In six patients with OCD, the ICRS scale of OCD type III lesions was used. In one study (Sharma et al., 2017), all patients were operated arthroscopically. The chondral flap of the OCD lesion was detected with a stainless steel cannula spongiosis screw. Platelet-rich plasma injections were used to increase the boiling. Ideal knee function was achieved by combining the chondral fragment with the main bone. The Tagner-Lysholm knee scoring system was used to assess knee function. In this study, the preoperative score was 52.8 and the postoperative score was 91.8. Because all chondral flaps of the osteochondral lesion were fixed in this study, this study showed that PRP was helpful in chondral flap healing.

PRP Applications in Delayed Bone Union

The use of PRP in the field of orthopedics and traumatology has gained more popularity in recent years. Andersen et al. stated that PRP accelerates bone fusion in their meta-analysis study on the effect of PRP on delayed fusion, but it is stated that more randomized controlled trials are needed to obtain more accurate results and to determine the appropriate dose and activator (Andersen et al., 2021).

Conclusion

In light of current data, PRP treatment is not a uniform treatment method, but considering the dosage at which it is applied, the frequency of administration, the presence of leukocytes and fibrin in its content, the variety of activators used, and a wide range of application areas, it is not surprising that very different results have been published in the literature. It will take time for the indications of PRP treatment, which is applied with increasing intensity in varying stages in many diseases in many branches, to settle. With qualified randomized controlled trials in specific areas of use, it will be revealed in which areas PRP can be used as a more effective treatment method in the future. It is obvious that more work needs to be done on this promising method.

References

Abel, M. E., Chiu, Y. S., Russell, T. R., & Volpe, P. A. (1993). Autologous fibrin glue in the treatment of rectovaginal and complex fistulas. *Diseases of the Colon &Rectum, 36*(5), 447–449. https://doi.org/10.1007/BF02050009.

Alessio-Mazzola, M., Felli, L., Trentini, R., Formica, M., Capello, A. G., Lovisolo, S., & Maffulli, N. (2022). Efficacy of autologous platelet-rich plasma injections for grade 3 symptomatic degenerative meniscal lesions: A 1-year follow-up prospective study. *Sports Health, 14*(2), 227–236. https://doi.org/10.1177/19417381211011074.

Belk, J. W., Kraeutler, M. J., Houck, D. A., Goodrich, J. A., Dragoo, J. L., & McCarty, E. C. (2021). Platelet-rich plasma versus hyaluronic acid for knee osteoarthritis: A systematic review and meta-analysis of randomized controlled trials. *The American Journal of Sports Medicine, 49*(1), 249–260. https://doi.org/10.1177/0363546520909397.

Belk, J. W., Kraeutler, M. J., Thon, S. G., Littlefield, C. P., Smith, J. H., & McCarty, E. C. (2020). Augmentation of meniscal repair with platelet-rich plasma: A systematic review of comparative studies. *Orthopaedic Journal of Sports Medicine, 8*(6). https://doi.org/10.1177/2325967120926145.

Camurcu, Y., Hakan, S., Ucpunar, H., Kockara, N., Cobden, A., & Duman, S. (2018). Single-dose intra-articular corticosteroid injection prior to platelet-rich plasma injection resulted in better clinical outcomes in patients with knee osteoarthritis: A pilot study. *Journal of Back and Musculoskeletal Rehabilitation*. Accessed 8 July 2018. https://doi.org/10.3233/BMR-171066.

Cervellin, M., de Girolamo, L., Bait, C., Denti, M., & Volpi, P. (2012). Autologous platelet-rich plasma gel to reduce donor-site morbidity after patellar tendon graft harvesting for anterior cruciate ligament reconstruction: A randomized, controlled clinical study. *Knee Surgery, Sports Traumatology, Arthroscopy, 20*(1), 114–120. https://doi.org/10.1007/s00167-011-1570-5.

Davey, M. S., Hurley, E. T., Withers, D., Moran, R., & Moran, C. J. (2020). Anterior Cruciate Ligament Reconstruction with Platelet-Rich Plasma: A Systematic Review of Randomized Control Trials. *Arthroscopy, 36(4)*, 1204-1210. https://doi.org/10.1016/j.arthro.2019.11.004.

Forogh, B., Mianehsaz, E., & Sajadi, S. (2015). Effect of single injection of platelet-rich plasma in comparison with corticosteroid on knee osteoarthritis: A double-blind randomized clinical trial. *Journal of Sports Medicine and Physical Fitness, 56(7–8)*, 901–908.

Franklin, S. P., Burke, E. E., & Holmes, S. P. (2017). The effect of platelet-rich plasma on osseous healing in dogs undergoing high tibial osteotomy. *PLoS One*. https://doi.org/10.1371/journal.pone.0177597.

Giuseffi, S. A., Replogle, W. H., & Shelton, W. R. (2015). Opening-wedge high tibial osteotomy: Review of 100 consecutive cases. *Arthroscopy: The Journal of Arthroscopic & Related Surgery, 31*, 2128–2137. 2018; https://doi.org/10.1016/j.rboe.2015.02.014.

Gosens, T., Den Oudsten, B. L., Van 'T Spijker, P., & Fievez, A. (2012). Pain and activity levels before and after platelet-rich plasma injection treatment of patellar tendinopathy: A prospective cohort study and the influence of previous treatments. *International Orthopaedics, 36(9)*, 1941-1946. https://doi.org/10.1007/s00264-012-1540-7.

Griffin, J. W., Hadeed, M. M., Werner, B. C., Diduch, D. R., Carson, E. W., & Miller, M. D. (2018). Platelet-rich plasma in meniscal repair: Does augmentation improve surgical outcomes? *Clinical Orthopaedics and Related Research, 473*, 1665–1672. https://doi.org/10.1007/s11999-015-4170-8.

Guerreiro, J. P. F., Danieli, M. V., Queiroz, A. O., Deffune, E., & Ferreira, R. R. (2015). Platelet-rich plasma (PRP) applied during total knee arthroplasty. *Revista Brasileira de Ortopedia, 50(2)*, 186–194. https://doi.org/10.1016/j.rboe.2015.02.014.

Guler, O., Mutlu, S., Isyar, M., Seker, A., Kayaalp, M. E., & Mahirogullari, M. (2015). Comparison of short-term results of intraarticular platelet-rich plasma (PRP) and hyaluronic acid treatments in early-stage gonarthrosis patients. *European Journal of Orthopaedic Surgery & Traumatology*, 25, 509–513. https://doi.org/10.1007/s00590-014-1517-x.

Hochberg, M. C., Altman, R. O. Y. D., & April, K. T. (2012). American College of Rheumatology 2012 recommendations for the use of nonpharmacologic and pharmacologic therapies in osteoarthritis of the hand, hip, and knee. *Arthritis Care & Research (Hoboken)*, 64(4), 465–474. https://doi.org/10.1002/acr.21596.

Joshi Jubert, N., Rodríguez, L., Reverté-Vinaixa, M. M., & Navarro, A. (2017). Platelet-rich plasma injections for advanced knee osteoarthritis: A prospective, randomized, double-blinded clinical trial. *Orthopaedic Journal of Sports Medicine*, 5(2), 2325967116689386. https://doi.org/10.1177/2325967116689386.

Kaminski, R., Kulinski, K., & Kozar Kaminska, K. (2018). A prospective, randomized, double-blind, parallel-group, placebo-controlled study evaluating meniscal healing, clinical outcomes, and safety in patients undergoing meniscal repair of unstable, complete vertical meniscal tears (bucket handle) augmented wit. *BioMed Research International*. https://doi.org/10.1155/2018/9315815.

Kanchanatawan, W., Arirachakaran, A., Chaijenkij, K., Prasathaporn, N., Boonard, M., Piyapittayanun, P., & Kongtharvonskul, J. (2016). Short-term outcomes of platelet-rich plasma injection for treatment of osteoarthritis of the knee. *Knee Surgery, Sports Traumatology, Arthroscopy*, 24(5), 1665-1777. https://doi.org/10.1007/s00167-015-3784-4.

Liddle, A. D., & Rodríguez-Merchán, C. (2015). Platelet-rich plasma in the treatment of patellar tendinopathy: A systematic review. *The American Journal of Sports Medicine*, 43(10), 2583-2590. https://doi.org/10.1177/0363546514560726.

Ma, J., Sun, J., Guo, W., Li, Z., Wang, B., & Wang, W. (2017). The effect of platelet-rich plasma on reducing blood loss after total knee arthroplasty: A systematic review and meta-analysis. *Medicine (Baltimore)*, 96(26), e7262. https://doi.org/10.1097/MD.0000000000007262.

Mangone, G., Orioli, A., Pinna, A., & Pasquetti, P. (2018). Infiltrative treatment with platelet-rich plasma (PRP) in gonarthrosis. *Revista Brasileira de Ortopedia*, 11, 607–615. https://doi.org/10.1016/j.rboe.2015.02.014.

Marmotti, A., Rossi, R., Castoldi, F., Roveda, E., Michielon, G., & Peretti, G. M. (2015). PRP and articular cartilage: A clinical update. *BioMed Research International*, 2015, 542502. https://doi.org/10.1155/2015/542502.

Mishra, A., Tummala, P., & King, A. (2009). Buffered platelet-rich plasma enhances mesenchymal stem cell proliferation and chondrogenic differentiation. Retrieved from https://www.ncbi.nlm.nih.gov/pubmed/19770183.

Morishita, M., Ishida, K., Matsumoto, T., Kuroda, R., Kurosaka, M., & Tsumura, N. (2014). Intraoperative platelet-rich plasma does not improve outcomes of total knee arthroplasty. *Journal of Arthroplasty*, 29, 2337–2341. https://doi.org/10.1016/j.arth.2014.04.007.

Muchedzi, T. A., & Roberts, S. B. (2017). A systematic review of the effects of platelet-rich plasma on outcomes for patients with knee osteoarthritis and following total knee arthroplasty. *Surgery*. https://doi.org/10.1016/j.surge.2017.08.004.

Murray, M. M., & Fleming, B. C. (2013). Use of a bioactive scaffold to stimulate anterior cruciate ligament healing also minimizes posttraumatic osteoarthritis after surgery. *American Journal of Sports Medicine*. https://doi.org/10.1177/0363546513483446.

Paoloni, J., De Vos, R. J., Hamilton, B., Murrell, G. A., & Orchard, J. (2011). Platelet-rich plasma treatment for ligament and tendon injuries. *Clinical Journal of Sport Medicine*, 21, 37-45. https://doi.org/10.1097/JSM.0b013e31820758c7.

Pujol, N., Salle De Chou, E., Boisrenoult, P., & Beaufils, P. (2014). Platelet-rich plasma for open meniscal repair in young patients: Any benefit? *Knee Surgery, Sports Traumatology, Arthroscopy*. https://doi.org/10.1007/s00167-014-3417-3.

Sampson, S., Gerhardt, M., & Mandelbaum, B. (2008). Platelet-rich plasma injection grafts for musculoskeletal injuries: A review. *Current Reviews in Musculoskeletal Medicine*, 1, 165-174. https://doi.org/10.1007/s12178-008-9032-5.

Sharma, D. K., Kumar, N., Lal, H., Sahu, B. K., & Saikia, S. S. (2018). Osteochondritis dissecans-Does platelet-rich plasma really help? *Journal of Clinical Orthopaedics and Trauma*, 9(2), 153–156. https://doi.org/10.1016/j.jcot.2017.09.020.

Sochacki, K. R., Safran, M. R., Abrams, G. D., Donahue, J., Chu, C., & Sherman, S. L. (2020). Platelet-rich plasma augmentation for isolated arthroscopic meniscal repairs leads to significantly lower failure rates: A systematic review of comparative studies. *Orthopaedic Journal of Sports Medicine*, 8(11). https://doi.org/10.1177/2325967120964534.

Steiner, M. E., Murray, M. M., & Rodeo, S. A. (2008). Strategies to improve anterior cruciate ligament healing and graft placement. *American Journal of Sports Medicine*, 36, 176–189. https://doi.org/10.1177/0363546507311690.

"Treatment of Osteoarthritis of the Knee" (2018). 2nd edition summary of recommendations. Retrieved from www.aaos.org/guidelines. Accessed August 8, 2018.

Vavken, P., Sadoghi, P., & Murray, M. M., Vavken, P. (2011). The effect of platelet concentrates on graft maturation and graft-bone interface healing in ACL reconstruction in human patients: A systematic review of controlled trials. *Arthroscopy*, 27(11), 1573–1583. https://doi.org/10.1016/j.arthro.2011.06.003.

Walters, B. L., Porter, D. A., Hobart, S. J., Bedford, B. B., Hogan, D. E., & McHugh, M. M. (2018). Effect of intraoperative platelet-rich plasma treatment on postoperative donor site knee pain in patellar tendon autograft anterior cruciate ligament reconstruction: A double-blind randomized controlled trial. *American Journal of Sports Medicine*, 46(8), 1827-1835. https://doi.org/10.1177/0363546518769295.

Wu, P. I.-K., Diaz, R., & Borg-Stein, J. (2016). Platelet-rich plasma. *Physical Medicine and Rehabilitation Clinics of North America*. https://doi.org/10.1016/j.pmr.2016.06.002.

Zhang, M., Zhen, J., Zhang, X., Yang, Z., Zhang, L., & Hao, D. (2018). Effect of autologous platelet-rich plasma and gelatin sponge for tendon-to-bone healing after rabbit anterior cruciate ligament reconstruction. *Arthroscopy*, 35, 1486-1497. https://doi.org/10.1016/j.arthro.2018.11.014.

Chapter 4

PRP Treatment for Hip

Özgür Mert Bakan*, MD
and Yüksel Laçin Avan, MD
Department of Orthopedics and Traumatology, Bakircay University Cigli Training and Research Hospital, Izmir, Turkiye

Abstract

Platelet-rich plasma (PRP) has gained recognition as a valuable treatment option in orthopedic medicine for accelerating tissue repair. This chapter focuses on the use of PRP in the treatment of hip disorders, including hip osteoarthritis, avascular necrosis of the femoral head, hamstring tendinopathy, adductor tendinopathy, and muscle strains around the hip. PRP is derived from the patient's own blood and contains various growth factors and bioactive molecules that promote tissue regeneration. In hip osteoarthritis, PRP injections have shown promising results in improving functional scores compared to traditional treatments, although no significant structural changes have been observed. In avascular necrosis of the femoral head, PRP has been used both as a nonsurgical injection and as an adjuvant in surgical procedures, demonstrating positive outcomes in select cases. For hamstring and adductor tendinopathies, PRP injections have yielded positive outcomes, reducing pain intensity and facilitating a faster return to activity. Additionally, PRP has shown promise in the treatment of adductor and hamstring tendinopathy, exhibiting a reduction in the size of the lesion and improved functional outcomes. Moreover, PRP has been used in the treatment of muscle strains around the hip. While PRP offers advantages such as simplicity and safety, image-guided methods are often required for accurate administration.

* Corresponding Author's Email: ozgurmertbakan@gmail.com.

In: Current Clinical Recommendations ...
Editors: Nazan Yurtcu and Emel Güler
ISBN: 979-8-89113-723-3

Although the use of PRP in other hip-related conditions is limited to case reports and small studies, it presents a promising avenue for future research and clinical applications.

Keywords: hip, platelet-rich plasma, osteoarthritis, muscle strain, tendinopathy

Introduction

In recent years, the field of orthopedic medicine has witnessed an increasing recognition and utilization of platelet-rich plasma (PRP) as a treatment modality for accelerating tissue repair. PRP is derived from the patient's own blood through a process involving centrifugation. This process effectively separates the platelet-rich component known as PRP. In musculoskeletal medicine, PRP has emerged as a viable therapeutic option with a solid safety profile. It harnesses the mobilization of cells derived from the circulation, including fibroblast-like cells responsible for matrix production, as well as inflammatory cells that release cytokines and growth factors (Kraeutler et al., 2016). A wide range of musculoskeletal conditions, such as rotator cuff tendinopathy, patellar tendinopathy, knee osteoarthritis, lateral epicondylitis, osteochondral lesions of the talus, plantar fasciitis, achilles injuries, and various other orthopedic conditions, have been successfully treated with PRP (Le et al., 2018). This section aims to provide an overview of the applications and outcomes of PRP in the management of hip disorders.

Main Body

PRP injection is a biological therapy with several advantages. It offers a straightforward and uncomplicated intra-articular injection procedure that can be conveniently performed at the doctor's office. The use of PRP is considered safe due to its use of the patient's own proteins and the proper concentration of bioactive molecules, which helps avoid potential negative effects and medication interactions. The existing literature does not report any serious side effects of PRP, and documented cases are mild and temporary, including bleeding, soreness, swelling, and bruising at the injection site.

However, the application of PRP to the hip joint is not without limitations. The need for image-guided methods, such as fluoroscopy and ultrasound, poses an important constraint. While this may seem restrictive, the literature often recommends performing all injections with basic imaging techniques such as ultrasound (US) for improved accuracy.

PRP has demonstrated efficacy in various hip pathologies, which are discussed below:

Hip Osteoarthritis

Hip osteoarthritis is a chronic and progressive disorder characterized by the degeneration of the hip joint's cartilage, leading to pain and restricted mobility. This condition significantly impacts the quality of life, particularly among the elderly population. Although conservative treatment methods, such as weight loss, activity modification, physical therapy, and pharmacological agents such as nonsteroidal anti-inflammatory drugs (NSAIDs) or opioids, are commonly used, they do not address the underlying cartilage pathology (Nouri et al., 2022). The effectiveness of glucosamine sulfate and chondroitin sulfate in the treatment of cartilage disorders remains a subject of debate. Intra-articular injections, including hyaluronic acid, corticosteroids, or PRP, provide a direct approach to treating hip osteoarthritis. In cases where these treatment options have failed, total hip arthroplasty is often necessary for advanced hip osteoarthritis.

Several studies in the literature have investigated the efficacy of PRP in treating hip osteoarthritis, demonstrating promising results. However, there is currently a lack of randomized controlled trials that specifically examine the effect of PRP on structural changes associated with osteoarthritis (Bennell et al., 2017). The underlying mechanisms by which PRP aids in osteoarthritis treatment are not yet fully understood, although it is believed to inhibit catabolic and inflammatory processes while promoting anabolic responses. PRP activation releases biologically active growth factors and molecules, including platelet-derived growth factor, transforming growth factor, type I insulin-like growth factor, and vascular endothelial growth factor (Battaglia et al., 2013). These proteins play crucial roles in tissue repair, such as inhibiting chondrocyte death, bone and blood vessel remodeling, inflammation control, and collagen synthesis. For instance, Nouri et al. conducted a study involving 105 patients with stage 2 and 3 hip osteoarthritis, dividing them into three groups receiving different treatments:

PRP, hyaluronic acid, and PRP combined with hyaluronic acid. Although functional scores improved in all groups compared to the pre-injection period, the PRP and PRP + hyaluronic acid groups exhibited significantly better functional improvement than the group treated with hyaluronic acid alone (Nouri et al., 2022). In a systematic review by Berney et al., which evaluated published prospective studies with a minimum follow-up period of three months, PRP injections demonstrated improved patient outcome scores at six and 12 months compared to hyaluronic acid alone. However, no significant difference was found between patients treated with PRP and those treated with hyaluronic acid alone (Berney et al., 2021). Consequently, current evidence does not support the routine use of intra-articular PRP injections for hip osteoarthritis treatment.

Avascular Necrosis of the Femoral Head

Avascular necrosis (AVN) of the femoral head is a type of osteonecrosis resulting from compromised blood supply to the proximal femur. It can occur due to various causes, including trauma or non-traumatic factors. PRP has been used in the treatment of AVN as a nonsurgical injection and as an intraoperative adjuvant during surgical procedures. For instance, Pak et al. reported a case of a 43-year-old man with grade 1 AVN of the femoral head treated with adipose-derived stem cells and PRP. The patient showed a significant improvement three months after receiving a weekly mixture of adipose-derived stem cells and PRP in the hip joint (Pak et al., 2014). Magnetic resonance imaging (MRI) showed a complete resolution of AVN. Studies have also reported the use of PRP for augmentation of arthroscopic core decompression in the AVN of the femoral head. Guadilla et al. described a surgical procedure involving core decompression of the necrotic areas of the femoral head, followed by the injection of fluid PRP into the perforation hole in patients with grade 1 or 2A AVN. In cases of grade 2B and 2C AVN, an iliac bone graft mixed with activated PRP was used. However, the outcomes of this surgical procedure have not been extensively studied in terms of patient outcomes (Guadilla et al., 2012). Martin et al. conducted a study involving 73 patients with AVN, where a mixture of PRP and autologous bone marrow aspirate concentrate was injected into the affected area after open decompression of the femoral head. The study found that out of the 73 patients, only 16 progressed to coxarthrosis and required arthroplasty (Martin et al., 2013). However, it is important to note that the majority of patients in this study had grade 1 AVN (57 out of 73), while only 16 had grade 2 AVN.

Hamstring Tendinopathy

Tendinopathy of the proximal hamstring tendon is a common cause of buttock pain and can result in significant discomfort and disability. PRP injections have shown promise in promoting healing when there is partial tendon involvement or tendinosis without retraction. Several randomized controlled trials have focused on hamstring injuries and have demonstrated positive outcomes with PRP injections. Hamilton et al. compared PRP, platelet-poor plasma (PPP), and no injection in professional athletes with MRI-positive hamstring injuries, alongside standard physical therapy (Hamilton et al., 2015). The PRP group exhibited a significantly shorter time to return to sport (mean of 21 days) compared to the PPP group (mean of 27 days). Another study by Hamid et al. compared PRP therapy plus a rehabilitation program with rehabilitation alone in patients with acute hamstring injuries (Hamid et al., 2014). A single injection of PRP, administered via Ultrasonography (US) guidance at an average of 4.6 days after injury, significantly reduced pain intensity and shortened the time to return to play (mean of 26.7 days) compared to the control group (mean of 42.5 days). Davenport et al. conducted a double-blind, randomized controlled trial focusing on proximal hamstring tendinopathy. They compared a single injection of PRP with autologous whole blood (WB) for the treatment of hamstring tendinopathy. No significant differences were found between the groups in hip functional scores at follow-up periods of 2, 6, and 12 weeks and 6 months (Davenport et al., 2015).

Adductor Tendinopathy

Adductor tendinopathy often occurs due to forceful movements or sudden changes in direction during certain athletic activities, resulting in pain in the groin. Treatment options include rest, activity restriction, and, in some cases, adductor tendon release surgery (Mei-Dan et al., 2013). PRP is frequently used in the management of adductor tendinopathy. Dallaudière et al. conducted a study on PRP treatment for tendinopathies, including hamstring and adductor longus tendinopathy. They observed significantly improved functional scores in patients after six weeks of PRP treatment. The US was also used to assess the size of the lesion at baseline and after six weeks, revealing a decrease in the size of the hamstring and adductor longus tendon lesions from an average of 21.2 mm to 2.6 mm (Dallaudière et al., 2014).

In addition to the aforementioned hip disorders, PRP has been used in the treatment of muscle strains involving the quadriceps, hamstrings, adductors, gluteus maximus, iliopsoas, and external oblique abdominal muscles (Hamilton et al., 2010; Kraeutler et al., 2016). While there are studies that demonstrate the use of PRP as a noninvasive injection for the treatment of osteitis pubis or as a postoperative adjuvant in pubic symphysis debridement, large case series are currently lacking (Park & Sussman, 2022).

Conclusion

PRP has emerged as a valuable therapeutic option for various hip disorders, providing a safe and effective approach to tissue repair and regeneration. The use of PRP in the treatment of hip osteoarthritis has shown favorable functional improvements, although its impact on structural changes remains uncertain. In avascular necrosis of the femoral head, PRP has demonstrated potential as both a nonsurgical and intraoperative adjuvant, warranting further investigation. For hamstring and adductor tendinopathies, PRP injections have yielded positive outcomes, reducing pain intensity and facilitating a faster return to activity. Additionally, PRP has shown promise in the treatment of adductor and hamstring tendinopathy, exhibiting a reduction in the size of the lesion and improved functional outcomes. While the evidence supporting PRP treatment for hip disorders is encouraging, larger randomized controlled trials are needed to validate its efficacy and establish standardized protocols. The ongoing research in this field holds promise for expanding the applications of PRP in hip-related conditions and enhancing patient outcomes.

References

Battaglia, M., Guaraldi, F., Vannini, F., Rossi, G., Timoncini, A., Buda, R., & Giannini, S. (2013). Efficacy of ultrasound-guided intra-articular injections of platelet-rich plasma versus hyaluronic acid for hip osteoarthritis. *Orthopedics*, *36*(12), e1501–e1508. https://doi.org/10.3928/01477447-20131120-13.

Bennell, K. L., Hunter, D. J., & Paterson, K. L. (2017). Platelet-Rich Plasma for the Management of Hip and Knee Osteoarthritis. *Current rheumatology reports*, *19*(5), 24. https://doi.org/10.1007/s11926-017-0652-x.

Berney, M., McCarroll, P., Glynn, L., & Lenehan, B. (2021). Platelet-rich plasma injections for hip osteoarthritis: a review of the evidence. *Irish journal of medical science*, *190*(3), 1021–1025. https://doi.org/10.1007/s11845-020-02388-z.

Dallaudière, B., Pesquer, L., Meyer, P., Silvestre, A., Perozziello, A., Peuchant, A., Durieux, M. H., Loriaut, P., Hummel, V., Boyer, P., Schouman-Claeys, E., & Serfaty, J. M. (2014). Intratendinous injection of platelet-rich plasma under US guidance to treat tendinopathy: a long-term pilot study. *Journal of vascular and interventional radiology: JVIR*, *25*(5), 717–723. https://doi.org/10.1016/j.jvir.2014.01.026.

Davenport, K. L., Campos, J. S., Nguyen, J., Saboeiro, G., Adler, R. S., & Moley, P. J. (2015). Ultrasound-Guided Intratendinous Injections With Platelet-Rich Plasma or Autologous Whole Blood for Treatment of Proximal Hamstring Tendinopathy: A Double-Blind Randomized Controlled Trial. *Journal of ultrasound in medicine : official journal of the American Institute of Ultrasound in Medicine*, *34*(8), 1455–1463. https://doi.org/10.7863/ultra.34.8.1455.

Guadilla, J., Fiz, N., Andia, I., & Sánchez, M. (2012). Arthroscopic management and platelet-rich plasma therapy for avascular necrosis of the hip. *Knee surgery, sports traumatology, arthroscopy : official journal of the ESSKA*, *20*(2), 393–398. https://doi.org/10.1007/s00167-011-1587-9.

Hamid, M. S. A., Mohamed Ali, M. R., Yusof, A., George, J., & Lee, L. P. (2014). Platelet-rich plasma injections for the treatment of hamstring injuries: a randomized controlled trial. *The American journal of sports medicine*, *42*(10), 2410–2418. https://doi.org/10.1177/0363546514541540.

Hamilton, B., Knez, W., Eirale, C., & Chalabi, H. (2010). Platelet enriched plasma for acute muscle injury. *Acta orthopaedica Belgica*, *76*(4), 443–448.

Hamilton, B., Tol, J. L., Almusa, E., Boukarroum, S., Eirale, C., Farooq, A., Whiteley, R., & Chalabi, H. (2015). Platelet-rich plasma does not enhance return to play in hamstring injuries: a randomised controlled trial. *British journal of sports medicine*, *49*(14), 943–950. https://doi.org/10.1136/bjsports-2015-094603.

Kraeutler, M. J., Garabekyan, T., & Mei-Dan, O. (2016). The use of platelet-rich plasma to augment conservative and surgical treatment of hip and pelvic disorders. *Muscles, ligaments and tendons journal*, *6*(3), 410–419. https://doi.org/10.11138/mltj/2016.6.3.410.

Le, A. D. K., Enweze, L., DeBaun, M. R., & Dragoo, J. L. (2018). Current Clinical Recommendations for Use of Platelet-Rich Plasma. *Current reviews in musculoskeletal medicine*, *11*(4), 624–634. https://doi.org/10.1007/s12178-018-9527-7.

Martin, J. R., Houdek, M. T., & Sierra, R. J. (2013). Use of concentrated bone marrow aspirate and platelet rich plasma during minimally invasive decompression of the femoral head in the treatment of osteonecrosis. *Croatian medical journal*, *54*(3), 219–224. https://doi.org/10.3325/cmj.2013.54.219.

Mei-Dan, O., Lopez, V., Carmont, M. R., McConkey, M. O., Steinbacher, G., Alvarez, P. D., & Cugat, R. B. (2013). Adductor tenotomy as a treatment for groin pain in professional soccer players. *Orthopedics*, *36*(9), e1189–e1197. https://doi.org/10.3928/01477447-20130821-23.

Nouri, F., Babaee, M., Peydayesh, P., Esmaily, H., & Raeissadat, S. A. (2022). Comparison between the effects of ultrasound guided intra-articular injections of platelet-rich plasma (PRP), high molecular weight hyaluronic acid, and their combination in hip osteoarthritis: a randomized clinical trial. *BMC musculoskeletal disorders*, *23*(1), 856. https://doi.org/10.1186/s12891-022-05787-8.

Pak, J., Lee, J. H., Jeon, J. H., & Lee, S. H. (2014). Complete resolution of avascular necrosis of the human femoral head treated with adipose tissue-derived stem cells and platelet-rich plasma. *The Journal of international medical research*, *42*(6), 1353–1362. https://doi.org/10.1177/0300060514546940.

Park, D. J., & Sussman, W. I. (2022). Osteitis Pubis Treated With Platelet-Rich Plasma: A Case Report. *Clinical journal of sport medicine : official journal of the Canadian Academy of Sport Medicine*, *32*(2), e172–e174. https://doi.org/10.1097/JSM.0000000000000875 .

Chapter 5

PRP Treatment for Avascular Necrosis

Serkan Erkuş[1,*], MD
and Tayfun Bacaksız[2], MD
[1]Department of Orthopedics and Traumatology, Private Medifema Hospital, Izmir, Turkiye
[2]Department of Orthopedics and Traumatology, Izmir Katip Çelebi University, Faculty of Medicine, Izmir, Turkey

Abstract

Avascular necrosis is the necrosis of bone tissue that can be due to many reasons. Today, a clear treatment algorithm has not been established yet. Platelet-rich plasma therapy is a method that has been widely used in regenerative medicine. Considering the mechanisms of action, it emerges as a method that can affect the histopathological changes due to avascular necrosis and ensure the appropriate differentiation of mesenchymal cells in the environment. Although the information in our literature is limited, the results are quite promising.

Keywords: avascular necrosis, PRP treatment in osteonecrosis, regenerative medicine

Introduction

Avascular necrosis is the necrosis of bone and bone marrow cells as a result of ischemia arising from different etiological reasons. In the continuation of

[*] Corresponding Author's Email: drserkanerkus@gmail.com.

In: Current Clinical Recommendations ...
Editors: Nazan Yurtcu and Emel Güler
ISBN: 979-8-89113-723-3

this destruction in the bone, a reactive bone formation process is observed. With reactive hyperemia and revascularization, necrotic tissues are removed from the surroundings, and bone development continues. During this cycle, the structural integrity of the trabecular bone tissue is impaired by partial resorption of the necrotic bone tissue. At this stage, a subchondral fracture may occur in necrosis adjacent to the joint (Glimcher & Kenzora, 1979). This collapse, which is defined as a subchondral fracture, results in the deterioration of joint function and loss of the natural histological quality of the joint. The size of the involved area and its relationship with the joint surface are crucial in the development of clinical symptoms. Some parts of bones in the body are more prone to avascular necrosis due to their anatomical and vascularization characteristics. However, it can be seen in all bone tissue. Cortical bone is usually not affected because of collateral vascularization. The femoral head, the femoral condyle, the talus, the scaphoid, and the metatarsal head can be counted among those that are frequently encountered (Lamb et al., 2019). When the etiology of avascular necrosis is examined, traumatic injuries, fractures, vascular injuries, drugs such as corticosteroids, long-term and excessive alcohol use, smoking, blood diseases such as sickle cell anemia, some chronic metabolic diseases such as Gaucher's disease and Caisson's disease, radiation treatments, chemotherapy, hyperlipidemia, and autoimmune diseases are often the causes.

Avascular necrosis, also called "osteonecrosis," usually does not give a clinical finding in the early stages. As the disease progresses, pain, especially with full weight-bearing, comes to the fore. Afterward, the complaint of pain is observed even at rest. There is a decrease in the range of motion of the joint and pain. In untreated cases, the area of necrosis may expand, and bone collapse may occur. The normal smooth shape feature of the bone structure is lost, and flattening occurs. As a result, severe arthritis becomes inevitable. Although the treatment options are similar, treatment options may differ depending on the bone involved, the area and size of the involvement, and etiological and patient-related factors. Medicines for pain control are applied in the early stages to reduce pain in the bone or joint. With the progression of the disease, interventional procedures such as core decompression, osteotomies, bone graft transplantation, and even joint replacement are applied according to the severity of the disease. The scope of application of regenerative medicine, which has become increasingly widespread in recent years, is a good option to support treatment.

Theoretical Perspectives

Regenerative medicine applications are methods that are effective in the repair and regeneration processes of tissues. Platelet-rich plasma (PRP) is one of these methods that is frequently applied. In general, it can be applied to all joints and musculoskeletal parts. In this section, information will be provided on the effectiveness of platelet-rich plasma (PRP) therapy in avascular necrosis in accordance with the current literature.

PRP treatment is a very modest procedure. When directly injecting into the affected area, cellular regeneration and damage repair, and wound healing are achieved. For osteonecrosis around the joint, the application is performed into the joint. Normally, our body increases the regional blood supply during the wound healing phase and platelet migration is provided to the zone. With PRP treatments, this pathway is copied and an application with a higher volume is realized. PRP treatment affects three basic mechanisms, especially in cases of avascular necrosis: 1) regrow bone and blood vessels, 2) prevent increased apoptosis, and 3) reduce inflammation in the affected area (Han et al., 2020). The autologous plasma of PRP contains platelets at concentrations above baseline. (Eppley et al., 2004). It also contains intense growth factors such as platelet-derived growth factor (PDGF), transforming growth factor-β (TGF-β), basic fibroblast growth factor (bFGF), endothelial growth factor (EGF), and vascular endothelial growth factor (VEGF). In this way, it directly affects the proliferation and differentiation of mesenchymal stem cells (Kuroda et al., 2015; Rackwitz et al., 2012). Growth factors have promotive effects on osteogenesis and angiogenesis separately (Nakamae et al., 2004; Radke et al., 2006; Suzuki et al., 2004). However, it has also been reported that some growth factors such as TGF-β may cause suppression in this process on their own (Broderick et al., 2005). While growth factors act synergistically, a balance is established in this complex process. In studies on the effects of PRP in the early stages of femoral head avascular necrosis, it is found that this diversity may provide an optimal environment (Brill, 2004; Han et al., 2020). Furthermore, the downregulation of IL-6 and IFN-γ release and its contribution to chondrogenic proliferation are among the other reported results (Bai et al., 2014; Suzuki et al., 2000).

Since PRP treatment is obtained from the person's own blood, the risk of rejection of the treatment by the system is low. This provides an advantage over other chemotherapeutic procedures applied in avascular necrosis. Persistent pain due to avascular necrosis is the result of inflammation. It is possible to suppress this ongoing inflammation with PRP. In this way, the patient can be treated and followed more easily. Although it seems like an advantageous treatment that can be applied theoretically, studies on the effectiveness of PRP methods are limited. In particular, PRP injections to be applied in the early stages when bone tissue can be repaired may provide an advantage.

PRP treatment in osteonecrosis is more effective when applied in combination with other methods rather than alone. It is applied intra-articularly and performs its effects in the synovial area. It is seen in the literature that PRP applications are performed more frequently, especially in the early period of osteonecrosis of the femoral head. PRP injection applied after core decompression rather than alone is a frequently applied method. There are randomized controlled studies showing that it provides better pain relief, midterm functional outcomes, and a decrease in the need for reoperation compared to the core decompression applications applied alone (Aggarwal et al., 2021; Grassi et al., 2020). In addition, the application of mesenchymal stem cells after core decompression is one of the preferred methods. It is possible to encounter clinical and radiological results reported for both bone marrow-derived mesenchymal stem cells (BmMSCs) and adipose-derived mesenchymal stem cells (AdMSCs). The purpose of this treatment is the transformation of mesenchymal stem cells into regenerative cells. In applications with BmMSCs, a significant decrease in the incidence of femoral head collapse, the need for total hip arthroplasty (THA) in the early period, and an improvement in Kerboul angles are noteworthy through this effect (Ha et al., 2006; Houdek et al., 2018). When PRP is supplementary to this treatment, it improves healing by showing osteoanagenic properties on MSCs. And this similar effect is also seen in applications combined with AdMSCs (Han et al., 2020). Moreover, one of the treatments performed in this patient group is the use of PRP together with a synthetic or autologous bone graft following the core decompression. Although there are limited data, successful results have been reported (Chen et al., 2020; D'Ambrosi et al., 2018; Han et al., 2020; Liang et al., 2023; Mont et al., 1998; Samy, 2016).

Accordingly, in the literature, it is seen that PRP applications for osteonecrosis in the field of orthopedics are limited in femoral head osteonecrosis. In the current literature review, there is also a case report that has been successfully applied in talar osteonecrosis. In this case, PRP was applied in addition to the stem cell with core decompression (Nevalainen et al., 2018). Likewise, there are a number of case series of medication-related osteonecrosis of the jaw (MRONJ) reflecting its applications in dentistry and Oromaxillofacial Surgery oral maxillofacial surgery (Cardoso et al., 2019; Souza Tolentino et al., 2019; Valente et al., 2019). The common conclusion of the studies is that it is a safe and effective adjuvant modality as in femoral head osteonecrosis (Egierska et al., 2023).

Conclusion

In light of current knowledge, PRP treatment is a very effective method in the early stages of osteonecrosis that can stimulate and accelerate healing and tissue regeneration in the musculoskeletal system. Applications alone are generally insufficient and its application in addition to other treatment methods is promising for osteogenesis and angiogenesis. It should be noted that this method is an adjunctive therapy. In the literature, there is almost no information other than proximal osteonecrosis of the femur. For this reason, more studies are still needed to provide helpful information. However, it is a rational approach to consider it among treatment options due to its positive effects and the fact that it is a method obtained from the patient's own blood.

References

Aggarwal, A. K., Poornalingam, K., Jain, A., & Prakash, M. (2021). Combining Platelet-Rich Plasma Instillation With Core Decompression Improves Functional Outcome and Delays Progression in Early-Stage Avascular Necrosis of Femoral Head: a 4.5- to 6-Year Prospective Randomized Comparative Study. *The Journal of Arthroplasty*, *36*(1), 54-61. https://doi.org/10.1016/j.arth.2020.07.010.

Bai, F., Tian, H. U. I., Niu, Z., Liu, M., Ren, G., Yu, Y., Sun, T., Li, S., & Li, D. (2014). Chimeric anti-IL-17 full-length monoclonal antibody is a novel potential candidate for the treatment of rheumatoid arthritis. *International Journal of Molecular Medicine*, *33*(3), 711-721. https://doi.org/10.3892/ijmm.2013.1611.

Brill, A. (2004). Differential role of platelet granular mediators in angiogenesis. *Cardiovascular Research*, *63*(2), 226-235. https://doi.org/10.1016/j.cardiores.2004.04.012.

Broderick, E., Infanger, S., Turner, T. M., & Sumner, D. R. (2005). Depressed Bone Mineralization Following High Dose TGF-β1 Application in an Orthopedic Implant Model. *Calcified Tissue International*, *76*(5), 379-384. https://doi.org/10.1007/s00223-004-0150-9.

Cardoso, C. L., Curra, C., Curi, M. M., Matsumoto, M. A., Argentino, C. D., Franzolin, S. d. O. B., Constantino, D., Barbarosa, D. N., & Ferreira JÚNior, O. (2019). Treatment of bisphosphonate-related osteonecrosis using platelet-rich plasma: microtomographic, microscopic, and immunohistochemical analyses. *Brazilian Oral Research*, *33*. https://doi.org/10.1590/1807-3107bor-2019.vol33.0050.

Chen, D. D., Lu, C., Yuwen, X., Li, H. H., Wang, Q. X., Yuan, X. C., & Hao, Y. Q. (2020). [Platelet-rich plasma combined with core decompression and bone grafting in the treatment of non traumatic necrosis of femoral head in ARCO stageII]. *Zhongguo Gu Shang*, *33*(11), 1048-1052. https://doi.org/10.12200/j.issn.1003-0034.2020.11.012.

D'Ambrosi, R., Biancardi, E., Massari, G., Ragone, V., & Facchini, R. (2018). Survival Analysis after Core Decompression in Association with Platelet-Rich Plasma, Mesenchymal Stem Cells, and Synthetic Bone Graft in Patients with Osteonecrosis of the Femoral Head. *Joints*, *06*(01), 016-022. https://doi.org/10.1055/s-0038-1626740.

Egierska, D., Perszke, M., Mazur, M., & Duś-Ilnicka, I. (2023). Platelet-rich plasma and platelet-rich fibrin in oral surgery: A narrative review. *Dental and Medical Problems*, *60*(1), 177-186. https://doi.org/10.17219/dmp/147298.

Eppley, B. L., Woodell, J. E., & Higgins, J. (2004). Platelet Quantification and Growth Factor Analysis from Platelet-Rich Plasma: Implications for Wound Healing. *Plastic and Reconstructive Surgery*, 1502-1508. https://doi.org/10.1097/01.Prs.0000138251.07040.51.

Glimcher, M. J., & Kenzora, J. E. (1979). Nicolas Andry award. The biology of osteonecrosis of the human femoral head and its clinical implications: 1. Tissue biology. *Clin Orthop Relat Res*(138), 284-309. https://www.ncbi.nlm.nih.gov/pubmed/445912.

Grassi, M., Salari, P., Massetti, D., Papalia, G. F., & Gigante, A. (2020). Treatment of avascular osteonecrosis of femoral head by core decompression and platelet-rich plasma: a prospective not controlled study. *International Orthopaedics*, *44*(7), 1287-1294. https://doi.org/10.1007/s00264-020-04628-4.

Ha, Y.-C., Jung, W. H., Kim, J.-R., Seong, N. H., Kim, S.-Y., & Koo, K.-H. (2006). Prediction of Collapse in Femoral Head Osteonecrosis: A Modified Kerboul Method with Use of Magnetic Resonance Images. *Journal of Bone and Joint Surgery*, *88*(suppl_3), 35-40. https://doi.org/10.2106/jbjs.F.00535.

Han, J., Gao, F., Li, Y., Ma, J., Sun, W., Shi, L., Wu, X., & Li, T. (2020). The Use of Platelet-Rich Plasma for the Treatment of Osteonecrosis of the Femoral Head: A Systematic Review. *BioMed Research International*, *2020*, 1-11. https://doi.org/10.1155/2020/2642439.

Houdek, M. T., Wyles, C. C., Collins, M. S., Howe, B. M., Terzic, A., Behfar, A., & Sierra, R. J. (2018). Stem Cells Combined With Platelet-rich Plasma Effectively Treat Corticosteroid-induced Osteonecrosis of the Hip: A Prospective Study. *Clinical Orthopaedics & Related Research*, *476*(2), 388-397. https://doi.org/10.1007/s11999.0000000000000033.

Kuroda, Y., Asada, R., So, K., Yonezawa, A., Nankaku, M., Mukai, K., Ito-Ihara, T., Tada, H., Yamamoto, M., Murayama, T., Morita, S., Tabata, Y., Yokode, M., Shimizu, A., Matsuda, S., & Akiyama, H. (2015). A pilot study of regenerative therapy using controlled release of recombinant human fibroblast growth factor for patients with pre-collapse osteonecrosis of the femoral head. *International Orthopaedics*, *40*(8), 1747-1754. https://doi.org/10.1007/s00264-015-3083-1.

Lamb, J. N., Holton, C., O'Connor, P., & Giannoudis, P. V. (2019). Avascular necrosis of the hip. *Bmj*, *365*, l2178. https://doi.org/10.1136/bmj.l2178.

Liang, D., Pei, J., Zhang, X., & Chen, X. (2023). Clinical outcomes of autologous platelet-rich plasma and bone marrow mononuclear cells grafting combined with core decompression for Association Research Circulation Osseous II–IIIA stage non-traumatic osteonecrosis of the femoral head. *International Orthopaedics*. https://doi.org/10.1007/s00264-023-05779-w.

Mont, M. A., Einhorn, T. A., Sponseller, P. D., & Hungerford, D. S. (1998). The trapdoor procedure using autogenous cortical and cancellous bone grafts for osteonecrosis of the femoral head. *The Journal of Bone and Joint Surgery. British volume*, *80-B*(1), 56-62. https://doi.org/10.1302/0301-620x.80b1.0800056.

Nakamae, A., Sunagawa, T., Ishida, O., Suzuki, O., Yasunaga, Y., Hachisuka, H., & Ochi, M. (2004). Acceleration of surgical angiogenesis in necrotic bone with a single injection of fibroblast growth factor-2 (FGF-2). *Journal of Orthopaedic Research*, *22*(3), 509-513. https://doi.org/10.1016/j.orthres.2003.10.001.

Nevalainen, M. T., Repo, J. P., Pesola, M., & Nyrhinen, J. P. (2018). Successful Treatment of Early Talar Osteonecrosis by Core Decompression Combined with Intraosseous Stem Cell Injection: A Case Report. *J Orthop Case Rep*, *8*(1), 23-26. https://doi.org/10.13107/jocr.2250-0685.982.

Rackwitz, L., Eden, L., Reppenhagen, S., Reichert, J. C., Jakob, F., Walles, H., Pulling, O., Tuan, R. S., Rudert, M., & Nöth, U. (2012). Stem cell- and growth factor-based regenerative therapies for avascular necrosis of the femoral head. *Stem Cell Research & Therapy*, *3*(1). https://doi.org/10.1186/scrt98.

Radke, S., Battmann, A., Jatzke, S., Eulert, J., Jakob, F., & Schütze, N. (2006). Expression of the angiomatrix and angiogenic proteins CYR61, CTGF, and VEGF in osteonecrosis of the femoral head. *Journal of Orthopaedic Research*, *24*(5), 945-952. https://doi.org/10.1002/jor.20097.

Samy, A. M. (2016). Management of osteonecrosis of the femoral head. *Indian Journal of Orthopaedics*, *50*(4), 359-365. https://doi.org/10.4103/0019-5413.185590.

Souza Tolentino, E., Castro, T. F., Michellon, F. C., Passoni, A. C. C., Ortega, L. J. A., Iwaki, L. C. V., & Silva, M. C. (2019). Adjuvant therapies in the management of medication-related osteonecrosis of the jaws: Systematic review. *Head & Neck*, *41*(12), 4209-4228. https://doi.org/10.1002/hed.25944.

Suzuki, M., Tetsuka, T., Yoshida, S., Watanabe, N., Kobayashi, M., Matsui, N., & Okamoto, T. (2000). The role of p38 mitogen-activated protein kinase in IL-6 and IL-8 production from the TNF-α- or IL-1β-stimulated rheumatoid synovial fibroblasts. *FEBS Letters*, *465*(1), 23-27. https://doi.org/10.1016/s0014-5793(99)01717-2.

Suzuki, O., Bishop, A. T., Sunagawa, T., Katsube, K., & Friedrich, P. F. (2004). VEGF-promoted surgical angiogenesis in necrotic bone. *Microsurgery*, *24*(1), 85-91. https://doi.org/10.1002/micr.10190.

Valente, N. A., Chatelain, S., Alfonsi, F., Mortellaro, C., & Barone, A. (2019). Medication-Related Osteonecrosis of the Jaw. *Journal of Craniofacial Surgery, 30*(4), 1095-1101. https://doi.org/10.1097/scs.0000000000005475.

Chapter 6

PRP Treatment for Lateral and Medial Epicondylitis

Ahmet Çağrı Uyar*, MD
Department of Orthopedics and Traumatology, University of Health Sciences, Kocaeli Derince Training and Research Hospital, Kocaeli, Turkiye

Abstract

Lateral epicondylitis (LE), also termed tennis elbow, is a tendonitis of the extensor carpi radialis brevis (ECRB) muscle. Involvement of the extensor carpi radialis longus and the extensor carpi ulnaris may also be observed. Its incidence in society is between 1% and 3% (Aksoy et al., 2022). Medial epicondylitis (ME), also known as golfer's elbow, occurs as a result of microtrauma and degeneration of the forearm flexor muscles at the common insertion point in the medial epicondyle of the elbow, which is similar to LE. It occurs between the fourth and sixth decades of life and affects both males and females equally (Amin et al., 2015).

Elbow epicondylitis is associated with excessive use combined with repetitive wrist flexion, extension, supination, and pronation movements. There are many treatment options for lateral and medial epicondylitis. The first choice is usually conservative treatment, and success is often achieved (Lenoir et al., 2019; Tarpada et al., 2018). Commonly used treatments include rest, activity modification, nonsteroidal anti-inflammatory drugs (NSAIDs), physiotherapy, injections (corticosteroids, platelet-rich plasma, prolotherapy), and orthotics. Surgical treatment can also be implemented in resistant cases (Aktaş et al., 2014; Lenoir et al., 2019).

---

* Corresponding Author's Email: ahmetcagriuyar@gmail.com.

In: Current Clinical Recommendations ...
Editors: Nazan Yurtcu and Emel Güler
ISBN: 979-8-89113-723-3

Platelet-rich plasma (PRP) injections are frequently used in tendon and ligament pathologies. The efficacy of PRP therapy in the treatment of elbow epicondylitis has been proven in many studies in the literature. PRP is a safe and effective treatment method in cases where lateral and medial epicondylitis cannot be treated with first-line treatments.

Keywords: lateral epicondylitis, medial epicondylitis, platelet-rich plasma, injection

Introduction

Lateral epicondylitis (LE), also known as tennis elbow, is tendonitis of the extensor carpi radialis brevis (ECRB) muscle. Involvement of the extensor carpi radialis longus and the extensor carpi ulnaris may also be observed. It is characterized by pain and tenderness around the lateral epicondyle of the elbow. The incidence in society is between 1% and 3% (Aksoy et al., 2022). It is more common in women between 40-60 years of age. It is associated with excessive use of repetitive wrist extension, supination, and pronation movements. It is frequently encountered in occupations that involve repetitive movements of the wrist and in racket sports such as tennis. The first preference in the treatment of LE is usually conservative treatment and success is often achieved (Lenoir et al., 2019).

Medial epicondylitis (ME), also known as golfer's elbow, is characterized by microtrauma and degeneration of the forearm flexor muscles at the common insertion point in the medial epicondyle of the elbow, which is similar to LE. It occurs between the fourth and sixth decades of life and affects both males and females equally (Amin et al., 2015).

There are various options for the treatment of lateral and medial epicondylitis. Commonly used treatments include rest, activity modification, nonsteroidal anti-inflammatory drugs (NSAIDs), physiotherapy, injections (corticosteroids, platelet-rich plasma, prolotherapy), and orthotics. Surgical treatment can also be implemented in resistant cases that do not improve with non-surgical treatments (Aktaş et al., 2014; Lenoir et al., 2019; Tarpada et al., 2018).

Platelet-rich plasma (PRP) injections are frequently used in tendon and ligament pathologies. It has been demonstrated to accelerate healing when administered locally in muscle and tendon diseases owing to its rich platelet, growth factors, and stoichins (Anitua et al., 2005).

Anatomy

The elbow joint consists of three joints, the humeroulnar, humeroradial, and proximal radioulnar joints, and is a stable joint due to the anatomical features of the structures that constitute the joint. The wrist and finger extensors and supinators are located at the elbow. These muscles are innervated by the radial nerve (Hutchinson & Wynn, 2004). The lateral epicondyle is the common insertion point of the forearm and hand extensors. Symptoms may occur in the lateral epicondyle as a result of strain at the insertion point of the brachioradialis, extensor carpi radialis, extensor carpi ulnaris, and extensor digitorum muscles.

The medial epicondyle is the insertion point of the forearm flexor group muscles. The tenoperiosteal junction of the flexor carpi ulnaris, flexor carpi radialis, flexor digitorum superficialis, and palmaris longus muscles is the area that is affected in medial epicondylitis.

Etiology

LE is an excessive use-related degenerative process associated with repetitive wrist extension, supination, and pronation movements. Repetitive microtrauma causes inflammation of the extensor tendon, resulting in fibrous adhesions that restrict movement and pain lateral to the elbow joint (Wadsworth, 1987). The most commonly affected muscle is the ECRB. Although LE is known as tennis elbow, only 10% of patients are tennis players. LE is most commonly seen in heavy manual laborers whose work requires repetitive fine motor movements (Haahr & Andersen, 2003; Lenoir et al., 2019).

Medial epicondylitis is related to microtrauma and degenerative processes resulting from repetitive movements of the forearm and wrist that affect the flexor muscle group (Amin et al., 2015; Tarpada et al., 2018). The overall prevalence is less than 1%. Although it has been associated with overhead throwing, golf, and tennis, it has been reported in soccer, weightlifting, and bowling players in the literature (Noyes et al., 1992).

Treatment Methods

Lateral epicondylitis and medial epicondylitis are often treated with conservative treatment modalities (Amin et al., 2015; Noyes et al., 1992; Tarpada et al., 2018; Haahr & Andersen, 2003; Lenoir et al., 2019). While spontaneous regression is observed in some cases, nonsteroidal anti-inflammatory drugs, physiotherapy, corticosteroid injections, extracorporeal shock therapy, and platelet-rich plasma injection are among the treatment methods (Aktaş et al., 2014; Filardo et al., 2016; Smidt et al., 2002). Although there are not enough data in the literature, orthoses such as forearm splinting are also used in treatment (Jafarian et al., 2009). Although LE and ME are mostly treated with conservative treatment methods, surgical treatment is required in a group of cases (Amin et al., 2015; Johns & Shridhar, 2020; Ma & Wang, 2020).

PRP (Platelet Rich-Plasma)

The practice of PRP (platelet-rich plasma) in chronic tendon and ligament diseases is being practiced more and more frequently in clinical practice. It is also among the methods that can be preferred in the treatment of lateral epicondylitis and medial epicondylitis in cases where treatment cannot be achieved with conservative treatment methods (Murray et al., 2015; Tarpada et al., 2018).

The patient may remain in a sitting or lying position during PRP injection in the treatment of LE. After the sterility procedures have been finalized, the insertion point of the forearm extensors in the lateral epicondyle is detected with the thumb. When palpation is performed, PRP injection is administered to the other sensitive points of the lesion starting from a point with intense tenderness. Similarly, in ME injection, the painful point of the lesion is determined with the thumb, and the injection is carried out to insertion of the flexor muscle group in the medial condyle. At this point, careful attention should be paid to the neighborhood of the ulnar nerve. The patient should be reminded that pain may occur 24-48 hours after injection. Intermittent ice practice and not using the affected arm for heavy work for one week are recommended.

Many studies in the literature report that PRP treatment can be implemented in cases where first-line treatments are inadequate (A. Mishra et al., 2012; Murray et al., 2015). In their controlled prospective study, Mirshra et al. performed PRP injection at 5 different points by making a single skin entry point around the ECRB tendon and compared the results with bupivacaine administered to the control group with a similar technique. In this study, they reported a higher improvement in the PRP group compared to the control group (A. Mishra et al., 2012). In two randomized controlled trials published by Gosens and Peerbooms, corticosteroid injection and PRP administration were compared. At four and eight weeks of early follow-up, the steroid group demonstrated greater improvement in terms of functional outcomes and pain scale compared to PRP. In long-term follow-up, it was reported that steroid efficacy decreased and the two-year long-term results of the PRP group were better (Gosens et al., 2011; Peerbooms et al., 2010). In two other prospective studies, long-term improvement on the pain scale was reported after PRP injection. In these two studies, it was reported that the increase in functional improvement continued in the long-term follow-up (Hechtman et al., 2011; A. K. Mishra et al., 2014).

Studies on PRP administration in the treatment of ME are quite limited compared to LE. It has been reported that conservative methods are often successful in the treatment of ME, but PRP practices are increasingly being used (Filardo et al., 2016; Tarpada et al., 2018).

Conclusion

The frequency of administration of platelet rich-plasma (PRP) therapy in tendon, muscle, and ligament injuries is increasing. The effectiveness of PRP therapy in the treatment of elbow epicondylitis has been reported in many studies in the literature. Platelet rich-plasma is a safe and effective treatment method in cases where lateral and medial epicondylitis cannot be treated with first-line treatments.

References

Aksoy, A., Gülcü, A., & Aslan, A. (2022). Comparison of the Effects of Different Treatment Methods Applied in Patients with Lateral Epicondylitis on Clinical Outcomes. *Acta Medica Alanya*. https://doi.org/10.30565/medalanya.1214401.

Aktaş, E., Yılmaz, B., Ataoğlu, B., Arıkan, M., Toğral, G., & İlikmen, M. (2014). The Efficacy of Platelet Rich Plasma Combined with Steroid Injection in the Treatment of Resistant Lateral Epicondylitis. *Acta Oncologica Turcica*, 47(3), 26–31. https://doi.org/10.5505/aot.2014.18480.

Amin, N. H., Kumar, N. S., & Schickendantz, M. S. (2015). Medial epicondylitis: evaluation and management. *The Journal of the American Academy of Orthopaedic Surgeons*, 23(6), 348–355. https://doi.org/10.5435/JAAOS-D-14-00145.

Anitua, E., Andía, I., Sanchez, M., Azofra, J., del Mar Zalduendo, M., de la Fuente, M., Nurden, P., & Nurden, A. T. (2005). Autologous preparations rich in growth factors promote proliferation and induce VEGF and HGF production by human tendon cells in culture. *Journal of Orthopaedic Research*, 23(2), 281–286. https://doi.org/10.1016/j.orthres.2004.08.015.

Filardo, G., di Matteo, B., Kon, E., Merli, G., & Marcacci, M. (2016). Platelet-rich plasma in tendon-related disorders: results and indications. *Knee Surgery, Sports Traumatology, Arthroscopy* 2016 26:7, 26(7), 1984–1999. https://doi.org/10.1007/S00167-016-4261-4.

Gosens, T., Peerbooms, J. C., van Laar, W., & den Oudsten, B. L. (2011). Ongoing positive effect of platelet-rich plasma versus corticosteroid injection in lateral epicondylitis: a double-blind randomized controlled trial with 2-year follow-up. *The American Journal of Sports Medicine,* 39(6), 1200–1208. https://doi.org/10.1177/0363546510397173.

Haahr, J. P., & Andersen, J. H. (2003). Physical and psychosocial risk factors for lateral epicondylitis: a population based case-referent study. *Occupational and Environmental Medicine*, 60(5), 322–329. https://doi.org/10.1136/OEM.60.5.322.

Hechtman, K. S., Uribe, J. W., Botto-vanDemden, A., & Kiebzak, G. M. (2011). Platelet-rich plasma injection reduces pain in patients with recalcitrant epicondylitis. *Orthopedics*, 34(2). https://doi.org/10.3928/01477447-20101221-05.

Hutchinson, M. R., & Wynn, S. (2004). Biomechanics and development of the elbow in the young throwing athlete. *Clinics in Sports Medicine*, 23(4), 531–544. https://doi.org/10.1016/J.CSM.2004.06.005.

Jafarian, F. S., Demneh, E. S., & Tyson, S. F. (2009). The immediate effect of orthotic management on grip strength of patients with lateral epicondylosis. *The Journal of Orthopaedic and Sports Physical Therapy*, 39(6), 484–489. https://doi.org/10.2519/JOSPT.2009.2988.

Johns, N., & Shridhar, V. (2020). Lateral epicondylitis: Current concepts. *Australian Journal of General Practice,* 49(11), 707–709. https://doi.org/10.31128/AJGP-07-20-5519.

Lenoir, H., Mares, O., & Carlier, Y. (2019). Management of lateral epicondylitis. *Orthopaedics & Traumatology: Surgery & Research,* 105(8), S241–S246. https://doi.org/10.1016/J.OTSR.2019.09.004.

Ma, K. L., & Wang, H. Q. (2020). Management of Lateral Epicondylitis: A Narrative Literature Review. *Pain Research & Management,* 2020. https://doi.org/10.1155/2020/6965381.

Mishra, A., Harmon, K., Woodall, J., & Vieira, A. (2012). Sports medicine applications of platelet rich plasma. *Current Pharmaceutical Biotechnology,* 13(7), 1185–1195. https://doi.org/10.2174/138920112800624283.

Mishra, A. K., Skrepnik, N. v., Edwards, S. G., Jones, G. L., Sampson, S., Vermillion, D. A., Ramsey, M. L., Karli, D. C., & Rettig, A. C. (2014). Efficacy of platelet-rich plasma for chronic tennis elbow: a double-blind, prospective, multicenter, randomized controlled trial of 230 patients. *The American Journal of Sports Medicine*, 42(2), 463–471. https://doi.org/10.1177/0363546513494359.

Murray, D. J., Javed, S., Jain, N., Kemp, S., & Watts, A. C. (2015). Platelet—Rich—Plasma Injections in Treating Lateral Epicondylosis: a Review of the Recent Evidence. *Journal of Hand and Microsurgery*, 7(2), 320. https://doi.org/10.1007/S12593-015-0193-3.

Noyes, F. R., DeMaio, M., Mangine, R. E., & Galloway, M. (1992). Rehabilitative techniques in the treatment of medial and lateral epicondylitis. *Orthopedics*, 15(9), 1089–1096. https://doi.org/10.3928/0147-7447-19920901-17.

Peerbooms, J. C., Sluimer, J., Bruijn, D. J., & Gosens, T. (2010). Positive effect of an autologous platelet concentrate in lateral epicondylitis in a double-blind randomized controlled trial: platelet-rich plasma versus corticosteroid injection with a 1-year follow-up. *The American Journal of Sports Medicine,* 38(2), 255–262. https://doi.org/10.1177/0363546509355445.

Smidt, N., van der Windt, D. A. W. M., Assendelft, W. J. J., Devillé, W. L. J. M., Korthals-de Bos, I. B. C., & Bouter, L. M. (2002). Corticosteroid injections, physiotherapy, or a wait-and-see policy for lateral epicondylitis: A randomised controlled trial. *Lancet,* 359(9307), 657–662. https://doi.org/10.1016/S0140-6736(02)07811-X.

Tarpada, S. P., Morris, M. T., Lian, J., & Rashidi, S. (2018). Current advances in the treatment of medial and lateral epicondylitis. *Journal of Orthopaedics*, 15(1), 107. https://doi.org/10.1016/J.JOR.2018.01.040.

Wadsworth, T. G. (1987). Tennis elbow: conservative, surgical, and manipulative treatment. *British Medical Journal (Clinical Research Ed.)*, 294(6572), 621–624. https://doi.org/10.1136/BMJ.294.6572.621.

Chapter 7

Platelet-Rich Plasma (PRP) Treatment for Achilles Tendinopathy

Anar Alakbarov[1,*], MD
and Vusala Garayeva[2], MD
[1]Department of Orthopedics and Traumatology,
Nakhchivan Diagnostic-Treatment Center, Nakhchivan, Azerbaijan
[2]Department of Radiology, Nakhchivan Diagnostic-Treatment Center,
Nakhchivan, Azerbaijan

Abstract

Achilles Tendinopathy is a common foot and ankle condition that cannot be easily treated. More than one treatment modality for the cure has been tried, such as physiotherapy, immobilization, injections, shockwave therapy, and surgical intervention. Among these treatments, injections, especially Platelet-Rich Plasma (PRP) treatment, are frequently used. It is obtained after centrifugation of blood and has a highly concentrated platelet content compared to plasma. Platelets are a natural human body product and have an important role in the clotting cascade, promoting the healing process of inflammatory tissue. Because PRP contains recovery speed-up autologous materials such as some cytokines and growth factors, it has recently become more popular in orthopedic practice, especially in the treatment of tendon injuries. Platelet-rich plasma (PRP) injections have been studied since the 1970s and are widely used for tendinopathies. More than a dozen studies have been conducted in recent years to assess the effectiveness of the Platelet-rich plasma injection method for Achilles tendon problems. However, there was still controversy about whether PRP injection had a

* Corresponding Author's Email: opr.dr.anar@hotmail.com.

In: Current Clinical Recommendations ...
Editors: Nazan Yurtcu and Emel Güler
ISBN: 979-8-89113-723-3

beneficial effect on Achilles tendinopathy and other tendinopathies. On the other hand, many articles in the literature support the success of the treatment and the positive impact of PRP on Achilles tendinopathy.

Keywords: platelet-rich plasma, PRP, achilles tendon, tendinopathy, treatment

Introduction

The Achilles tendon (AT) is anatomically located in the calf and is not only the largest but also the strongest tendon in the body. It is the conjugation of the gastrocnemius (two-headed) and soleus muscle tendons (Figure 1). Because of its anatomical position and functional mission, it is prone to injury, such as tendinopathy. Intrinsic and extrinsic factors are the cause of Achilles tendinopathy. The tendinopathy mechanisms of the Achilles tendon are still unclear, but some intrinsic factors are considered to cause this situation. These factors are age and sex of patients, systemic diseases, tendon vascularity impairment, body weight and height, gastrocnemius-soleus dysfunction, pes cavus, lateral ankle instability, and genetic predisposition. Extrinsic factors are overuse and some drug usage (Wagnan et al., 2014).

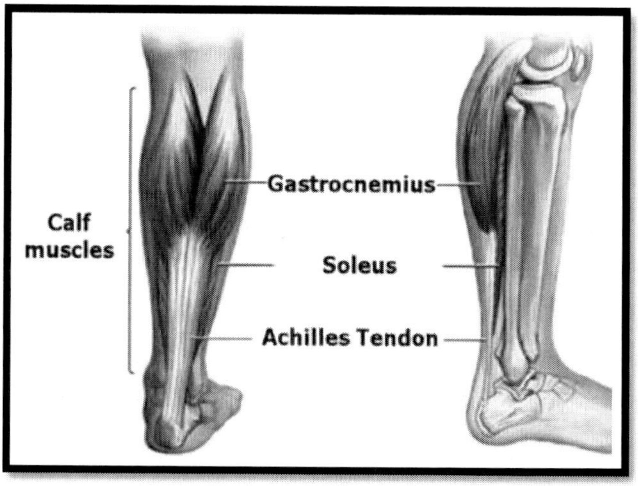

Figure 1. Anatomical illustration of Achilles tendon (Mobile Physical Therapy, 2019).

Normal and healthy Achilles tendon contains tenocytes and tenoblasts specialized fibroblasts that secrete collagen. Approximately 70% of the dry weight of the tendon is collagen (nearly 95% of collagen is type I), and about 2% is elastin fibers. The remaining parts are cells, neurovascular structures, glycosaminoglycans, and proteoglycans. The general meaning of tendinopathy is failure of the healing response, with degeneration, proliferation, and improper arrangement of tendon cells (tenocytes), disruption of collagen fibers, and non-collagenous matrix enhancement. Typically and normally, collagen fibers are arranged in a parallel fashion and tightly bundled, but collagen fibers lose their parallel orientation in the tendinopathic areas, and their diameter decreases. Microscopically, collagen microtears occur, and fibers are surrounded by erythrocytes, fibrin, and fibronectin deposits (Mafulli et al., 2019). Degenerative collagen fibers are loose, waviness increases, and type I collagen replaces type III (reparative) collagen. Various types of degeneration have been described in the electron microscope, such as 1-hypoxic degeneration, 2-myxoid or mucoid degeneration, 3-lipoid degeneration, 4-hyaline degeneration, 5-fibrinoid degeneration, 6-fibrocartilaginous and bony metaplasia, and 7-calcification (Longo et al., 2009). All of these degeneration types lead to a tendon injury in the tendinopathic area (Figure 2).

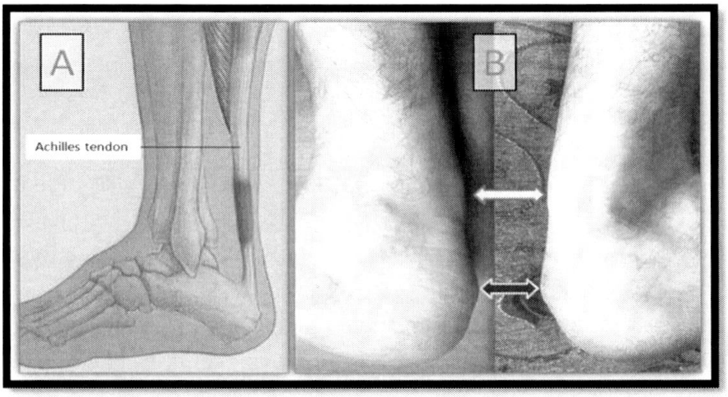

Figure 2. Illustration and clinical photo of Achilles tendinopathy location. A– Illustration from https://www.mayoclinic.org/diseases-conditions/achilles-tendinitis/symptoms-causes/syc-20369020, B – The clinical photo of the patient represents both non–insertional tendinosis - thickening and degeneration 3–6 cm proximally to the calcaneal insertion (up–white arrow) and insertional tendinosis (down–black arrow) classification and thickening at the calcaneal insertion (Author's own archive).

Some essential tools may help distinguish Achilles tendinopathy from other conditions during the physical examination. One of these tools is the Victorian Institute of Sports Assessment–Achilles (VISA-A) questionnaire specifically measures the severity of Achilles tendinopathy (Robinson et al., 2001). The questionnaire assesses function, pain, and activity, which provides a user-friendly, valid, and reliable index for the severity of Achilles tendinopathy (Figure 3 and Figures 4-A, 4-B, 4-C).

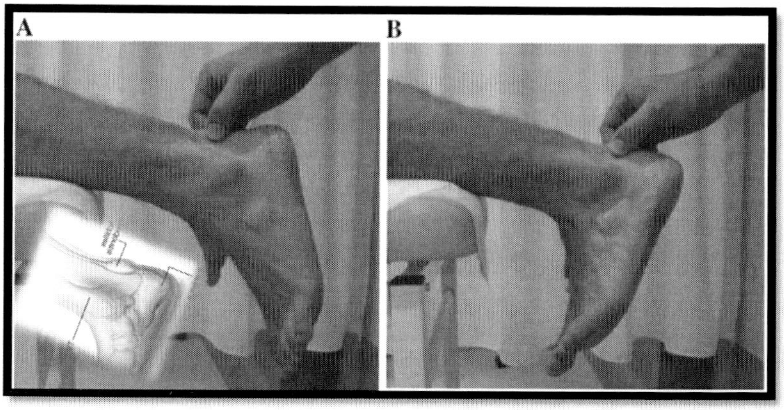

Figure 3. Royal London Hospital Test.
A- The physician (tester) finds the tendon tender area at the outset. B- The patient actively plantarflexes and dorsiflexes the ankle, and the tender area of the tendon is palpated by the physician again for determining the increasing pain (Robinson et al., 2001; Mayo Clinic, n.d.).

As with clinical examination and history, imaging is also indispensable for diagnosis. The ankle roentgenogram (especially in the lateral view) can help detect bony abnormalities. It is routinely obtained from patients who have symptoms lasting longer than six weeks to disclose any abnormal calcification or ossification. The presence of a posterior heel spur (calcaneal insertion calcification) is diagnostic of insertional Achilles tendinopathy.

Ultrasonography is well correlated with histopathological findings, but it is operator-dependent and an interactive capability is a major advantage of ultrasonography. Grey-scale ultrasonography (G-s USG) can detect neovascularity and may be tears (Figures 5-A and 5-B).

Victorian Institute of Sports Assessment–Achilles (VISA-A) questionnaire. VISA-A Questionnaire: A index of the severity of Achilles tendinopathy (in this questionnaire, the term pain refers specifically to pain in the Achilles region). 10

1. For how many minutes do you have stiffness in the Achilles region on first getting up?

100 mins **0 mins**

0 1 2 3 4 5 6 7 8 9 10

2. Once you are warmed up for the day, do you have pain when stretching the Achilles tendon fully over the edge of a step? (keeping knee straight)

pain

0 1 2 3 4 5 6 7 8 9 10

3. After walking on flat ground for 30 minutes, do you have pain within the next 2 hours?

(if unable to walk on flat ground for 30 minutes because of pain, score 0 for this question)

pain

0 1 2 3 4 5 6 7 8 9 10

4. Do you have pain walking downstairs with a normal gait cycle?

pain

0 1 2 3 4 5 6 7 8 9 10

Figure 4A. The Victorian Institute of Sports Assessment–Achilles (VISA-A) questionnaire specifically measures the severity of Achilles tendinopathy.

5. Do you have pain during or immediately after doing 10 (single leg) heel raises from a flat surface? If you cannot perform a heel raise, please check here: [ ], and indicate level of pain in attempting a heel raise.

pain

0 1 2 3 4 5 6 7 8 9 10

6. How many single leg hops can you do without pain? If you cannot perform a single leg hop, please check here:

pain

0 1 2 3 4 5 6 7 8 9 10

7. Are you currently undertaking a sport or other physical activity? Please indicate what type of physical activity or

exercise: ______________________

0 Not at all

4 Modified training/exercise

7 Full training/exercise, though not at the same level as pre-injury

10 Full training/exercise, as the same or higher level than when Achilles symptoms began (pre-injury)

Figure 4B. The Victorian Institute of Sports Assessment–Achilles (VISA-A) questionnaire specifically measures the severity of Achilles tendinopathy.

8. Please complete EITHER A, B, or C in this question:

- If you have NO PAIN while undergoing Achilles tendon loading sports/exercise/activity, please complete question 8a only.

- If you have SOME PAIN while undertaking Achilles tendon loading sports/exercise/activity, please complete question 8b only.

- If you have PAIN THAT STOPS YOU from completing Achilles tendon loading sports/exercise/activity, please complete question 8c only.

A. If you have NO PAIN while undertaking Achilles tendon loading sport/exercise/activity, for how long can you participate in activity?

NIL	1-10 mins	11-20 mins	21-30 mins	>30 mins
0	7	14	21	30

B. If you have SOME PAIN while undertaking Achilles tendon loading sport/exercise/activity, but it does not stop you from completing your training/

NIL	1-10 mins	11-20 mins	21-30 mins	>30 mins
0	7	14	21	30

C. If you have pain that STOPS YOU from completing your Achilles tendon loading activity, for how long can you participate in this activity before

having to stop?

NIL	1-10 mins	11-20 mins	21-30 mins	>30 mins
0	7	14	21	30

Figure 4C. The Victorian Institute of Sports Assessment–Achilles (VISA-A) questionnaire specifically measures the severity of Achilles tendinopathy.

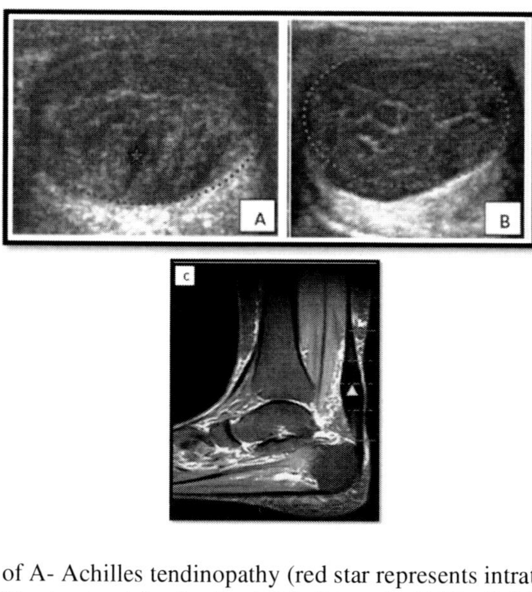

Figure 5. USG of A- Achilles tendinopathy (red star represents intratendinous tear), B- Normal Achilles tendon (after healing) (Madhi et al., 2020), C- MRI of Achilles tendinopathy (yellow triangle shows the tendinopathic area) (Owens et al., 2011).

MRI (magnetic resonance imagining) is more sensitive than ultrasonography to detect incomplete rupture of the tendon, but it is used when ultrasonography is unclear. MRI provides more detailed information about the internal human morphology and especially soft tissue and bone pathologies. It is superior to other imaging modalities regarding pre-operative planning and follow-up advantages (Figure 5-C). On MRI images, the scoring of tendinopathy can also be performed. This scoring system is important for physicians to use the same language to classify pathology and manage the disease (Figure 6).

Computed tomography is not used routinely because radiography (X-ray) is sufficient for first-step imaging.

Once the diagnosis of Achilles tendinopathy has been obtained after physical examination and imaging, various modalities can be selected for the treatment. One of these modalities is PRP treatment.

Achilles Tendinopathy Grade.

Grade 0	Hypertrophy, with homogeneous signal
Grade 1	Hypertrophy, with isolated signal changes in <25% of tendon
Grade 2	Hypertrophy, with signal changes in more than 1 area, or diffuse changes in >25% of tendon
Grade 3	Severe hypertrophy, <50% tendon signal changes, with interstitial tear
Grade 4	Severe thickening, >50% of tendon with abnormal signal, partial tendon tear

Figure 6. Scoring system of Achilles tendinopathy on MRI (Oloff et al., 2015).

PRP is obtained from blood after centrifugation. After taking a certain amount of blood (generally 10 mL) from the patient's peripheral vein system, it is prepared for centrifugation in a particular container and placed on the spin device.

In general, PRP production is obtained after two spins (most kit require two spins). One spin is for separation, and the second is for concentration. The speed in rotations per minute (RPM) and duration (spin time) are two main indicators and factors of the spins. The spin rate of the device should be adjusted between 1000 to 3600 RPM, and the time last 4 to 15 minutes to separate blood. Deciding on the amount of spin and time depends on the protocol to be selected, the type of device, the type of container, and the amount of platelets to be obtained (Gaveda et al., 2010; Lui et al., 2019).

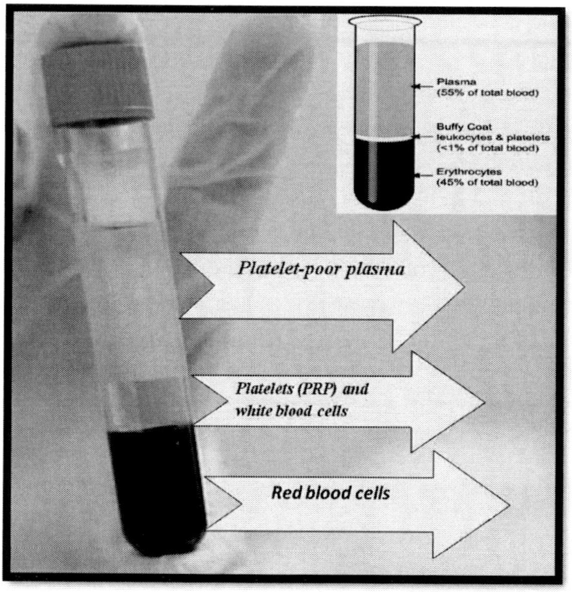

Figure 7. The PRP container includes three layers of blood after the centrifugation procedure.

After centrifugation of the blood in the container, it is separated into three distinct layers. The first and upper parts are platelet-poor plasma, the second and middle are buffy coat-white blood cells (platelet-rich plasma), and the third and lower are red blood cells (Figure 7). Because of the large amount of platelet, the buffy coat layer is a more convenient and recommended part of centrifuged blood for PRP therapy. The concentration of platelet that is assumed to be the most effective is above 100,000/mm3. Sabarish et al. obtained large amounts of platelet after lower spin rates and predicted that high spin rates could cause platelet disintegration and clumping (Sabarish et al., 2015). Generally, the concentration of platelet in the PRP is 2 (two) to 6 (six) times higher than the normal blood sample.

Anticoagulants are used to block the coagulation cascade (prevent coagulation) of blood in the container. The most commonly used chemical is anticoagulant citrate dextrose-A (ACD-A) in commercial kits. The anticoagulant citrate dextrose-A (ACD-A) maintains a pH of 7.2, optimal for citrate binding to calcium to block coagulation. Because of the suppression effect of platelet degranulation, ethylenediaminetetraacetic acid (EDTA) is not recommended. Due to the spontaneous aggregation effect of platelets in some individuals, heparin is also not recommended (Dhurat et al., 2014).

After preparation of PRP, it can be injected directly into the affected area (around pain), especially in the superficial part of the body, or USG can be used as a guide to injection (Figure 8).

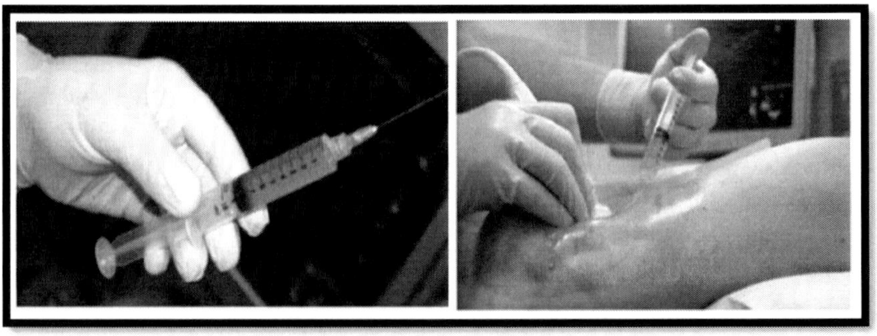

Figure 8. Injection of PRP into the Achilles tendinopathy area with the USG guided (Kaux, 2016).

Discussion

Achilles tendinopathy is commonly the mid-portion and chronic degeneration of the tendon. The etiology is not well understood, but overuse of tendons, trauma, rheumatologic diseases, and some drugs (especially steroid medication) are thought to be risk factors. Repetitive overload is considered to cause microtears, and failure of the normal healing process results in tendinopathy. It has been shown that tendinopathy generally occurs at 2-6 cm proximal to the calcaneal attachment region of the Achilles tendon due to relatively decreased blood flow in the accepted hypo-vascular area (Courville et al., 2009).

Non-operative and operative treatments are widely used for Achilles tendinopathy. Besides conservative treatments, PRP has a special place because it is an autologous blood component and essentially is a new entity. PRP undertakes the role of coagulation cascade activation and several factors releasing that recruit injured tendons, tenocytes, and other cells, which promotes the healing process (Nurden et al., 2011). After injection of PRP, some growth factors and cytokines such as PDGF (platelet-derived growth factor), VEGF (vascular endothelial growth factor), TGFB-1 (transforming growth factor-beta 1), FBGF (fibroblast growth factor), HGF (hepatocyte growth factor), IGF (insulin-like growth factor), CGF (connective tissue growth factor), and EGF (epidermal growth factor) were secreted and acted as chemo-attractants for reparative cells, modulate angiogenesis (new vessel production) and neovascularization (perfusion), enhance local production of collagen, and block cylco-oxygenase-2 (COX-2) enzyme production, which provides anti-inflammatory effects (Monto et al., 2012). Despite these effects, there is no consensus among the authors about the effectiveness of PRP in Achilles tendinopathy in the orthopedic literature at the current date.

Traditional non-operative treatment of Achilles tendinopathy has a 25% failure rate so numerous surgical procedures have been reported in the literature such as operative debridement of off-grade tissues, allograft augmentation, and autogenous flexor digitorum longus or flexor hallucis longus tendon transfer (Monto et al., 2012). Therefore, Madhi et al. have not shown any promising results with surgical treatments, including debridement or tendon transfer (Madhi et Al., 2020). Because of the varying clinical outcomes of these surgical interventions, PRP therapy was predicted and accepted to be relevant and favorable for Achilles tendinopathy. The advantages of PRP are that it is an autologous substance, free of transmissible diseases, a small volume of blood is enough for the procedure, it is safe and is well or easily accepted by patients and surgeons. Furthermore, it is a relatively cheaper and more tolerable treatment method than other treatments (Guelfi et al., 2015). Because PRP is autologous blood, it has no immunogenic reactions or other serious adverse effects. Regarding safety, there have been no reports of infection after PRP injection or any condition leading to hospitalization. The only mentioned side effect reported was injection-related pain (Nauwelaers et al., 2020). Whether PRP injection is done under USG (USG guided) or injected directly, the injection point is still a challenging topic. It can be done directly to the most affected area (puncture location), around the affected area, between the tendon and the peritendinous space, or the thickest part of the tendon. But the consensus in the articles is that PRP should be injected into the 'injured area' without further specification. (Nauwelaers et al., 2020). Besides PRP injection, saline, and dry injections can be used to heal Achilles tendinopathy. Injection of saline or stimulation with a dry needle provides inflammation and bleeding in the affected area of the Achilles tendon (Wang et al., 2019). This is why saline and dry injections are compared with PRP injections and designed as control groups (in randomized control trials) in the literature. However, eccentric calf training treatment is also used to heal Achilles tendinopathy, and it is also compared as a control marker with PRP in the articles, but it is not interventional therapy, so it is different from saline and dry injections. By the way, Murphy et al. found that VISA-A scores are substantially less than in intense eccentric calf training compared to using PRP, and they claimed that PRP can be a successful treatment for Achilles tendinopathy (Murphy et al., 2019).

According to Murawski et al. PRP injection improves patient satisfaction and relieves pain in the condition of tendon degeneration (Murawski et al., 2014). On the other hand, an eccentric exercise program which was used for chronic mid-portion Achilles tendinopathy as a treatment, a comparison of saline injection and PRP injection did not significantly improve activity and pain in patients. Thus, the authors did not recommend PRP injection therapy for CMAT-chronic mid-portion Achilles tendinopathy (De Vos et al., 2010). Although Monto et al. found that the PRP injection group returned to especially sporting activities twice as the placebo group in the six months follow-up, in the end, they concluded that the PRP injection had no more effectiveness than the placebo as a saline injection in the Achilles tendinosis treatment. (Monto et al., 2012). This opinion is supported by meta-analyses and systematic reviews of studies that PRP injection therapy has no clinical benefit or treatment advantages compared to a saline injection or eccentric loading program (Collins et al., 2021).

Vithran et al. also published a systemic review and meta-analysis in 2023 and screened 405 articles initially, but they selected only eight high-quality papers that met their criteria. The study showed moderate evidence that the PRP injection therapy effect was not superior to saline or eccentric treating therapy regarding patient satisfaction, pain reduction (VAS score), return to activity –especially sports, and VISA–A scores of patients at 6 and 24 weeks. Although it was not statistically significant, they found that in the PRP-treated group, the Achilles tendon thickness is greater than in the placebo group at 12 weeks of treatment. The only acceptable result was at 12 weeks, the VAS score was better in the PRP group than in the placebo group. With these findings, they conclude that PRP injections are not a good option as a non-surgical therapy for Achilles tendinopathy, and they did not recommend PRP injection (Vithran et al., 2023).

Finally, it should be taken into account that many variables can affect results after PRP therapy, such as the patient's medical condition and chronic disorders, hematologic individuality (patient leukocyte count and platelet count), PRP preparation procedure, device-brand selection, number of injections, application individuality, and stage of degeneration (Owens et al., 2011). And despite all this discussion, PRP therapy is still one of the treatment choices and the most widely used option for Achilles tendinopathy.

Conclusion

Achilles tendinopathy is a common medical condition, especially in active individuals. Although its etiology is not well understood and multifactorial, both extrinsic and intrinsic factors play a role in the etiology. The failed healing response is the main cause of Achilles tendinopathy after degeneration and histopathological changes. The first chosen treatment for Achilles tendinopathy should be conservative modalities such as patient education, ice application, pain killers, and exercise therapy such as eccentric training. If conservative therapy is going to be insufficient, then additional treatments like invasive intervention could be considered. Invasive interventions generally contain surgery and injection therapy. In the beginning surgery can be more brutal and have possible adverse effects. Moreover, surgery may sometimes be unsuccessful. In light of these facts, non-invasive therapies such as pharmaceutical (injection therapy and Glyceryl Trinitrate (GTN) patch) and non-pharmaceutical (extracorporeal shock-wave therapy-ESWT) therapies should be considered first. Platelet-rich plasma (PRP) is derived from an individual's blood and classified among pharmaceutical therapies. PRP is obtained from blood by centrifugation (autologous concentration of platelets), so it is biological augmentation therapy and has no significant side effects. Although its exact pathways and healing mechanisms remain unclear, PRP may stimulate the healing process by the release of signaling substances at the injured tendon. That is why it is widely used in orthopedic clinics. But the current literature is still ambiguous and has no evidence-based study about its effect. There are many supportive and unsupportive articles in the orthopedic literature because it has no standardized PRP kit, preparation or application. Also, the results may be affected by individual differences and blood quality. Finally, the efficacy of PRP for Achilles tendinopathy remains highly debated according to current evidence, so more studies are needed to make a decision.

References

Collins, T., Alexander, D., & Barkatali, B. (2021). Platelet-rich plasma: a narrative review. *EFORT Open Reviews*, 6(4), 225. https://doi.org/10.1302/2058-5241.6.200017.

Courville, X. F., Coe, M. P., & Hecht, P. J. (2009). Current concepts review: noninsertional achilles tendinopathy. *Foot & Ankle International*, 30, 1132–1142. https://doi.org/10.3113/FAI.2009.1132.

De Vos, R. J., Weir, A., van Schie, H. T. M., Bierma-Zeinstra, S. M. A., Verhaar, J. A. N., Weinans, H., & Tol, J. L. (2010). Platelet-rich plasma injection for chronic achilles tendinopathy. *JAMA*, 303(2), 144. https://doi.org/10.1001/jama.2009.1986.

Dhurat, R., & Sukesh, M. (2014). Principles and methods of preparation of platelet-rich plasma: A review and author's perspective. *Journal of Cutaneous and Aesthetic Surgery*, 7(4), 189. https://doi.org/10.4103/0974-2077.150734.

Gaweda, K., Tarczynska, M., & Krzyzanowski, W. (2010). Treatment of achilles tendinopathy with platelet-rich plasma. *International Journal of Sports Medicine*, 31(08), 577–583. https://doi.org/10.1055/s-0030-1255028.

Guelfi, M., Pantalone, A., Vanni, D., Abate, M., Guelfi, M. G. B., & Salini, V. (2015). Long-term beneficial effects of platelet-rich plasma for non-insertional achilles tendinopathy. *Foot and Ankle Surgery*, 21(3), 178–181. https://doi.org/10.1016/j.fas.2014.11.005.

Kaux, J.-F. (2016). Platelet-rich plasma for treating chronic tendinopathy. *ASPETAR Sports Medicine Journal*, 5(1), 118-122.

Longo, U. G., Ronga, M., & Maffulli, N. (2018). Achilles tendinopathy. *Sports Medicine and Arthroscopy Review*, 26(1), 16–30. https://doi.org/10.1097/jsa.0000000000000185.

Liu, C., Yu, K., Bai, J., Tian, D., & Liu, G. (2019). Platelet-rich plasma injection for the treatment of chronic achilles tendinopathy. *Medicine*, 98(16), e152. https://doi.org/10.1097/md.0000000000015278.

Madhi, M. I., Emmanuel, O., Khamdan, K., & Trigkilidas, D. (2020). The use of PRP in treatment of Achilles tendinopathy: A systematic review of literature. *Annals of Medicine and Surgery*. https://doi.org/10.1016/j.amsu.2020.04.042.

Maffulli, N., Longo, U. G., Kadakia, A., & Spiezia, F. (2019). Achilles tendinopathy. *Foot and Ankle Surgery*, 26(3), 240-249. https://doi.org/10.1016/j.fas.2019.03.009.

Magnan, B., Bondi, M., Pierantoni, S., & Samaila, E. (2014). The pathogenesis of Achilles tendinopathy: A systematic review. *Foot and Ankle Surgery*, 20(3), 154–159. https://doi.org/10.1016/j.fas.2014.02.010.

Mayo Clinic. (n.d.). Achilles tendon. Retrieved from https://sportsmedicine.mayoclinic.org/condition/achilles-tendon/.

Mobile Physical Therapy. (2019). CALF MUSCLE: Details and Exercise. Retrieved from https://mobilephysiotherapyclinic.in/calf-muscle-details-and-exercise/.

Monto, R. R. (2012). Platelet rich plasma treatment for chronic Achilles tendinosis. *Foot & Ankle International*, 33(5), 379–385. https://doi.org/10.3113/fai.2012.0379.

Murawski, C. D., Smyth, N. A., Newman, H., Kennedy, J. G. (2014). A single platelet-rich plasma injection for chronic midsubstance Achilles tendinopathy: a retrospective preliminary analysis. *Foot Ankle Spec.*, 7(5), 372-6. https://doi.org10.1177/1938640014532129.

Murphy, M. C., Travers, M. J., Chivers, P., Debenham, J. R., Docking, S. I., Rio, E. K., Gibson, W. (2019). Efficacy of heavy eccentric calf training for treating mid-portion Achilles tendinopathy: a systematic review and meta-analysis. *Br J Sports Med.*, 53(17), 1070-1077. https://doi.org/10.1136/bjsports-2018-099934.

Nauwelaers, A.-K., Van Oost, L., & Peers, K. (2020). Evidence for the use of PRP in chronic midsubstance Achilles tendinopathy: A systematic review with meta-analysis. *Foot and Ankle Surgery*. https://doi.org/10.1016/j.fas.2020.07.009.

Nurden, A. (2011). Platelets, inflammation and tissue regeneration. *Thromb. Haemostasis*, 105(Suppl 1), S13-33. https://doi.org/10.1160/THS10-11-0720.

Oloff, L., Elmi, E., Nelson, J., & Crain, J. (2015). Retrospective analysis of the effectiveness of platelet-rich plasma in the treatment of Achilles tendinopathy. *Foot & Ankle Specialist*, 8(6), 490–497. https://doi.org/10.1177/1938640015599033.

Owens, R. F., Ginnetti, J., Conti, S. F., & Latona, C. (2011). Clinical and magnetic resonance imaging outcomes following platelet-rich plasma injection for chronic midsubstance Achilles tendinopathy. *Foot & Ankle International*, 32(11), 1032–1039. https://doi.org/10.3113/fai.2011.1032.

Robinson, J. M., Cook, J. L., Purdam, C., Visentini, P. J., Ross, J., Maffulli, N. (2001). The VISA-A questionnaire: a valid and reliable index of the clinical severity of Achilles tendinopathy. *Br J Sports Med.*, 35, 335–41. https://doi.org/10.1136/bjsm.35.5.335.

Sabarish, R., Lavu, V., & Rao, S. R. (2015). A comparison of platelet count and enrichment percentages in the platelet-rich plasma (PRP) obtained following preparation by three different methods. *J Clin Diagn Res*, 9, ZC10–ZC12. https://doi.org10.7860/JCDR/2015/11011.5536.

Vithran, A. D. T., Xie, W., Opoku, M., Essien, A. E., He, M., Li, Y. (2023). The efficacy of platelet-rich plasma injection therapy in the treatment of patients with Achilles tendinopathy: A systematic review and meta-analysis. *J. Clin. Med.*, 12(3), 995. https://doi.org/10.3390/jcm12030995.

Wang, Y., Han, C., Hao, J., Ren, Y., & Wang, J. (2019). Efficacy of platelet-rich plasma injections for treating Achilles tendonitis. *Der Orthopäde*. https://doi.org/10.1007/s00132-019-03711-y.

Chapter 8

PRP Treatment for Low Back Pain

Mustafa Karademir*, MD
Department of Neurosurgery, Sivas Cumhuriyet University, Faculty of Medicine, Sivas, Turkiye

Abstract

Low back pain (LBP) is a common disorder that contributes significantly to social and economic loss. A significant portion of the population suffers from this disease, one of the most-seen musculoskeletal disorders. LBP can be associated with myofascial pain, facet joint pain, sacroiliac joint pain, discogenic pain, spinal stenosis, or failed back surgery. Platelet-rich plasma (PRP) is one of the novel treatment methods for LBP. PRP is plasma that contains concentrated platelets from autologous blood. Platelets contain cytokines and growth factors, thought to speed up the repair processes of the body. As a result, they may help manage inflamed nerves associated with lumbar neuropathic pain and canal stenosis. PRP is platelet sequestration in the plasma component of autologous blood that releases various intermediaries and growth factors. All these procedures ultimately result in tissue repair and LBP treatment. PRP is an efficient and less invasive method of treating LBP in routine clinical practice.

Keywords: epidural PRP injection, fascet pain, low back pain, lumbalgia, platelet-rich plasma

* Corresponding Author's Email: krdmr58@gmail.com.

In: Current Clinical Recommendations ...
Editors: Nazan Yurtcu and Emel Güler
ISBN: 979-8-89113-723-3

Introduction

Low back pain (LBP) is a common disorder that contributes significantly to social and economic morbidity and loss of physical activity. Various types of LBP range from localized to generalized. Pain in the back can sometimes radiate to other parts of the body, including the buttocks, legs, and abdomen. There are three types of LBP: axial, radicular, and referral. The intensity of back pain varies from person to person. It is one of the main reasons why young people restrict their physical activity. A significant portion of the population suffers from this disease, one of the most expensive musculoskeletal conditions. On the pathophysiology of this process, many things participate. They include facet arthropathy, ligamentum flavum hypertrophy, posterior longitudinal ligament ossification, congenital stenosis of the neural foramen, ligamentous laxity, and subluxation. Disc degeneration leading to herniation is another. History, physical examination, and, occasionally, patient imaging can help distinguish the etiology of LBP. Myofascial pain, especially after trauma or repetitive motion damage, is a typical musculoskeletal problem. LBP can be associated with myofascial pain, facet joint pain, sacroiliac joint pain, discogenic pain, spinal stenosis, or failed back surgery. A multidisciplinary and rational treatment strategy is also most useful in chronic LBP and may include integrative clinical, psychological, physical, and surgical procedures (Baig et al., 2021; Urits et al., 2019).

Anatomy and Pathophysiology

The intervertebral disc (IVD) is essential for the ability of the spinal column to move. The discs, located between adjacent vertebrae and acting as shock absorbers, improve the strength and flexibility of the spine and the absorption of different mechanical stresses. The IVD comprises a gelatinous nucleus pulposus (NP) and a collagenous annulus fibrosus (AF). Collagen type II and a few chondrocyte-like cells are present in NP, which is 85% water. It resists axial compression and has a high proteoglycan and water content. The cartilaginous end plate of each vertebra is where the 15–50 concentric lamellae of the annulus fibrosus are joined and is composed of type I collagen and a few fibroblasts, giving it a high tensile force. Because IVD is avascular and depends on oxygen and nutrient diffusion from blood supply to end plates, the nutritional pathway of the disc is fragile. Degeneration and cellular apoptosis are the result of the reduced ability of IVD to maintain matrix and cell turnover because of the lack of end plate permeability. As a result of the degradation of proteoglycan and aggrecan during maturation, glycosaminoglycans are lost, and the osmotic pressure decreases. This interferes with the ability of the IVD to support weight, which causes the disc to lose height and causes the nuclear contents to bulge posteriorly through a damaged or thinner annulus and an inadequate posterior longitudinal ligament. Desiccation and loss of hydration can cause the end plate and annulus to be under more stress, leading to discogenic pain. Due to disturbed enzyme activity, collagen type II fibers become more denatured. Aggrecan molecules, which have been demonstrated to prevent neural degeneration, also deteriorate in aging discs, causing neural irritation and persistent LBP. Moreover, a loaded degenerative disc's loss of disc height might result in aberrant facet joint hypertrophy, eventually resulting in osteoarthritic alterations and spinal stenosis. Due to these physiological changes, IVDs are more sensitive to herniation, most frequently through radial fibers (Knezevic et al., 2017).

Etiology of Low Back Pain

The etiology of LBP can frequently be distinguished based on the medical history of the patient, physical examination, and imaging. Myofascial pain is a common musculoskeletal condition, especially after trauma or repetitive stress damage. Myofascial trigger points in the fascia, tendons, and muscles that result myofascial pain; they cause a symptomatic pain response when stimulated. Physical examination may indicate localized painful sites in a taut band, restricted range of motion, and detection of pain in the patient (Partanen et al., 2010).

Facet-mediated pain is caused by a multifactorial process associated with IVD degeneration, which leads to lumbar facet joint hypertrophy. Facet joint osteoarthritic changes or increased axial or rotational stress within the facet joint capsule can cause LBP. Patients often describe their LBP as deep and stabbing pain and numbness that may have a one-sided or two-sided distribution. LBP can extend to one or both hips, groin, and thighs, but usually, the pain ends above knee level (Bogduk, 2008).

LBP may originate in the sacroiliac joint, a synovial joint with increased sensory innervation. Pain around the sacroiliac joint generally occurs in the upper hips or lower back. However, several clinical examination findings, such as instant palpation pain over the sacroiliac joint, diagnose sacroiliac joint pain (Foley & Buschbacher, 2006).

Discogenic pain is another widely known factor in LBP. IVD is responsible for 39% of the factors that cause LBP. Internal disc disruption is entirely caused by the degradation of the disc and nuclear component. It can be exacerbated by the growth of radial fissures that spread from the nucleus into the annulus (Comer & Conaghan, 2009).

Spinal stenosis is a disorder that develops when degenerative changes in the spine result in fewer open spaces for neurological and vascular parts. Lumbar spinal stenosis symptoms include gluteal and lower extremity pain. There are several stimulating and relaxing aspects. Provocative characteristics include good exercises such as walking and positional changes such as lumbar extension, which cause neurogenic symptoms of claudication. Healing with resting, seating, and lumbar flexion are examples of palliative features (Koc et al., 2009).

Patients who had one or more spinal surgeries risk developing lumbar post-laminectomy syndrome, often known as persistent or recurrent LBP with or without radicular symptoms. All intraoperative issues include poor surgical technique, incorrect spinal level or location surgery, and failure to perform the intended surgery (Chan & Peng, 2011).

What Is PRP, and How Does It Affect LBP?

Novel therapeutic alternatives for LBP are being investigated. Platelet-rich plasma (PRP) is one of those treatment methods. PRP is plasma that contains concentrated platelets from autologous blood. PRP supporters call it a bridge between conservative treatment and surgery. Platelets contain cytokines and growth factors, thought to speed up the repair processes of the body. As a result, they may help manage inflamed nerves associated with lumbar neuropathic pain and canal stenosis. PRP is platelet sequestration in the plasma component of autologous blood that releases various intermediaries and growth factors when stimulated by an exogenous mediator (Marx, 2004). Essential growth factors such as platelet-derived growth factor (PDGF), transforming growth factor-beta (TGF-β), insulin-like growth factor 1(IGF-1), vascular endothelial growth factor (VEGF), and epithelial growth factor (EGF) are widely distributed in platelets. They facilitate healing when discharged from degranulated platelets and are crucial for chemotaxis, migration, angiogenesis, cell proliferation, and differentiation. All of these procedures ultimately result in tissue repair and LBP treatment. These functions are also supported by several cytokines, chemokines, and metabolites generated by activated platelets (Navani et al., 2017).

PRP Treatment for Myofascial Pain Syndrome

Due to its form and anatomical location, the lumbar multifidus (MLF) muscle helps stabilize the spine. Its tiny fibers and large cross-sectional area support the function of the muscle in stabilizing the spine rather than moving it. Previously, it has been conclusively demonstrated that the multifidus muscle and LBP are related to decreased muscle size and cross-sectional area in persistent LBP without segmental disc degeneration. Injections of platelet-rich plasma have been shown to impact LMF muscle in one investigation. A previous study detected a statistically substantial improvement in all pain ratings after intramuscular injection of PRP into patients. The overall success rate was 71.2%, which shows that PRP injections in the MLF muscle can be an effective and reasonably priced method of treating LBP (Hussein & Hussein, 2016). Another study showed that PRP injections significantly improved patients' myofascial pain (Ediz et al., 2021).

Intra-Facet and Ligament Injections

PRP is a concentrated form of growth factors and inflammatory mediators that speed up the repair of wounded tissues. By injecting many growth factors, PRP has been used autogenously to reduce LBP associated with facet joint degeneration and improve recovery. PRP is one biologic that is becoming more widely available and affordable for people who may not respond to regular medical therapies. However, there currently needs to be more scientific support regarding the use of biologics such as PRP. Facet injections of PRP are beneficial in investigations; however, neither long-term follow-up nor comparisons to the radiofrequency of medial branches have been made regarding clinical alleviation or functional capacity (Patel et al., 2022). In a trial, 19 patients with lumbar facet joint conditions were included, and under X-ray fluoroscopic guidance, autologous PRP was injected into the lumbar facet joints. Nine patients (47.37%) reported significant pain relief immediately, 14 patients (73.68%) after one week, and fifteen patients (78.95%) after 1-3 months (Wu et al., 2017).

PRP Injection in Sacroiliac Joint Dysfunction

Injection of PRP for LBP related to sacroiliac joint dysfunction may be a helpful treatment method. The patient enters the interventional procedure room for sacroiliac injection using this method and lies on the fluoroscopy table. After preparing a typical sterile solution, the local anesthetic application is performed. The application is performed by inserting a 20-gauge spinal needle into the sacroiliac joint. The correct needle location is determined by anterior-posterior fluoroscopic imaging. The clinical outcomes for those who received PRP as sacroiliac joint injection improved significantly compared to the previous literature (Mohi Eldin et al., 2019).

Epidural PRP Injections

Interlaminar epidural PRP injections have received significant research on their role in the treatment of radicular pain from disc herniation, spinal stenosis, axial back pain without disc herniation, and failed back surgery syndrome. The ligamentum flavum is passed through the interlaminar technique to inject PRP into the epidural space. The capacity to treat bilateral radicular pain and the requirement of less PRP volume are benefits of this technique. Moreover, there is a greater possibility that PRP injections reach nearby spinal levels. Studies support the use of this approach to treat LBP, including discogenic pain, postoperative pain, and radicular symptoms by disc herniation (Bhatia & Chopra, 2016). In a preliminary trial, the efficacy and safety of PRP and corticosteroids in caudal epidural injections was tested for patients with LBP guided by fluoroscopy. Injections of corticosteroids into the caudal epidural space under fluoroscopic supervision and autologous PRP are equally safe and therapeutically efficient for patients with LBP. Nevertheless, PRP is preferable to corticosteroids for a longer pain-relieving impact and improved quality of life (Ruiz-Lopez & Tsai, 2020).

Intradiscal PRP Injections

The primary reason for discogenic LBP is IVD degeneration in the lower back. The external surface of the annulus is affected by sympathetic fibers and vertebral sinusoidal nerves; however, IVD does not include any vascular tissues (Zhang et al., 2022). The NP, AF, and bone end plates that connect the IVD to the vertebral body contribute to the stability of the segmental.

Proinflammatory cytokines, such as tumor necrosis factor-alpha (TNF-α) and IL-1, increase significantly during the disc degeneration process, which disturbs the extracellular matrix (ECM) of IVD tissues hemostasis by increasing the levels of matrix metalloproteinases (MMPs), nitric oxide, and aggrecans. The use of autologous cells, such as PRP, multipotent adipose cells, and mesenchymal stem cells from the bone marrow cells, to treat degenerative disc disorders has recently gained popularity. PRP, which has elevated levels of growth factors and is thought to enhance healing and tissue development, has been extensively explored to treat musculoskeletal problems, including LBP (Everts et al., 2020). After receiving conservative treatment for 2 to 6 months, most patients with LBP had considerable improvements; however, 20% of patients continue to have LBP (Lee et al., 2016). Therefore, they may help the treatment of irritated radicular nerves in lumbar disc herniation, spinal canal stenosis, and failed back surgery.

Conclusion

In standard clinical practice, PRP is an efficient and less invasive method of treating LBP. It was reported to have more successful results after PRP applications. Further randomized clinical trials should verify these hopeful outcomes.

References

Baig, M. Z., Abdullah, U. E. H., Muhammad, A., Aziz, A., Syed, M. J., & Darbar, A. (2021). Use of Platelet-Rich Plasma in Treating Low Back Pain: A Review of the Current Literature. *Asian Spine Journal*, *15*(1), 117–126. https://doi.org/10.31616/asj.2019.0161.

Bhatia, R., & Chopra, G. (2016). Efficacy of Platelet Rich Plasma via Lumbar Epidural Route in Chronic Prolapsed Intervertebral Disc Patients-A Pilot Study. *Journal of*

Clinical and Diagnostic Research : JCDR, 10(9), UC05. https://doi.org/10.7860/JCDR/2016/21863.8482.

Bogduk, N. (2008). Evidence-informed management of chronic low back pain with facet injections and radiofrequency neurotomy. *The Spine Journal, 8*(1), 56–64. https://doi.org/10.1016/J.SPINEE.2007.10.010.

Chan, C. wern, & Peng, P. (2011). Failed back surgery syndrome. *Pain Medicine (Malden, Mass.), 12*(4), 577–606. https://doi.org/10.1111/J.1526-4637.2011.01089.X.

Comer, C., & Conaghan, P. G. (2009). Tackling persistent low back pain in primary care. *The Practitioner, 253*(1721), 32–34, 3. https://europepmc.org/article/med/19873857.

Ediz, L., Çağaç, A., & Delen, V. (2021). The efficacies of medicinal leech therapy and platelet-rich plasma injection added to muscle stretching exercises in treating myofascial pain syndrome. *Eastern Journal of Medicine, 26*(1), 109–116. https://doi.org/10.5505/ejm.2021.06025.

Foley, B. S., & Buschbacher, R. M. (2006). Sacroiliac joint pain: anatomy, biomechanics, diagnosis, and treatment. *American Journal of Physical Medicine & Rehabilitation, 85*(12), 997–1006. https://doi.org/10.1097/01.PHM.0000247633.68694.C1.

Hussein, M., & Hussein, T. (2016). Effect of autologous platelet leukocyte rich plasma injections on atrophied lumbar multifidus muscle in low back pain patients with mono segmental degenerative disc disease. *SICOT-J, 2*. https://doi.org/10.1051/SICOTJ/2016002.

Knezevic, N. N., Mandalia, S., Raasch, J., Knezevic, I., & Candido, K. D. (2017). Treatment of chronic low back pain - New approaches on the horizon. *Journal of Pain Research, 10*, 1111–1123. https://doi.org/10.2147/JPR.S132769.

Koc, Z., Ozcakir, S., Sivrioglu, K., Gurbet, A., & Kucukoglu, S. (2009). Effectiveness of physical therapy and epidural steroid injections in lumbar spinal stenosis. *Spine, 34*(10), 985–989. https://doi.org/10.1097/BRS.0B013E31819C0A6B.

Marx, R. E. (2004). Platelet-Rich Plasma: Evidence to Support Its Use. *Journal of Oral and Maxillofacial Surgery, 62*(4), 489–496. https://doi.org/10.1016/j.joms.2003.12.003.

Mohi Eldin, M., Sorour, O. O., Hassan, A. S. A., Baraka, M., & Ahmed, M. F. (2019). Percutaneous injection of autologous platelet-rich fibrin versus platelet-rich plasma in sacroiliac joint dysfunction: An applied comparative study. *Journal of Back and Musculoskeletal Rehabilitation, 32*(3), 511–518. https://doi.org/10.3233/BMR-181366.

Navani, A., Li, G., & Chrystal, J. (2017). Platelet-Rich Plasma in Musculoskeletal Pathology: A Necessary Rescue or a Lost Cause? *Pain Physician, 20*(3), E345–E356. https://doi.org/10.36076/ppj.2017.e356.

Partanen, J. V., Ojala, T. A., & Arokoski, J. P. A. (2010). Myofascial syndrome and pain: A neurophysiological approach. *Pathophysiology : The Official Journal of the International Society for Pathophysiology, 17*(1), 19–28. https://doi.org/10.1016/J.PATHOPHYS.2009.05.001.

Patel, A., Koushik, S., Schwartz, R., Gritsenko, K., Farah, F., Urits, I., Varrassi, G., Viswanath, O., & Shaparin, N. (2022). Platelet-Rich Plasma in the Treatment of

Facet Mediated Low Back Pain: A Comprehensive Review. *Orthopedic Reviews*, *14*(3), 1–6. https://doi.org/10.52965/001c.37076.

Ruiz-Lopez, R., & Tsai, Y. C. (2020). A Randomized Double-Blind Controlled Pilot Study Comparing Leucocyte-Rich Platelet-Rich Plasma and Corticosteroid in Caudal Epidural Injection for Complex Chronic Degenerative Spinal Pain. *Pain Practice : The Official Journal of World Institute of Pain*, *20*(6), 639–646. https://doi.org/10.1111/PAPR.12893.

Urits, I., Viswanath, O., Galasso, A. C., Sottosani, E. R., Mahan, K. M., Aiudi, C. M., Kaye, A. D., & Orhurhu, V. J. (2019). Platelet-Rich Plasma for the Treatment of Low Back Pain: A Comprehensive Review. *Current Pain and Headache Reports*, *23*(7). https://doi.org/10.1007/s11916-019-0797-6.

Wu, J., Zhou, J., Liu, C., Zhang, J., Xiong, W., Lv, Y., Liu, R., Wang, R., Du, Z., Zhang, G., & Liu, Q. (2017). A Prospective Study Comparing Platelet-Rich Plasma and Local Anesthetic (LA)/Corticosteroid in Intra-Articular Injection for Treating Lumbar Facet Joint Syndrome. *Pain Practice*, *17*(7), 914–924. https://doi.org/10.1111/papr.12544.

Chapter 9

PRP Treatment for Neuronal Injury

Ayşe Yağmur Çolak*, MD
Department of Neurology, Tepecik Training and Research Hospital, Izmir, Turkiye

Abstract

Platelet-rich plasma (PRP) has been actively practiced in treatment for the last 30 years because of the indication of its effect on the healing process of tissue and nerve damage. PRP has shown an effective role in the healing process of nerve damage by accelerating axonal regeneration. The mechanism of action occurs through the effect of regulating inflammation and increasing the angiogenesis and growth factors released from alpha granulations of platelets, especially axonal regeneration, such as platelet-derived growth factor (PDGF), vascular endothelial growth factor (VEGF), transforming growth factor-beta (TGF-β), epidermal growth factor (EGF), and insulin-like growth factor (IGF). Platelets and growth factors physiologically released from platelets have an important role in the healing processes of nerve damage. Therefore, it has been considered that it might be useful to apply PRP to the area of nerve damage. Hence, PRP has been practiced in cases where neuronal damage is observed, such as nerve injuries, nerve damage as the reason for crushing, carpal tunnel syndrome, and polyneuropathy in treatment. While there are studies indicating that PRP is effective in these diseases, there are also in vitro, animal, and clinical testing indicating that it has no effect. Therefore, there is a need for more studies evaluating the efficiency of PRP in nerve damage.

Keywords: PRP, nerve damage, carpal tunnel syndrome, neuropathic pain

* Corresponding Author's Email: dryagmurcolak@hotmail.com.

In: Current Clinical Recommendations ...
Editors: Nazan Yurtcu and Emel Güler
ISBN: 979-8-89113-723-3

Introduction

Platelet-rich plasma (PRP) is an autologous blood product obtained by centrifuging whole blood. After the centrifuge process, plasma with a higher platelet component is taken. The mechanism of action on the nerve damage in this plasma with a high level of platelets is related to the fact that some growth factors released from the alpha granules of platelets increase axonal regeneration. Besides increasing axonal regeneration, the main mechanisms of action of PRP on the nervous system are that it prevents neuronal apoptosis and increases neuroprotection, stimulates vascular regeneration and regulates the inflammatory response (Sánchezet al., 2017).The therapeutic factors released from the alpha granules of platelets are mainly; platelet-derived growth factor (PDGF), ADP, ATP, calcium, serotonin, platelet factor 4, fibronectin, β-thromboglobulin, von Willebrand factor (vWF), fibrinogen, factor V and XIII, transforming growth factor-beta (TGF-β), vascular endothelial growth factor (VEGF), epithelial growth factor (EGF), basic fibroblast growth factor (FGF-β), fibroblast growth factor-2 (FGF-2), platelet factor 4 (PF4), insulin-like growth factor-1 (IGF-1), platelet-derived angiogenesis factor (PDAF) (Peterson et al., 2010; Kakudo et al., 2014). PRP is used for the treatment of carpal tunnel syndrome, nerve injury, acute and chronic neuropathic pain, and polyneuropathy with these growth factors.

Peripheral Nerve Damage

Peripheral nerve damage is an important disease that is common and reduces the quality of life. While it can be seen as localized trauma, such as nerve entrapment related to nerve injury or anatomical structures, it can also occur generalized with autoimmune causes or metabolic causes such as diabetes. The observed nerve entrapments can be indicated mainly as cubital tunnel syndrome, carpal tunnel syndrome, and dorsal interosseous syndrome (pronator teres syndrome). As a result of the high incidence of entrapment neuropathies, although the effect of PRP on all peripheral nerve damage has been researched in recent years, studies on carpal tunnel syndrome have been focused at the forefront.

Carpal Tunnel Syndrome

Carpal tunnel syndrome (CTS) is the most common mononeuropathy (Ghasemi-rad et al., 2014). It occurs due to pressure of the median nerve along the carpal tunnel. It is prominently presented on the front face of the first three fingers and in the palm with numbness, pain, and weakness. In its advanced stages, aseptic inflammation, permanent nerve damage, and atrophy can progress (Alfonso et al., 2014). Conservative treatments such as splint application and corticosteroid injection are preferred in the foreground. Alternative treatments have been studied, as treatment methods do not provide complete recovery, including surgical operations. It has been considered that growth factors released from alpha granulations of platelets, whose mechanism of action was mentioned previously, have a positive effect on axonal regeneration. Therefore, studies on the efficiency of PRP in the treatment of CTS have been recently conducted. In a study conducted by Raeissadat et al. on 41 female patients in 2018, cases with mild or moderate carpal tunnel syndrome were included in the study, and at the end of this study no significant differences were found in the treatment of pain, severity of symptoms, functional status, and electrophysiological parameters (Malahias et al., 2019). However, in a study by Malahias et al. in 2015, 14 patients were taken in the study and an increase in functional capacity and a decrease in pain score were confirmed after injection of PRP (Malahias et al., 2019). In a single-blind, non-randomized study conducted by Wu et al. in 60 patients, a decrease in the level of pain and disability was found compared to the control group during a 6-month follow-up of patients practicing PRP (Wu et al., 2017). In a prospective and randomized controlled single-blind study conducted by Shen et al. in 2019, 52 patients were evaluated, and it was observed that PRP practice resulted in a better postoperative outcome (Boston carpal tunnel questionnaire-BCTQ) and neurophysiological recovery (Shen et al., 2019). However, there have also been different studies conducted that the PRP has a positive efficiency in the treatment of peripheral neuropathy (Sánchez et al., 2017; Farrag et al., 2007; Sariguney et al., 2008; Ding et al., 2009; Cho et al., 2009; Giannessi et al.,2014; Park & Kwon, 2014). The latest study on carpal tunnel syndrome of PRP was conducted by Jiang et al. (Jiang et al., 2022). All studies up to 2021 were included in this meta-analysis. As a result of this analysis, it was observed that PRP caused a significant decrease in the symptom severity scale (SSS) during short-term follow-up. In medium-term follow-ups, significant recovery was found in parameters such as visual analog scale (VAS), SSS, functional status scale (FSS), sensory peak latency (SPL), and cross-sectional area (CSA) in the PRP group. In long-term follow-ups, it was observed that only a decrease in the SSS score was detected, similar to the short-term follow-up. Even though there are some studies that PRP is effective in the treatment of carpal tunnel syndrome, more studies are needed.

Nerve Injury

Traumatic peripheral nerve injury is one of the leading causes of nerve damage and is a significant cause of disability and impairment (Robinson et al., 2000). After nerve injury, the management of the healing process is essential. The long duration of this process causes muscle atrophy and joint contractures and, in addition to motor loss, also causes neuropathic pain, resulting in loss of work force. The gold standard in nerve injury is direct nerve repair performed with epineural microstructures (Grinsell et al., 2014). In patients under the age of 25, if the repair is performed within 2-3 months after trauma and the nerve gap is less than 2 cm, the chances of success of direct nerve repair increase (Karabeg et al., 2009; Andelkovic et al., 2017). In addition to direct nerve repair, the efficiency of PRP is being tested in vitro, in animal testing, and in clinical research. In an in vitro study conducted by Takeuchi et al., a rat brain-spinal cord organ culture was examined, and it was detected that PRP increases axon regeneration through VEGF and IGF-1 (Takeuchi et al., 2012). Furthermore, in another in vitro study, it was shown that the release of IGF-1 and PDGF from PRP increases the proliferation and migration of Schwann cells involved in peripheral nerve regeneration (Pereira et al., 2020). Another mechanism is the regulation of inflammation as a result of increasing macrophage aggregation.

Different results have been obtained in animal testing conducted on the positive effect of PRP on axonal regeneration. In the study by Pişkin et al. on sciatic nerve regeneration, there was no positive effect of platelet gel use on axon regeneration (Piskin et al., 2009). On the other hand, other studies have shown that PRP causes more thickening in the axon myelin layer, faster axon regeneration, and longer-term axon regeneration (Ding et al., 2009; Cho et al., 2010; Hiraizumi et al., 1996; Elgazzar et al., 2008). As a result of a simple injury to the peripheral nerve, an average 3 mm long nerve gap occurs between the stumps formed at both nerve ends. As a physiological mechanism, the previously mentioned growth factors fill this gap and regeneration begins. However, if the nerve gap is longer than 3 mm, polymerized pure fibrin can be used to bridge to induce axon regeneration. In a recent study, a 12 cm-long nerve gap was bridged with a PRP-filled collagen tube, and recovery in motor and sensory symptoms was found during follow-up (Kuffler et al., 2011). Moreover, this newly developed technique was found to be superior to performing PRP in combination with acellular nerve grafts practiced for nerve injuries with a maximum length of 1.5 cm, only performing nerve grafts (Giannessi et al., 2014; Zheng et al., 2014).

Neuropathic Pain

Pain related to tissue damage can be neurological due to the primary effect of the damage or neuropathic in relation to the damage caused to neuroceptive neurons despite recovery of the damage (Kuffler, 2013). Neuropathic pain is related to spontaneous ectopic activity that develops with hyperexcitability of the nociceptive neuron. This activity can continue independently of tissue healing (Campbell et al., 2006). Although the affected area is small, the hyperalgesia caused by it can affect the person widely and reduce the quality of life (Devor et al., 2006). It can be related to nerve damage that occurs in the peripheral or central nervous system. Peripheral nerve damage can occur for a variety of reasons. Inflammation, cuts, crushing, amputation, infection, or metabolic damage are some of these causes. When tissue damage occurs as a result of one or more of these causes, platelet-rich plasma is physiologically infiltrated instead of the wound. With the start of the healing process of the wound, the probability of developing neurological pain decreases (Sanchez-Gonzalez et al.,2012). The first study on the analgesic effect of PRP was conducted by Everts et al. in 2008 and confirmed a decrease in the pain scale applied after shoulder surgery and a decrease in the need for opioid use (Everts et al., 2007). In a randomized controlled double-blind study by Semenov et al., it was found that the application of PRP, which was performed in terms of pain treatment after tonsillectomy operation, did not provide an advantage over placebo (Semenov et al., 2007). In another study, it was stated that it can indirectly cause a decrease in neuropathic pain, while highlighting that the direct role of PRP in the treatment of neuropathic pain is doubtful (Maffulli et al., 2012).

In some animal models, PRP has been shown to cause a reduction in neuropathic pain by increasing axon regeneration with growth factors containing or through stem cells containing (Elgazzar et al., 2008; Emel et al., 2011; Wu et al., 2012). The gap between the two injured ends of the nerve caused by nerve damage and the time elapsed after trauma are negatively effective in the recovery of nerve damage. In a recently developed technique, it has been shown that nerve recovery can be induced after an average of 3 years by placing a collagen tube filled with PRP between both nerve endings (Kuffler et al., 2011). It is considered that the efficiency of PRP on neuropathic pain in in vitro studies, animal testing, and clinical research results that differ may be related to the use of PRP in different concentrations.

Conclusion

Peripheral nerve damage occurs frequently in clinical practice. Although surgery is the gold standard in cases such as nerve injuries, different methods are being tested to accelerate healing. In the last 20 years, clinical testing has focused on finding that PRP is rich in growth factors and has a positive effect on nerve regeneration in in vitro and animal testing. Because PRP treatment is a promising treatment for nerve regeneration, many studies have been conducted on it in recent years. These studies focus on compression neuropathies such as nerve injury, and carpal tunnel syndrome. At the same time, studies on the neuropathic pain reduction of PRP have been conducted for the reasons of the frequent occurrence of neuropathic pain and a significant decrease in quality of life. Even though the studies conducted on these points have shown conflicting results, it has been concluded that PRP can be useful for neuronal damage when evaluated in consideration of recent meta-analyses. There is a need for clinical research to be conducted in larger populations in the future.

References

Alfonso, C., Jann, S., Massa, R., & Torreggiani, A. (2010). Diagnosis, treatment and follow-up of the carpal tunnel syndrome: A review. *Neurological Sciences, 31*(3), 243-252. https://doi.org/10.1007/s10072-009-0213-9.

Andelkovic, S. Z., Lesic, A. R., Bumbasirevic, M. Z., & Rasulic, L. G. (2017). The outcomes of 150 consecutive patients with digital nerve injuries treated in a single center. *Turkish Neurosurgery, 27*, 289-293. https://doi.org/10.5137/1019-5149.JTN.15106-15.0.

Campbell, J. N., & Meyer, R. A. (2006). Mechanisms of neuropathic pain. *Neuron, 52,* 77-92. https://doi.org/10.1016/j.neuron.2006.09.021.

Cho, H. H., Jang, S., Lee, S. C., Jeong, H. S., Park, J. S., Han, J. Y., Lee, K. H., & Cho, Y. B. (2010). Effect of neural-induced mesenchymal stem cells and platelet-rich plasma on facial nerve regeneration in an acute nerve injury model. *Laryngoscope, 120,* 907. https://doi.org/10.1002/lary.20860.

Devor, M. (2006). Sodium channels and mechanisms of neuropathic pain. The Journal of Pain, 7, S3-S12. https://doi.org/10.1016/j.jpain.2005.09.006.

Ding, X. G., Li, S. W., Zheng, X. M., Hu, L. Q., Hu, W. L., & Luo, Y. (2009). The effect of platelet-rich plasma on cavernous nerve regeneration in a rat model. *Asian Journal of Andrology, 11*, 215. https://doi.org/10.1038/aja.2008.37.

Elgazzar, R. F., Mutabagani, M. A., Abdelaal, S. E., & Sadakah, A. A. (2008). Platelet-rich plasma may enhance peripheral nerve regeneration after cyanoacrylate reanastomosis: A controlled blind study on rats. *International Journal of Oral and Maxillofacial Surgery, 37,* 748. https://doi.org/10.1016/j.ijom.2008.05.010.

Emel, E., Ergun, S. S., Kotan, D., Gursoy, E. B., Parman, Y., Zengin, A., & Nurten, A. (2011). Effects of insulin-like growth factor-I and platelet-rich plasma on sciatic nerve crush injury in a rat model. *Journal of Neurosurgery, 114,* 522-528. https://doi.org/10.3171/2010.9.JNS091928.

Everts, P. A., De Vilee, R. J. J., Mahoney, C., Van Erp, A., Oosterbos, C. J. M., Stellenboom, M., Knape JT, & van Zundert A. (2007). Exogenous application of platelet-leukocyte gel during open subacromial decompression contributes to improved patient outcome. *European Surgical Research, 40,* 203-210. https://doi.org/10.1159/000110862.

Farrag, T. Y., Lehar, M., Verhaegen, P., Carson, K. A., & Byrne, P. J. (2007). Effect of platelet-rich plasma and fibrin sealant on facial nerve regeneration in a rat model. *The Laryngoscope, 117*(1), 157-165. https://doi.org/10.1097/01.mlg.0000249726.98801.77.

Ghasemi-rad, M., Nosair, E., Vegh, A., Mohammadi, A., Akkad, A., Lesha, E., Mohammadi MH, Sayed D, Davarian A, Maleki-Miyandoab T, & Hasan A. (2014). A handy review of carpal tunnel syndrome: From anatomy to diagnosis and treatment. *World Journal of Radiology, 6*(6), 284. https://doi.org/10.4329/wjr.v6.i6.284.

Giannessi, E., Coli, A., Stornelli, M. R., Miragliotta, V., Pirone, A., Lenzi, C., Burchielli S, Vozzi G, De Maria C, & Giorgetti M. (2014). An autologously generated platelet-rich plasma suturable membrane may enhance peripheral nerve regeneration after neurorraphy in an acute injury model of sciatic nerve neurotmesis. *Journal of Reconstructive Microsurgery, 30*(09), 617-626. https://doi.org/10.1055/s-0034-1372483.

Grinsell, D., & Keating, C. (2014). Peripheral nerve reconstruction after injury: A review of clinical and experimental therapies. *BioMed Research International, 2014,* 698256. https://doi.org/10.1155/2014/698256.

Hiraizumi, Y., Fujimaki, E., Transfeldt, E. E., Kawahara, N., Fiegel, V. D., Knighton, D., Sung, J. H. (1996). The effect of the platelet derived wound healing formula and the nerve growth factor on the experimentally injured spinal cord. *Spinal Cord, 34,* 394. https://doi.org/10.1038/sc.1996.71.

Jiang, J., Xing, F., Luo, R., & Liu, M. (2022). Effectiveness of Platelet-Rich Plasma for Patients With Carpal Tunnel Syndrome: A Systematic Review and Meta-Analysis of Current Evidence in Randomized Controlled Trials. *Frontiers in Pharmacology, 13,* 834213. https://doi.org/10.3389/fphar.2022.834213.

Kakudo, N., Morimoto, N., Kushida, S., Ogawa, T., & Kusumoto, K. (2014). Platelet-rich plasma releasate promotes angiogenesis in vitro and in vivo. *Medical Molecular Morphology, 47*(2), 83-89. https://doi.org/10.1007/s00795-013-0045-9.

Karabeg, R., Jakirlic, M., & Dujso, V. (2009). Sensory recovery after forearm median and ulnar nerve grafting. *Medical Archives, 63*, 97-99.

Kuffler, D. P., Reyes, O., Sosa, I. J., & Santiago-Figueroa, J. (2011). Neurological recovery across a 12-cm-long ulnar nerve gap repaired 3.25 years post trauma: Case report. *Neurosurgery, 69,* E1321-E1326. https://doi.org/10.1227/NEU.0b013e31822a9fd2.

Kuffler, D. P. (2013). Platelet-rich plasma and the elimination of neuropathic pain. *Molecular Neurobiology, 48,* 315. https://doi.org/10.1007/s12035-013-8494-7.

Maffulli, N., & Del Buono, A. (2012). Platelet plasma rich products in musculoskeletal medicine: Any evidence? *The Surgeon, 10,* 148-150. https://doi.org/10.1016/j.surge.2011.03.004.

Malahias, M. A., Chytas, D., Mavrogenis, A. F., Nikolaou, V. S., Johnson, E. O., & Babis, G. C. (2019). Platelet-rich plasma injections for carpal tunnel syndrome: A systematic and comprehensive review. *European Journal of Orthopaedic Surgery & Traumatology, 29*(1), 1-8. https://doi.org/10.1007/s00590-018-2278-8.

Park, G. Y., & Kwon, D. R. (2014). Platelet-rich plasma limits the nerve injury caused by 10% dextrose in the rabbit median nerve. *Muscle & Nerve, 49*(1), 56-60. https://doi.org/10.1002/mus.23863.

Pereira, C. T., Paxton, Z. J., & Li, A. I. (2020). Involvement of PDGF-BB and IGF-1 in activation of human Schwann cells by platelet-rich plasma. *Plastic and Reconstructive Surgery, 146*(6), 825e-827e. https://doi.org/10.1097/PRS.0000000000007406.

Peterson, J. E., Zurakowski, D., Italiano, J. E. Jr., Michel, L. V., Fox, L., Klement, G. L., & Folkman, J. (2010). Normal ranges of angiogenesis regulatory proteins in human platelets. *American Journal of Hematology, 85*, 487. https://doi.org/10.1002/ajh.21732.

Piskin, A., Kaplan, S., Aktaş, A., Ayyildiz, M., Raimondo, S., Aliç, T., Bozkurt, H. H., & Geuna, S. (2009). Platelet gel does not improve peripheral nerve regeneration: An electrophysiological, stereological, and electron microscopic study. *Microsurgery, 29*(2), 144-153. https://doi.org/10.1002/micr.20599.

Robinson, L. R. (2003). Traumatic injury to peripheral nerves. *Suppl Clin Neurophysiol, 57*, 173.

Sanchez-Gonzalez, D. J., Mendez-Bolaina, E., & Trejo-Bahena, N. I. (2012). Platelet-rich plasma peptides: Key for regeneration. *International Journal of Peptides, 2012*, 532519. https://doi.org/10.1155/2012/532519.

Sánchez, M., Anitua, E., Delgado, D., Prado, R., Sánchez, P., Fiz, N., Guadilla J, Azofra J, Pompei O, Orive G, Ortega M, Yoshioka T, & Padilla S. (2017). Ultrasound-guided plasma rich in growth factors injections and scaffolds hasten motor nerve functional recovery in an ovine model of nerve crush injury. *Journal of Tissue Engineering and Regenerative Medicine, 11*(5), 1619-1629. https://doi.org/10.1002/term.2079.

Sariguney, Y., Yavuzer, R., Elmas, C., Yenicesu, I., Bolay, H., & Atabay, K. (2008). Effect of platelet-rich plasma on peripheral nerve regeneration. *Journal of Reconstructive Microsurgery, 24*(03), 159-167. https://doi.org/10.1055/s-2008-1076752.

Semenov, F. V., & Iakobashvili, I. (2007). Usage of platelet-enriched plasma as hemostatic and analgesic medication in tonsillectomy. *Vestnikotorinolaringologii, 48*-50.

Shen, Y. P., Li, T. Y., Chou, Y. C., Ho, T. Y., Ke, M. J., Chen, L. C., & Wu, Y. T. (2019). Comparison of perineural platelet-rich plasma and dextrose injections for moderate carpal tunnel syndrome: A prospective randomized, single-blind, head-to-head comparative trial. *Journal of Tissue Engineering and Regenerative Medicine, 13*(11), 2009-2017. https://doi.org/10.1002/term.2950.

Takeuchi, M., Kamei, N., Shinomiya, R., Sunagawa, T., Suzuki, O., Kamoda, H., Ohtori S, & Ochi M. (2012). Human platelet-rich plasma promotes axon growth in brain-spinal cord coculture. *NeuroReport, 23*(12), 712-716. https://doi.org/10.1097/WNR.0b013e3283567196.

Wu, C. C., Wu, Y. N., Ho, H. O., Chen, K. C., Sheu, M. T., & Chiang, H. S. (2012). The neuroprotective effect of platelet-rich plasma on erectile function in bilateral cavernous nerve injury rat model. *The Journal of Sexual Medicine, 9*, 2838. https://doi.org/10.1111/j.1743-6109.2012.02881.x.

Wu, Y. T., Ho, T. Y., Chou, Y. C., Ke, M. J., Li, T. Y., Huang, G. S., & Chen, L. C. (2017). Six-month efficacy of platelet-rich plasma for carpal tunnel syndrome: A prospective randomized, single-blind controlled trial. *Scientific Reports, 7,* 1. https://doi.org/10.1038/s41598-017-00224-6.

Zheng, C., Zhu, Q., Liu, X., Huang, X., He, C., Jiang, L., & Quan, D. (2014). Improved peripheral nerve regeneration using acellular nerve allografts loaded with platelet-rich plasma. *Tissue Engineering Part A*, *20*, 3228. https://doi.org/10.1089/ten.TEA.2013.0729.

Chapter 10

PRP Treatment for the Diabetic Foot

Salih Metin*, MD

Department of Family Medicine, Bursa City Hospital, University of Health Science, Bursa, Turkiye

Abstract

Diabetes mellitus is a metabolic and chronic disease caused by the combination of a sedentary lifestyle and genetic factors. Increasing life expectancy, the increase in the elderly population, and the fight against diabetes and its complications are becoming important social problems. Despite known debridement, antibiotherapy, and surgical approaches, amputations due to diabetic foot threaten human health and cause an increase in the resources allocated by the states to health. Therefore, there is a need for new treatment approaches besides known and established treatments. Platelet-rich plasma (PRP) treatments, which are encouraging right now, have given satisfactory results in the treatment of patients with diabetic foot. The isolated and combined development of ischemic and neurological processes on different grounds from patient to patient in the formation of diabetic ulcer complicates a single treatment approach. With the understanding that there is no disease, there is a patient, a detailed examination of each patient, and a detailed examination of the formation of the diabetic foot appear to be effective in the wound healing of PRP, which is started on an appropriate basis, and in preventing the loss of limb of the patient. For this treatment to become widespread, it needs to be tested in larger populations and a timeline of proven literature.

---

* Corresponding Author's Email: slhmtn@hotmail.com.

In: Current Clinical Recommendations ...
Editors: Nazan Yurtcu and Emel Güler
ISBN: 979-8-89113-723-3

Keywords: diabetic foot, platelet rich plasma, diabetic vascular complication, current treatment approaches

Introduction

Diabetes Mellitus (DM) is a chronic disease that causes many micro- and macro-complications, leading to hyperglycemia due to the deficiency or ineffectiveness of the insulin hormone secreted from the pancreas, leading to disorders in carbohydrate, protein, and fat metabolism. In 2014, 8.5% of adults 18 years and older had diabetes (WHO, 2022). It is responsible for approximately 1.5 million deaths annually (GBD 2019 Collaborators, 2020). The processes that are effective in the death process of DM occur through micro- and macro-complications. Among microvascular complications, there are retinopathy, nephropathy, and neuropathy. Macrovascular complications renovascular, cerebrovascular, coronary artery disease, peripheral vascular disease, and diabetic foot ulcers can be shown.

The occurrence of many disorders at the microvascular level of DM has different effects on the body at the macro-level. Autonomic neuropathy, disruption of the functioning of the sebaceous and sweat glands, adversely affects the regulation of the temperature in the foot. As a result, it causes anhidrosis and hyperkeratosis on the plantar aspect of the foot. After the development of motor neuropathy, paralysis, atrophy, and fibrosis of the intrinsic muscles of the feet develop, and flexor and extensor balance is impaired in the foot secondary to these. The tissue under the metatarsal head becomes thinner, and the risk of pressure ulcer increases with increasing the load on this area. With sensory neuropathy, which is another neuropathy, fissures, and ulcers occur in areas that are exposed to heavy loads, along with factors such as repetitive stress and trauma as a result of loss of sensation (Cavanagh et al., 2005). Microorganisms enter damaged tissues in these areas, and the infectious process is added to the process. Due to the defect in glucose regulation, the functions of immune system cells decrease and resistance to microorganisms becomes difficult (Cavanagh et al., 2005). Diabetic foot occurs when sensory neuropathy and immune system disorder are isolated or all together on the predisposing ground of autonomic neuropathy and motor neuropathy (Brem et al., 2004). It is thought that 60% of patients with DM have peripheral neuropathy. About 90% of diabetic ulcer patients have peripheral neuropathy (Tesfaye et al., 1996).

The lifetime risk of developing diabetic foot in patients with DM is 15% (Lauterbach et al., 2010). Diabetic ulcer is responsible for more than half of non-traumatic lower extremity amputations (Moxey et al., 2011). While the majority (60-80%) of foot ulcers heal, 10-15% persist and 5-24% go to amputation within 6-18 months of initial assessment (Alexiadou & Doupis, 2012). Reasons such as aging and duration of diabetes from the first diagnosis increase the risk of foot ulceration and limb amputation (Malgrange et al., 2003). Considering the negative impact on the patient's quality of life and health system, the treatment and prevention of diabetic foot diagnosis is very important.

Previous diabetic foot ulceration or amputation, diabetic or non-diabetic visual impairment, diabetic nephropathy, poor glycemic control, and smoking are other risk factors for diabetic foot ulcers other than age and duration of diabetes (Alexiadou & Doupis, 2012). Some studies on diabetics have shown that foot ulcers are more common in men than in women (Prompers et al., 2007). It has been shown that sociodemographic factors such as low education and socioeconomic status, and difficulties in accessing health services increase the likelihood of foot ulcers (Benotmane et al., 2000).

To roughly classify diabetic foot ulcers: neuropathic in the absence of vascular ischemia but in the presence of peripheral diabetic neuropathy; ischemic in the absence of diabetic peripheral neuropathy and in the presence of a vascular complication such as peripheral vascular disease. In the presence of both vascular ischemic and peripheral neuropathy, it is called a neuro-ischemic diabetic ulcer (Alexiadou & Doupis, 2012). Apart from this rough classification, many scales and classification methods have been developed to categorize foot ulcers by size, presence of infection, size, extent, and ischemia. The Meggitt-Wagner classification is one of the most widely used classifications for foot ulcers (Table 1) (Alexiadou & Doupis, 2012). There are other accepted and effective classification systems for diabetic foot ulcers (Schaper, 2004).

Regardless of which classification method is used in the evaluation of diabetic foot ulcer, all classification systems should guide the selection of the right treatment, ensure the correct follow-up of the healing process, and provide meaningful communication in consultations between branches.

Table 1. Meggitt–Wagner classification of foot ulcers

Grade	Definition
0	Completely epithelialized pre/post ulcerative lesion
1	Ulcer that does not extend to the superficial subcutaneous
2	Ulcer extending between the exposed tendon and bone without abscess or osteomyelitis
3	Deep ulcer with abscess or osteomyelitis
4	Localized gangrene of the toes or forefoot
5	Wide gangrenous foot

The gold standard for the treatment of diabetic foot ulcers includes wound debridement, treatment of wound infection with appropriate antibiotics, revascularization when indicated, and surgical procedures to drain the ulcer (Doupis & Veves, 2008). It has been reported that other methods such as hyperbaric oxygen therapy, the use of advanced wound care products, and negative pressure wound therapy (NPWT) can be used as additional treatments in diabetic foot treatment (Hinchliffe et al., 2008).

The Importance of Platelet-Rich Plasma

Initiates the healing process after surgical intervention and trauma in the natural healing process of the body. Activation of platelets with biologically active proteins provides hemostasis by forming a platelet plug and ensuring blood coagulation. A hematoma containing 95% red blood cells, 4% platelets, and 1% white blood cells occurs naturally. With the use of PRP, hematomas can be formed with 95% platelet, 4% red blood cell, and 1% white blood cell compositions (Anitua et al., 2004; Marx, 2001).

Platelet-rich plasma contains a complement of active secretory proteins and coagulation factors. Biologically, it contains close to 30 proteins. Theseare platelet-derived growth factor (PDGF), interleukin-1, platelet-derived angiogenesis factor, vascular endothelial growth factor (VEGF), epidermal growth factor (EGF), transforming growth factor (TGF)-β1, TGF-β2, platelet factor IV, osteocalcin, osteonectin, fibrinogen, fibronectin, vitronectin, insulin-like growth factor (IGF), and thrombospondin (Anitua et al., 2004; Kevy et al., 2001; Marx, 2001).

Autologous PRP is plasma enriched with platelets taken from the patient himself in a limited volume. Whole blood is separated from platelet-poor plasma, red and white blood cells, and platelets by centrifugation. Ascorbic acid or 10% calcium citrate solution is used as anticoagulant and the fibrin skeleton is formed through the thrombin formation pathway, which is platelet concentrate. Activation of the fibrin pathway and the release of concentrated growth factors lead to accelerated wound healing (Anitua et al., 2004; Ogino et al., 2005).

Platelet-derived growth factor is the only growth factor approved by the FDA as a 10% diabetic wound healing accelerator in a phase 3 trial on humans (d'Hemecourt, 1998; Smiell et al., 1999). The topical application of platelet-derived growth factor has been shown to accelerate the healing of diabetic wounds by accelerating granulation tissue formation and epithelialization (Lacci & Dardik, 2010). PDGF secreted from endothelial cells, megakaryocytes, and fibroblasts is a growth factor that has a critical importance in wound healing (Raslan et al., 2017).

Extracellular matrix deposition includes activation of immune cells and fibroblasts by the actions of collagen synthesis, matrix metalloproteinase, and tissue inhibitory synthesis and angiogenesis of metalloproteinase (Hosgood, 1993). Platelet-derived growth factor is a potent stimulator of fibroblast growth and is involved in all its stages, including angiogenesis, fibrin formation, and re-epithelialization (Hosgood, 1993). Platelet-derived growth factor is stable and has been shown to be resistant to temperature and pH changes compared to other proteins (Pierce et al., 1991). This property provides a metalloproteinase-rich environment against destructive proteases if you try to inhibit the activation of PDGF. TGF-β is a potent inhibitor of immune reactivity (Pfeilschifte et al., 1990).

It attracts macrophages with the secretion of additional cytokines, enhances fibroblasts, induces smooth muscle cell chemotaxis, synthesis and deposition of bone matrix with type 1 collagen TGF-β also promotes angiogenesis and extracellular matrix formation (Bennett et al., 2003). Although TGF-β1 has not been tested in human experiments, it is the predominant form in wound healing, while TGF-β2 has been clinically shown to contribute to the healing of diabetic wounds in human experiments. TGF-β1 has been tested in baby rabbits and has been shown to accelerate wound healing with the formation of new granulation tissue and to accelerate the establishment of a new epithelium (Wu et al., 1999). Many different cells secrete VEGF or fibroblast growth factor 4, PDGF, TNF-α, IGF, and some interleukin, which regulate its production (Neufeld et al., 1999). VEGF indirectly increases the permeability of capillaries, creates leakage and creates extracellular tissue plasma, stimulates endothelial growth, and promotes angiogenesis (PFEILSCHIFTE et al., 1990). What distinguishes

VEGF from PDGF is that it has no effect on macrophages, smooth muscle, and fibroblasts, it but only binds to endothelial cells and acts (Corral et al., 1999). Wound healing has not yet been studied in human clinical trials examining the effects of VEGF, but studies in rabbits have shown that it accelerates tissue formation by doubling granulation in ischemic wounds (Corral et al., 1999).

Epiderma growth factor (EGF) is a cytokine that has been shown to stimulate and accelerate wound repair by angiogenesis and collagen deposition in the wound, found in fibroblasts and epithelial cells (Diegelmann & Evans, 2004; PFEILSCHIFTE et al., 1990). EGF is stimulating for fibroblasts, endothelial cells, and keratinocytes, and also stimulates re-epithelialization, increases angiogenesis, and provides synthesis and transformation of the extracellular matrix (Bennett et al., 2003).

The mechanism of action of PRP has been mentioned in detail above. If we talk about the production of PRP, we will try to explain in some simple steps.

Platelet Gel Preparation

Platelet concentrates are prepared from autologous 20 mL of peripheral blood and centrifuged at 1500 rpm for 5 minutes using a compact table top centrifuge to obtain platelet-poor plasma (PPP), RBC, and PRP. This plasma is then centrifuged and centrifuged at 3,500 rpm for 5 minutes to collect the platelets as pellets. At the bottom of the centrifuge tube, it forms pellets, which is diluted in 3 mL of plasma and is considered PRP, while the remaining plasma is considered PPP. In PRP, platelet count is measured, and calcium chloride and thrombin ensure the release of growth factor from platelets.

Preparation of Thrombin

Homologous thrombin is obtained by centrifuging 5 ml of blood taken into a blood test tube at 3200 rpm for 10 minutes. The serum is then separated and 50 mL of 10% calcium gluconate is added, previously incubated at 37°C for 15-30 minutes. Finally, the supernatant is ready to be activated into PRP platelet gel containing thrombin precursors.

Activation of Platelet Gel

By adding platelet concentrate, the product is activated at the bedside. 2 mL of thrombin and 2 mL of 10% calcium chloride are added to a sterile 10 cm Petri dish; the concentrate thus obtained is gently mixed and allowed to rest. The concentrate becomes a gelatinous disc, which is rested for 10-15 min until a platelet gel forms. The gel is applied on the wound after washing. It is covered with a sterile, non-absorbent dressing with 0.9% normal saline solution. The most appropriate method of application for the patient is to remove necrotic tissues, if any, as shown in the figure, and apply the PRP gel using the principle of more comfortable absorption by healthy tissues (Figure 1) (Ahmed et al., 2017).

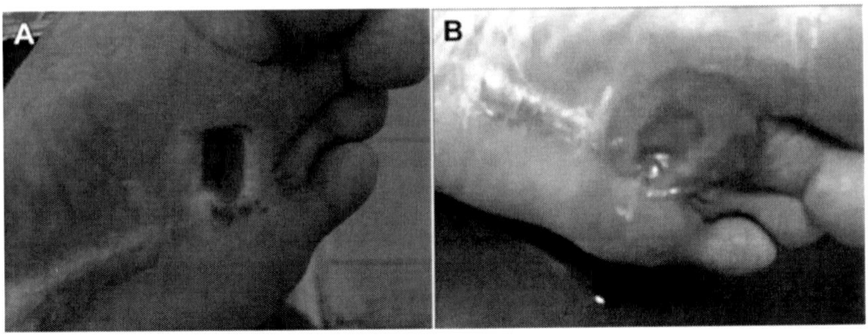

Figure 1. Wound before (A) and after (B) platelet gel application.

In a study, it was reported that wound healing was achieved in 68% of the group in which PRP gel was not used and in the group treated with traditional methods, and in 86% of the group in which PRP gel was applied to the diabetic foot wound for 3 months. In the same study, the initial state of the wound before PRP at the 2nd week and the 3rd week after PRP is shown in Figure 2 below (Ahmed et al., 2017).

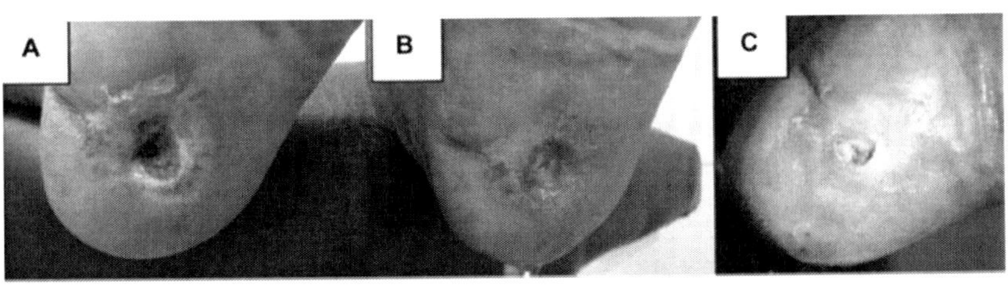

Figure 2. (A) Wound treated with PRP: (A) before application, (B) 2 weeks, and (C) 3 weeks after.

Many case series, case reports, descriptive studies, and comparative studies with interventions have shown that PRP is recommended for wound healing in diabetic foot ulcer (Ahmed et al., 2017; Driver, 2006; Scimeca et al., 2010; Tzeng et al., 2013). Many of these studies are advisory in nature, and in an intervention study conducted by measuring and recording the wound site with a controlled intervention study, it was reported that the wound healed faster than the normal group (Ahmed et al., 2017). Evidence seems to continue to emerge that it accelerates wound healing and delays amputation. In another study investigating the benefits of a PRP application, the epithelialization state before PRP application (Figure 3) and after 7 weeks is shown in Figure 4 (Scimeca et al., 2010).

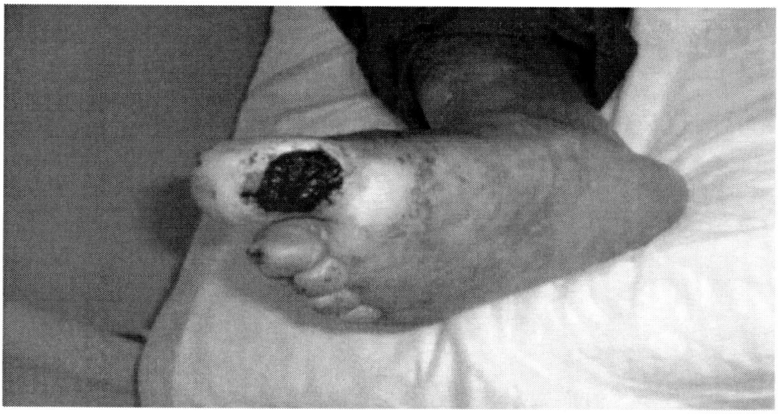

Figure 3. Foot wound of a diabetic patient before PRP.

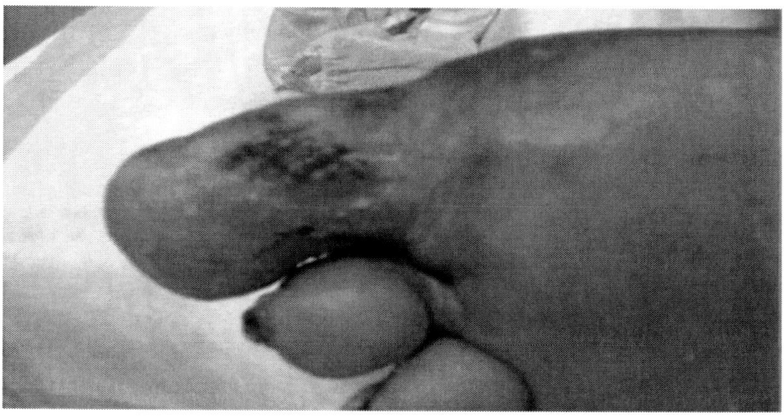

Figure 4. 4 weeks later PRP.

In another study conducted on a group of patients with diabetes mellitus, at the end of an eight-month follow-up, healing was observed in diabetic foot wounds without reopening in patients with small ulcers (2–5.5 cm2) compared to patients with large ulcers (8.5-12.5 cm^2) (Babaei et al., 2017). These results confirm that the PRP procedure can be easily performed on patients with diabetic foot ulcers at many clinics at a low cost. However, for large non-healing ulcers in patients with diabetes, skin grafting is mandatory as the definitive procedure for wound healing (Chen et al., 2010). In another study conducted in 35 patients, it was reported that wound healing was statistically significant in wounds between 0.5 cm^2 and 7 cm^2, that is, in relatively small wounds, which supports previous studies (Dougherty, 2008).

Eight-fold concentrations of early-activating platelet concentrates from whole blood may be useful because they have a mitogenic and chemotactic role for many cytokines that promote coagulation and wound healing (Eppley et al., 2004). Optimistic and promising results have also been reported in diabetic foot wounds with platelet-rich concentrated PRP, which has been used and shown to be beneficial in other chronic wounds (Crovetti et al., 2004; Everts et al., 2006; Falanga, 2005; Hom et al., 2007).

Conclusion

In light of many things we have mentioned and the literature we have scanned, it can be said that especially when caught at an early stage, PRP offers extra solutions for the treatment of diabetic foot ulcers, which is a complication of DM, as in many diseases. For this reason, while patients diagnosed with DM are followed up in primary care, adding loss of sensation and control of wounds to routine visits will provide the opportunity for early diagnosis. Primary care preventive medicine practices are the basic medical services in which chronic diseases are routinely followed, followed against complications, and an early warning system, such as an early warning system, in the development of possible complications despite all kinds of precautions, ensuring that the patient receives the necessary treatment at a higher level. With the increase in life expectancy, unhealthy diets, sedentary lifestyles, and many more factors inviting people, the number of individuals with chronic diseases will increase rapidly in our world. Alternative processes should be tried quickly and new hopes should be gained instead of stereotypical treatments with limited effectiveness, without DM and its complications, which lead to this increase, do not burden our health system.

References

Ahmed, M., Reffat, S. A., Hassan, A., & Eskander, F. (2017). Platelet-rich plasma for the treatment of clean diabetic foot ulcers. *Annals of vascular surgery*, *38*, 206-211. https://doi.org/10.1016/j.avsg.2016.04.023.

Alexiadou, K., & Doupis, J. (2012). Management of diabetic foot ulcers. *Diabetes Therapy*, *3*(1), 1-15. https://doi.org/10.1007/s13300-012-0004-9.

Anitua, E., Andia, I., Ardanza, B., Nurden, P., & Nurden, A. T. (2004). Autologous platelets as a source of proteins for healing and tissue regeneration. *Thrombosis and haemostasis*, *91*(01), 4-15. https://doi.org/10.1160/TH03-07-0440.

Babaei, V., Afradi, H., Gohardani, H., Nasseri, F., Azarafza, M., & Teimourian, S. (2017). Management of chronic diabetic foot ulcers using platelet-rich plasma. *Journal of wound care*, *26*(12), 784-787. https://doi.org/ 10.12968/jowc.2017.26.12.784.

Bennett, S., Griffiths, G., Schor, A., Leese, G., & Schor, S. (2003). Growth factors in the treatment of diabetic foot ulcers. *Journal of British Surgery*, *90*(2), 133-146. https://doi.org/10.1002/bjs.4019.

Benotmane, A., Mohammedi, F., Ayad, F., Kadi, K., & Azzouz, A. (2000). Diabetic foot lesions: etiologic and prognostic factors. *Diabetes & metabolism*, *26*(2), 113-117.

Brem, H., Sheehan, P., & Boulton, A. J. (2004). Protocol for treatment of diabetic foot ulcers. *The American journal of surgery*, *187*(5), S1-S10. https://doi.org/10.1016/ S0002-9610(03)00299-X.

Cavanagh, P. R., Lipsky, B. A., Bradbury, A. W., & Botek, G. (2005). Treatment for diabetic foot ulcers. *The Lancet*, *366*(9498), 1725-1735. https://doi.org/10.1016/ S0140-6736(05)67699-4.

Chen, T. M., Tsai, J. C., & Burnouf, T. (2010). A novel technique combining platelet gel, skin graft, and fibrin glue for healing recalcitrant lower extremity ulcers. *Dermatologic Surgery*, *36*(4), 453-460. https://doi.org/10.1111/j.1524-4725.2010.01480.x.

Corral, C. J., Siddiqui, A., Wu, L., Farrell, C. L., Lyons, D., & Mustoe, T. A. (1999). Vascular endothelial growth factor is more important than basic fibroblastic growth factor during ischemic wound healing. *Archives of surgery*, *134*(2), 200-205. https://doi.org/10.1001/archsurg.134.2.200.

Crovetti, G., Martinelli, G., Issi, M., Barone, M., Guizzardi, M., Campanati, B., Moroni, M., & Carabelli, A. (2004). Platelet gel for healing cutaneous chronic wounds. *Transfusion and Apheresis Science*, *30*(2), 145-151. https://doi.org/10.1016/j.transci. 2004.01.004.

d'Hemecourt, P. (1998). Sodium carboxymethylcellulose aqueous-bared gel vs. becaplermin gel in patients with nonhealing lower extremity diabetic ulcers. *Wounds*, *10*, 69-75. https://doi.org/10.2147/cia.s1106.

Diegelmann, R. F., & Evans, M. C. (2004). Wound healing: an overview of acute, fibrotic and delayed healing. *Front biosci*, *9*(1), 283-289. https://doi.org/10.2741/1184.

Dougherty, E. J. (2008). An evidence-based model comparing the cost-effectiveness of platelet-rich plasma gel to alternative therapies for patients with nonhealing diabetic foot ulcers. *Advances in Skin & Wound Care,* 21(12), 568-575. https://doi.org/10.1097/01.ASW.0000323589.27605.71.

Doupis, J., & Veves, A. (2008). Classification, diagnosis, and treatment of diabetic foot ulcers. *Wounds: a compendium of clinical research and practice*, *20*(5), 117-126.

Driver, V. R. (2006). Autologel Diabetic Foot Ulcer Study Group. A prospective, randomized controlled trial of autologous platelet-rich plasma gel for the treatment of diabetic foot ulcers. *Ostomy. Wound Manage.*, *52*, 68-87.

Eppley, B. L., Woodell, J. E., & Higgins, J. (2004). Platelet quantification and growth factor analysis from platelet-rich plasma: implications for wound healing. *Plastic and reconstructive surgery*, *114*(6), 1502-1508. https://doi.org/10.1097/01.prs.0000138251.07040.51.

Everts, P. A., Devilee, R. J., Brown Mahoney, C., Eeftinck-Schattenkerk, M., Box, H. A., Knape, J. T., & Van Zundert, A. (2006). Platelet gel and fibrin sealant reduce allogeneic blood transfusions in total knee arthroplasty. *Acta Anaesthesiologica Scandinavica*, *50*(5), 593-599. https://doi.org/10.1111/j.1399-6576.2006.001005.x.

Falanga, V. (2005). Wound healing and its impairment in the diabetic foot. *The Lancet*, *366*(9498), 1736-1743. https://doi.org/10.1016/S0140-6736(05)67700-8.

GBD 2019 Collaborators (Institute for Health Metrics and Evaluation) (2020). *Global Burden of Disease Study 2019 Results.* https://vizhub.healthdata.org/gbd-results/.

Hinchliffe, R., Valk, G., Jeffcoate, W., Apelqvist, J., Armstrong, D., & Bakker, K. (2008). Specific guidelines on wound and wound-bed management. *Diabetes/metabolism research and reviews (Print)*, *24*. https://doi.org/10.1002/dmrr.854.

Hom, D. B., Linzie, B. M., & Huang, T. C. (2007). The healing effects of autologous platelet gel on acute human skin wounds. *Archives of facial plastic surgery*, *9*(3), 174-183. https://doi.org/10.1001/archfaci.9.3.174.

Hosgood, G. (1993). Wound healing: the role of platelet-derived growth factor and transforming growth factor beta. *Veterinary surgery*, *22*(6), 490-495. https://doi.org//10.1111/j.1532-950X.1993.tb00426.x.

Kevy, S., Jacobson, M., Blasetti, L., & Fagnant, A. (2001). Preparation of growth factor enriched autologous platelet gel. Proceedings of the 27th Annual meeting of Service Biomaterials.

Lacci, K. M., & Dardik, A. (2010). Platelet-rich plasma: support for its use in wound healing. *The Yale journal of biology and medicine*, *83*(1), 1.

Lauterbach, S., Kostev, K., & Kohlmann, T. (2010). Prevalence of diabetic foot syndrome and its risk factors in the UK. *Journal of wound care*, *19*(8), 333-337. https://doi.org/10.12968/jowc.2010.19.8.77711.

Malgrange, D., Richard, J., Leymarie, F., & Foot, F. W. G. o. t. D. (2003). Screening diabetic patients at risk for foot ulceration. A multi-centre hospital-based study in France. *Diabetes & metabolism*, *29*(3), 261-268. https://doi.org/10.1016/S1262-3636(07)70035-6.

Marx, R. E. (2001). Platelet-rich plasma (PRP): what is PRP and what is not PRP? *Implant dentistry*, *10*(4), 225-228. https://doi.org/10.1097/00008505-200110000-00002.

Moxey, P., Gogalniceanu, P., Hinchliffe, R., Loftus, I., Jones, K., Thompson, M., & Holt, P. (2011). Lower extremity amputations—a review of global variability in incidence.

Diabetic Medicine, *28*(10), 1144-1153. https://doi.org/10.1111/j.1464-5491.2011.03279.x.

Neufeld, G., Cohen, T., Gengrinovitch, S., & Poltorak, Z. (1999). Vascular endothelial growth factor (VEGF) and its receptors. *The FASEB journal*, *13*(1), 9-22.

Ogino, Y., Ayukawa, Y., Tsukiyama, Y., & Koyano, K. (2005). The effect of platelet-rich plasma on the cellular response of rat bone marrow cells in vitro. *Oral Surgery, Oral Medicine, Oral Pathology, Oral Radiology, and Endodontology*, *100*(3), 302-307. https://doi.org/ 10.1016/j.tripleo.2005.03.007.

Pfeılschıfte, J., Oechsner, M., Naumann, A., Gronwald, R. G., Mınne, H. W., & Zıegler, R. (1990). Stimulation of bone matrix apposition in vitro by local growth factors: a comparison between insulin-like growth factor I, platelet-derived growth factor, and transforming growth factor β. *Endocrinology*, *127*(1), 69-75. https://doi.org/10.1210/endo-127-1-69.

Pierce, G. F., Mustoe, T. A., Altrock, B. W., Deuel, T. F., & Thomason, A. (1991). Role of platelet-derived growth factor in wound healing. *Journal of cellular biochemistry*, *45*(4), 319-326. https://doi.org/10.1002/jcb.240450403.

Prompers, L., Huijberts, M., Apelqvist, J., Jude, E., Piaggesi, A., Bakker, K., Edmonds, M., Holstein, P., Jirkovska, A., & Mauricio, D. (2007). High prevalence of ischaemia, infection and serious comorbidity in patients with diabetic foot disease in Europe. Baseline results from the Eurodiale study. *Diabetologia*, *50*(1), 18-25. https://doi.org/
10.1007/s00125-006-0491-1.

Raslan, M. M., Milad, N. M., & Abd AlAziz, A. (2017). Effect of autologous platelet-rich plasma in the promotion of healing of chronic ulcers. *International Surgery Journal*, *5*(1), 15-19. https://doi.org//10.18203/2349-2902.isj20175484.

Schaper, N. (2004). Diabetic foot ulcer classification system for research purposes: a progress report on criteria for including patients in research studies. *Diabetes/Metabolism Research and Reviews*, *20*(S1), S90-S95. https://doi.org/10.1002/dmrr.464.

Scimeca, C. L., Bharara, M., Fisher, T. K., Kimbriel, H., & Armstrong, D. G. (2010). Novel use of platelet-rich plasma to augment curative diabetic foot surgery. *Journal of Diabetes Science and Technology*, *4*(5), 1121-1126. https://doi.org/10.1177/193229681000400510.

Smiell, J. M., Wieman, T. J., Steed, D. L., Perry, B. H., Sampson, A. R., & Schwab, B. H. (1999). Efficacy and safety of becaplermin (recombinant human platelet-derived growth factor-BB) in patients with nonhealing, lower extremity diabetic ulcers: a combined analysis of four randomized studies. *Wound Repair and Regeneration*, *7*(5), 335-346. https://doi.org/10.1046/j.1524-475x.1999.00335.x.

Tesfaye, S., Stevens, L., Stephenson, J., Fuller, J., Plater, M., Ionescu-Tirgoviste, C., Nuber, A., Pozza, G., & Ward, J. (1996). Prevalence of diabetic peripheral neuropathy and its relation to glycaemic control and potential risk factors: the EURODIAB IDDM Complications Study. *Diabetologia*, *39*(11), 1377-1384. https://doi.org/10.1007/
s001250050586.

Tzeng, Y.-S., Deng, S.-C., Wang, C.-H., Tsai, J.-C., Chen, T.-M., & Burnouf, T. (2013). Treatment of nonhealing diabetic lower extremity ulcers with skin graft and autologous platelet gel: a case series. *BioMed Research International, 2013*. https://doi.org/10.1155/2013/837620.

WHO. (2022). *Diabetes*. https://www.who.int/news-room/fact-sheets/detail/diabetes.

Wu, L., Xia, Y.-P., Roth, S. I., Gruskin, E., & Mustoe, T. A. (1999). Transforming growth factor-β1 fails to stimulate wound healing and impairs its signal transduction in an aged ischemic ulcer model: importance of oxygen and age. *The American journal of pathology*, *154*(1), 301-309. https://doi.org/10.1016/s0002-9440(10)65276-5.

Chapter 11

The Use of Platelet-Rich Plasma in Hair Diseases

İsmail Kaba[*]**, MD**

Department of Family Medicine, Nilüfer District Health Directorate, Bursa, Turkiye

Abstract

Hair diseases vary both in clinic, pathogenesis, and treatment form according to the types of treatment sought for various reasons. In cases of hair diseases, patients consult the doctor, especially with cosmetic concerns. Patients prefer treatment options with fast results. There are many different treatment options such as medical treatment, transplantation, and platelet-rich plasma (PRP) in these diseases. In this section, we examine the use of PRP in hair diseases, the mechanism of action of PRP, and its effectiveness on hair diseases. PRP is a plasma compound with high platelets in the content obtained by centrifugation of blood taken from the patient's own venous blood. PRP has advantages such as a low level of side effects in hair diseases, easy to apply, safe treatment process, and relatively easy to solve the side effects that may occur. PRP has been used in hair diseases with successful results in various diseases such as androgenetic alopecia, alopecia areata female hair loss, and cicatricial alopecia. PRP is used in combination with medical treatment or in medical treatment of hair diseases.

Keywords: PRP, hair diseases, alopecia

[*] Corresponding Author's Email: drismailkaba61@gmail.com.

In: Current Clinical Recommendations ...
Editors: Nazan Yurtcu and Emel Güler
ISBN: 979-8-89113-723-3

Introduction

What Is Platelet-Rich Plasma?

Platelet–rich plasma (PRP) is a plasma compound obtained by centrifugation of venous whole blood and containing high concentrations of platelets, its use has been increased in recent years (De Pascale et al., 2015).

PRP is defined as high concentrations of platelets found in blood plasma. As a procedure, the PRP patient is isolated from blood taken from their own body by a phlebotomy (the process of taking blood from the vein) and into a tube containing a citrate or EDTA-based anticoagulant. The blood sample is subjected to centrifugation, and as a result of the removal of red blood cells and immune cells, a high concentration of thrombocytes is obtained in plasma (Kuşpınar, 2023).

After activating the high concentration platelets obtained with variable activators (thrombin, calcium, adp, collagen), a platelet-rich plasma compound is obtained that can be applied to the patient (Kuşpınar, 2023).

Since 1987, PRP has been tested as an alternative medicine method in the treatment of various diseases (Ferrari et al., 1987).

Plasma rich in platelet has a wide range of uses today, from wound healing to urologic diseases, from dermatological diseases to physical treatment, as described in other chapters of this book.

In this section, we will talk about the use and effectiveness of platelet-rich plasma in hair diseases.

Advantages of Using Platelet-Rich Plasma

The main advantages of PRP are that the level of side effects of PRP is low, that it is easy to apply, that the effect provided in repeated procedures is relatively long, that the treatment process is safe, and that the solution of the side effects that may occur is relatively easy, that similar results can be obtained from the experienced practitioner due to the fact that it is an application-based procedure and that the patient does not take an effective role in the treatment.

Platelet-Rich Plasma Complications

Even though PRP is a safe treatment with few side effects, it has some contraindications that should be considered as with any procedure.

Absolute contraindications to PRP include critical thrombocytopenia, thrombocytoregulation, hemodynamicscency, sepsis, local infection, and the patient who does not want to take risks. Nsaid use within 48 hours is one of the relative contraindications, and other related contraindications are glucocorticoid injection at the site of treatment within one month, systemic glucocorticoid use within two weeks, cancer, especially bone or hematolymphoid cancers, anemia, thrombocytopenia (low thrombocyte level) (Hesseler & Shyam, 2020).

Sensitivity, itching, burning, pain, erythema, ecchymosis, small hematomas, secondary infections, and allergic reactions that may occur are the most common complications of PRP in the PRP application area (Yildirim et al., 2018).

In Which Hair Diseases PRP Is Used

PRP is used mainly in hair diseases such as androgenic alopecia, female pattern hair loss, alopecia areata, cicatricial alopecia. Although there are studies showing that PRP is effective in these diseases, which we will examine in detail, there are also studies showing that there is no effectiveness.

Pathogenes of Hair Diseases

Hair diseases are an important application area in developed countries and countries where health tourism is popular, such as our country. When we examine the pathogenesis of hair diseases, an important part of the applications is androgenetic alopecia.

Androgeneticalopecia (AGA) is a type of hair loss with varying severity and frequency in which a genetic predisposition with different defined mechanisms is at the forefront (Sahin).

The level of the clinical course of androgenetic alopecia, which is a slow progression over the years, varies from person to person. The first symptoms usually appear during adolescence. Hair loss in men can start from the area we call the frontal area, vertex (m pattern), or temporal area. Due to hair loss in these areas, patients often consult family physicians or dermatology polyclinics as the first application.

Patients with androgenic alopecia often present without symptoms due to cosmetic concerns.

Use of PRP in Androgenic Alopecia

PRP can stimulate the differentiation of stem cells into hair follicle cells by regulating the translational activity of cells-caten. In addition, it is known that due to the FGF-7 (fibroblast growth factor-7) that it contains prolongs the anagen phase of the hair growth cycle and increases cell survival by inhibiting apoptosis, hair follicles become more bleeding due to the increased in perifollicular vascularp leplexus with increased levels of in VEGF and PDGF, which have angiogenic potential (Yildirim et al., 2018).

PRP is also preferred in the treatment of androgeneticalopecia because PRP is a less invasive and reliable procedure than other treatment options. Although the frequency of application varies on the basis of the practitioner in PRP, the application periods, which are generally preferred, are preferred as 6-8 with 2-4 weeks of aelic (Schiavone et al., 2014).

In androgenetic alopecia, the effect of dihydrotestosterone on undermalpapila cells suppresses the canonic want signal, causing defective hair growth and a delayed hair cycle. Therefore, hair loss is slightly higher in patients with high conversion of testosterone to dihydrotestosterone. As with inhibition of the 5 alpha reductase enzyme that converts testosterone to dihydrotestosterone, we can also achieve the effect with the PRP process, which stimulates hair growth by activating the signal of wnt/β-catine, and PRP activates this signal, stimulating the proliferation and differentiation of hair follicle cells and stimulating the start of the new hair cycle (Paichitrojjana & Paichitrojjana, 2022).

The most important issue in treating such patients is to take a detailed history. When selecting the treatment options of the patient after anamnesis by the physician, the patient's subjective factors, continuity of treatment, ease of access to treatment, and compliance with treatment should also be taken into consideration. The treatment option can be quite complicated for hair diseases. Especially in hair diseases, the expectation of patients is to get very fast results. If these expectations are met in a short time, turning to alternative physicians or treatments is a situation that we frequently encounter.

Therefore, all stages of the process should be clearly explained to patients who will decide to apply the platelet-rich plasma treatment after the diagnosis, and the treatment should begin as such. Other medical treatment options should be well examined and appropriate patients should be selected for practice.

Female Pattern Hair Loss (FPHL)

In studies involving 92 patients from 6 randomized controlled clinical trials conducted to investigate the efficacy of PRP in female hair loss, it was found that PRP has a positive effect on FPHL treatment by increasing hair thickness and density (Torabi et al., 2020).

Two meta-analysis studies have recently confirmed the efficacy of the treatment with PRP and FPHL. The first study of 776 female participants showed that PRP had a good therapeutic effect on FPHL in hair density when compared to the control groups (Zhou et al., 2021).

Alopecia Areata

The lifetime risk of alopecia areata is estimated to be approximately 2% of the population, with no incidence difference between genders (Paichitrojjana & Paichitrojjana, 2022). Alopecia areata is an important hair loss disease that is encountered in the clinic. As in other hair diseases, the use of PRP in alopecia areata is a method preferred by clinicians.

Use of PRP in Alopecia Areata

It has been thought that the growth factors contained in PRP may be effective in alopeciata because it stimulates angiogenesis, proliferation, and differentiation in hair follicles, increases the anagen phase, stimulates hair growth, and mainly because of its local anti-inflammatory effect (Gupta et al., 2017).

PRP is known to have a strong anti-inflammatory effect. PRP reduces local tissue inflammation and suppresses cytokine release, making it potentially beneficial in the treatment of inflamed hair loss such as alopecia areata.

In a study of 45 patients with alopecia areata, intralesional PRP or triamcinolonasenite or placebo injections were applied to one-half of the patient's scalp, but the other half of the patient's scalp was not treated. As a result of the study, PRP was shown to significantly increase hair regrowth and ki-67 levels (a marker of cell proliferation) compared to triamcinolonase or placebo injection (Trink et al., 2013).

In the treatment of alopecia areata, several randomized controlled trials have shown that treatment with PRP can stimulate hair growth to the same extent as triamcinolone intralesional injection (Paichitrojjana & Paichitrojjana, 2022).

The therapeutic effect of intralesional PRP injections in alopecia areata was compared with triamcinolonocene in two recent studies. A study found that the final score of alopecia violence mediator (salt) showed significantly lower levels in both groups compared to basic levels (p = 0.025 and p = 0.008), that there were no significant differences between the two treatment methods in terms of clinical recovery (Fawzy et al., 2021).

Conversely, three randomized-controlled clinical trials found different results showing that PRP was significantly less effective than intralesional steroids, according to the mac donald hull and norris rating system, hair growth percentage, and a decrease in salt score relative to baseline, respectively (Agrawal et al., 2018; Kapoor et al., 2020; Ranpariya et al., 2019).

In a study in which PRP and intralesional trimcinolone treatment was applied to one half of the scalp and only intralesional triamcinolotonide treatment was applied to the other half, more hair growth and larger hair diameter hair growth were observed in the half treated with combined therapy (Mubki, 2016).

A prospective study on the efficacy of PRP treatment in 20 cases of chronic alopecia areata who did not respond to conventional treatment for 2 years also found that all patients with chronic alopecia areata were successfully treated with PRP, with only one patient having a recurrence after one year (Singh, 2015).

Successful PRP treatment has also been reported in a patient with corticosteroid-resistant aphasia alopecia area who experiences hair growth again after PRP injections and in a patient with alopecia (Donovan, 2015). Therefore, PRP can be used as an alternative treatment in patients who do not respond to standard treatment. PRP can also be used as an adjuvant treatment for alopecia areata for patients who do not want conventional treatment or steroid therapy.

When these and similar studies increase and when sufficient studies are performed on a large scale, we will be able to talk more about the effectiveness of PRP.

Cicatricial Alopecia

Cicatricial alopecia is a type of scarring alopecia caused by different inflammatory conditions, physical trauma, burns, or serious infections that lead to the destruction of the hair follicles and subsequent scarring (Paichitrojjana & Paichitrojjana, 2022).

The goal of treatment in cicatricial alopecia is to stop the progression of the disease by using different anti-inflammatory drugs such as topical steroids, intralesional triamcinolone acetonide injection, and immunomodulatory agents to prevent further hair loss and scarring. However, there is no effective treatment to encourage hair regrowth in the fibrotic region, which may occur in the normal flow of the defect (Kanti et al., 2018).

Effective treatment of cicatricial alopecia with PRP is possible due to various cytokines and growth factors with anti-inflammatory and proangiogenic effects, such as TGFB and TGF1 in platelet granules. But we believe that more clinical research is required in order to produce more evidence that it may be effective in the treatment of cadastral alopecia (Alves & Grimalt, 2020).

Mechanism of Action of PRP in Hair Diseases

VEGF plays an important role as a powerful hair growth stimulant through induction of angiogenesis (Yildirim et al., 2018).

Igf-1 induces and prolongs the anagen phase of the hair growth cycle while stimulating the proliferation of cyclic ki67+basal keratinoides (Yildirim et al., 2018).

In addition, PRP can induce the proliferation of dermalpapilla (dp) cells by activating extracellular signal-bound kinase (erk), fibroblast growth factor 7 (FGF-7), beta-catenin, and akt signal (an anti-apoptotic signal molecule) (Yildirim et al., 2018).

In vitro, human dermalpapilla cells cultured with PRP, the expression of the bcl-2 protein (an anti-apoptotic protein) also increases. Therefore, it has been clearly demonstrated that PRP can increase hair follicle cell survival through anti-apoptotic effects and stimulate hair growth by prolonging the anagen phase of the hair cycle. (Yildirim et al., 2018).

The number of platelets is an important factor in the effectiveness of PRP. In terms of hair density, follicle diameter, and thermal hair density, PRP treatment with a higher number of platelets outperforms the procedure with a lower number of platelets.

What Kind of Treatment Option Is PRP

The majority of patients who apply for PRP consist of patient groups that started with medical treatments and left the treatment for various reasons. In PRP, the use of PRP is becoming widespread due to the fact that the practitioner is a physician and the patient has an active role in many stages, unlike other treatment methods.

The aim of PRP treatment is to stop follicular miniaturization and increase hair density (Şahin et al., 2021).

PRP is most commonly used in alopecia and androgenoptia as hair diseases.

Conclusion

The selection of all these treatments according to their effectiveness and side effects is made in cooperation with the clinician and the patient. Due to the ease of application of patient satisfaction in hair diseases in the recent period, the PRP option is one of the first choices both as a clinician preference and as a patient preference.

PRP can be used as a new therapeutic option for hair loss, including androgenetic alopecia and female pattern hair loss, or as a supplement to hair transplantation. In terms of side effect profile comparison to steroid use, PRP can also be considered a very safe, highly effective, safer, and alternative treatment for alopecia areata.

In some studies, there is also evidence that PRP can improve clinical symptoms in some types of cadastral alopecia. However, more work is required to determine the treatment regime, including the protocols, including the standardization of the PRP treatment preparation, the amount of dose applied and the dose dates, the injection technique, the number and interval of optimal treatment sessions.

References

Agrawal, P., Jerajani, H. R., & Jindal, S. (2018). Intralesional platelet rich plasma therapy vs intralesional triamcinolone acetonide for the treatment of alopecia areata. *MGM J Med Sci*, *5*(2), 68-75. https://doi.org/10.5005/jp-journals-10036-1187.

Alves, R., & Grimalt, R. (2020). Platelet-rich plasma and its use for cicatricial and non-cicatricial alopecias: a narrative review. *Dermatology and Therapy*, *10*(4), 623-633. https://doi.org/10.1007/513555-020-00408-5.

De Pascale M. R., Sommese, L., Casamassimi, A., & Napoli, C. (2015). Platelet derivatives in regenerative medicine: an update. *Transfusion medicine reviews*, 29(1), 52-61. https://doi.org/10.1016/j.tmrv.2014.11.001.

Donovan, J. (2015). Successful treatment of corticosteroid-resistant ophiasis-type alopecia areata (AA) with platelet-rich plasma (PRP). *JAAD Case Reports*, *1*(5), 305-307. https://doi.org/10.1016/j.jdcr.2015.07.004.

Fawzy, M. M., Abdel Hay, R., Mohammed, F. N., Sayed, K. S., Ghanem, M. E. D., & Ezzat, M. (2021). Trichoscopy as an evaluation method for alopecia areata treatment: A comparative study. *Journal of Cosmetic Dermatology*, *20*(6), 1827-1836.

Ferrari, M., Zia, S., Valbonesi, M., Henriquet, F., Venere, G., Spagnolo, S., Grasso, M. A., & Panzani, I. (1987). A new technique for hemodilution, preparation of autologous platelet-rich plasma and intraoperative blood salvage in cardiac surgery. *The International journal of artificial organs*, *10*(1), 47-50. https://doi.org/10.1177/039139888701000111.

Gupta, A. K., Carviel, J., & Abramovits, W. (2017). Treating alopecia areata: current practices versus new directions. *American journal of clinical dermatology*, *18*, 67-75. https://doi.org/10.1007/s40257-016-0230-4.

Hesseler, M. J., & Shyam, N. (2020). Platelet-rich plasma and its utilities in alopecia: a systematic review. *Dermatologic Surgery*, *46*(1), 93-102. https://doi.org/10.1097/DSS.0000000000001965 31211715.

Kanti, V., Röwert-Huber, J., Vogt, A., & Blume-Peytavi, U. (2018). Cicatricial alopecia. *JDDG: Journal der Deutschen Dermatologischen Gesellschaft*, *16*(4), 435-461. https://doi.org/10.1111/ddg.13498.

Kapoor, P., Kumar, S., Brar, B. K., Kukar, N., Arora, H., & Brar, S. K. (2020). Comparative evaluation of therapeutic efficacy of intralesional injection of triamcinolone acetonide versus intralesional autologous platelet-rich plasma injection in alopecia areata. *Journal of Cutaneous and Aesthetic Surgery*, *13*(2), 103.

Kuşpınar, G. (2023). *Sıçan In Vivo Prematür Ovaryan Yetmezliği Modelinde Intraovaryan Plateletten Zengin Plazma Uygulamasının Ovaryan Foliküllerin Gelişimine Etkisi* [The Effect of Intraovarian Platelet-Rich Plasma Injection on the Development of Ovarian Follicles in the Rat In Vivo Model of Premature Ovarian Failure](Doctoral dissertation). Bursa Uludag University, Bursa, Turkiye.

Mubki, T. (2016). Platelet-rich plasma combined with intralesional triamcinolone acetonide for the treatment of alopecia areata: a case report. *Journal of Dermatology & Dermatologic Surgery*, *20*(1), 87-90. https://doi.org/10.1016/j.jdds.2015.11.002.

Paichitrojjana, A., & Paichitrojjana, A. (2022). Platelet rich plasma and its use in hair regrowth: a review. *Drug Design, Development and Therapy*, 635-645. https://doi.org/10.18203/issn.2455-4529.

Ranpariya, R. H., Gupta, S. B., Deora, M. S., Agrawal, P. V., Mathur, R., & Raheja, A. (2019). Intralesional triamcinolone acetonide versus platelet rich plasma: a comparative study in the treatment of alopecia areata of scalp. *Int J Res Dermatol*, *5*(3), 521-7. https://doi.org/10.18203/issn.2455-4529.İntJResDermatol20193223.

Schiavone, G., Raskovic, D., Greco, J., & Abeni, D. (2014). Platelet-rich plasma for androgenetic alopecia: a pilot study. *Dermatologic Surgery*, *40*(9), 1010-1019. https://doi.org/10.1097/01.DSS.0000452629.76339.2b.

Singh, S. (2015). Role of platelet-rich plasma in chronic alopecia areata: our centre experience. *Indian Journal of Plastic Surgery*, *48*(01), 057-059. https://doi.org/10.4103/0970-0358.155271.

Şahin, G., Özdemir, H., & Aydın, F. (2021). Androgenetik Alopesi [Androgenetic Alopecia]. *Uludağ Üniversitesi Tıp Fakültesi Dergisi*, *47*(1), 141-149. https://doi.org/10.32708/uutfd.857676.

Torabi, P., Behrangi, E., Goodarzi, A., & Rohaninasab, M. (2020). A systematic review of the effect of platelet-rich plasma on androgenetic alopecia of women. *Dermatologic Therapy*, *33*(6), e13835. https://doi.org/10.1111/dth.13835 32588941.

Trink, A., Sorbellini, E., Bezzola, P., Rodella, L., Rezzani, R., Ramot, Y., & Rinaldi, F. (2013). A randomized, double-blind, placebo-and active-controlled, half-head study to evaluate the effects of platelet-rich plasma on alopecia areata. *British Journal of Dermatology*, *169*(3), 690-694. https://doi.org/10.1111/bjd.12397.

Yildirim, M. E. C., Ince, B., Uyanik, O., Okur, M. I., & Dadaci, M. (2018). Development of Hyperalgesia in Patients Treated with Autologous Platelet Rich Plasma Due to Androgenetic Alopecia. *Selcuk University Medical Journal*, *34*(3). https://doi.org/10.30733/std.2018.01051.

Zhou, S., Qi, F., Gong, Y., Zhang, C., Zhao, S., Yang, X., & He, Y. (2021). Platelet-rich plasma in female androgenic alopecia: a comprehensive systematic review and meta-analysis. *Frontiers in Pharmacology*, *12*, 642980. https://doi.org/10.3389/fphar.2021.642980 341408.

Chapter 12

PRP Treatment for Dental Application

Samir Goyushov*
Department of Periodontology, Istanbul Aydin University, Istanbul, Turkiye

Abstract

Platelet concentrates collected from the patient's blood were first presented over 20 years ago. The aim of this technique was to collect the maximum number of platelets and growth factors and implement them during surgery. This relatively "new" regenerative method could surely be applied to various clinical procedures in dentistry with favorable results and low risks. The PRF membrane helps in the wound healing process, protecting the surgical area and stimulating soft tissue repair. When PRF is mixed with bone graft, it may attract stem cells and provide neo-angiogenesis. The following chapter attempts to summarize the significant literature regarding the technique of PRF application, focusing on its preparation, advantages, and disadvantages of using it in dental procedures.

Keywords: platelet concentrates, dentistry, dental implant, maxillary sinus augmentation

Introduction

Approximately twenty years have passed since platelet concentrations were first introduced. Autologous platelet concentrates (Platelet-Rich Plasma

* Corresponding Author's Email: samir.goyush@gmail.com.

In: Current Clinical Recommendations ...
Editors: Nazan Yurtcu and Emel Güler
ISBN: 979-8-89113-723-3

(PRP) and Platelet-Rich Fibrin (PRF) are used in several dental treatments, predominantly in oral and maxillofacial surgery. These concentrates comprise high levels of growth factors, naturally derived from blood. Growth factors are the key elements in wound healing, particularly in soft and hard tissue regeneration. We focus specifically on their properties for intraoral wound healing and their application in different fields of dentistry.

Wound Healing

An autologous concentrate of human platelets has been widely used in dentistry for several years. Using platelet concentrations enhances the healing process in hard and soft tissues. Platelets are involved primarily in wound healing through clot formation and the release of growth factors that initiate and support wound healing. The growth factors released by platelets initiate and accelerate wound healing. The interaction between various cell types and growth factors leads to the efficient repair of wounds. Scientists continue to understand different growth factors and their participation in different phases of wound healing. Growth factors are natural biological mediators that determine essential cellular events involved in soft tissue repair by binding to specific cell surface receptors (Giannobile, 1996). After attachment, growth factors initiate signaling pathways inside cells. Those processes result in intracellular gene activation, which changes the cellular activity and phenotype (Anusaksathien & Giannobile, 2002). Platelet concentrates derived from whole blood were first presented at the beginning of the last century. The aim of the concept was to use human blood proteins as a source of growth factors accomplished of supporting new vessel formation which was considered a necessity for tissue regeneration [5-prf book]. The first generation of platelet concentrates (platelet-rich plasma) was established in dentistry by clinician scientist Marx et al. (Marx, 2004). Since then, platelet concentrates have been widely applied in different fields of dentistry, especially in oral and maxillofacial surgery. Depending on the recognized blood cell content and fibrin network design, various platelet concentrates were classified in the literature into four principal categories: pure platelet-rich plasma (P-PRP), leukocyte- and platelet-rich plasma (L-PRP), pure platelet-rich fibrin (P-PRF), and leukocyte- and platelet-rich fibrin (L-PRF). Despite the increasing clinical achievement of PRP in the initial years after presentation, various limitations were reported that hampered its healing potential. Because of the long-lasting preparation procedure, anticoagulant factors were used to prevent clotting. Anticoagulant factors, such as bovine thrombin or CaCl2, were known inhibitors of wound healing. Another limitation of PRP was its liquid nature, which required its combination with other "unnatural" products such as bone substitutes derived from animal products or human cadavers.

To summarize, the above-mentioned several limitations of PRP in the dentistry field have forced the authors to investigate new methods for successful regeneration. Therefore, a second-generation platelet concentrate named platelet-rich fibrin (PRF) was developed with shorter preparation times and without any anticoagulant agent that was considered 100% autologous and natural.

The PRF protocol was established using a simpler 1-cycle centrifugation protocol demanding 12 minutes at 2700 rpm. The resulting product after high centrifugation speed consists of the following three layers (Figure 1):

- an overlaying liquid containing platelet-poor plasma (PPP)
- platelet-rich fibrin (PRF) and concentrated growth factors (CGF) in the middle
- red corpuscle at the bottom (RBC)

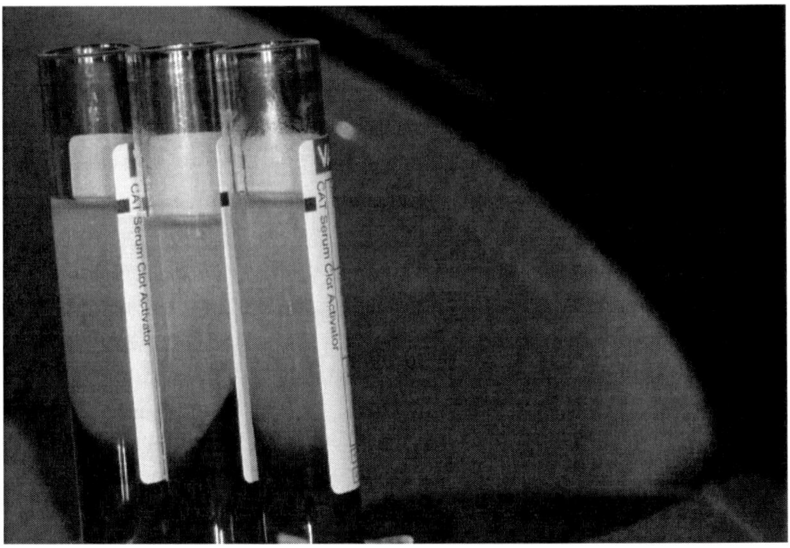

Figure 1. Processed blood tubes with a tabletop centrifuge (Author's own archive, taken by Furkan Yavaş and Serap Kaşıkcı).

As no anticoagulants were used, the blood coagulation process begins as soon as it encounters the tube glass surface, and the three-dimensional fibrin scaffold termed PRF came into existence. According to the current literature, PRF contains all three crucial principles for tissue regeneration. Attending as a three-dimensional fibrin scaffold, it embraces blood cells and slow-releasing grow factors. Over the past decade, PRF has gained extraordinary popularity in a variety of dental procedures. In dentistry, PRF has been applied for the treatment of extraction sockets, endodontic treatments, root coverages, wound closure, and regeneration of periodontal defects, in implantology. Therefore, the purpose of this chapter is to report the current state of knowledge and clinical potential of PRF in different dental procedures.

Platelet Concentrations in Regenerative Endodontics

Despite the fact that endodontic treatments are an invasive and difficult procedure, especially in complex anatomies, the success rate is very high (López-Valverde et al., 2023). Calcium hydroxide is considered the traditional material for apexification. However, long-term calcium hydroxide application may result in various complications such as reduced dentinal wall hardness and root fracture (Grigoratos et al., 2001). To overcome the weaknesses of the apexification method with calcium hydroxide, mineral trioxide aggregate (MTA) was introduced for the apical closure. After the application of the MTA technique, the root length and wall thickness remain stable. Because of these possible complications of different materials, regenerative/revitalization endodontic procedures have gained popularity. Treatments that contain biomaterials that boost the healing and repair of the pulp dentin complex after reestablishing the infectious or contaminated tooth tissue are called regenerative procedures. Platelet concentrates have also been suggested as a potential scaffold for regenerative endodontic treatments (Figure 2). PRF is considered a tremendous autogenous biomaterial for the regeneration of the pulp-dentin complex. There have been published preclinical studies that support the role of PRF in reparative dentin formation (Hotwani & Sharma, 2014). The application of suitable scaffolds is a crucial component of well-designed regenerative endodontic treatment (ElSheshtawy et al., 2020). Platelet concentrates have been used in regenerative procedures due to their rich substance with important growth factors leads to predictable outcomes. The disadvantage of PRF in endodontic treatments is its manipulation to insert the root canal. Some clinicals use only blood clots inside the canal to make a natural scaffold. However, compared to the blood clot, the concentration of platelets and growth factors in autologous platelet concentrates is much higher. Studies are needed to explore the complete mechanism of action of platelet concentrates for endodontic regeneration both *in vitro* and *in vivo*.

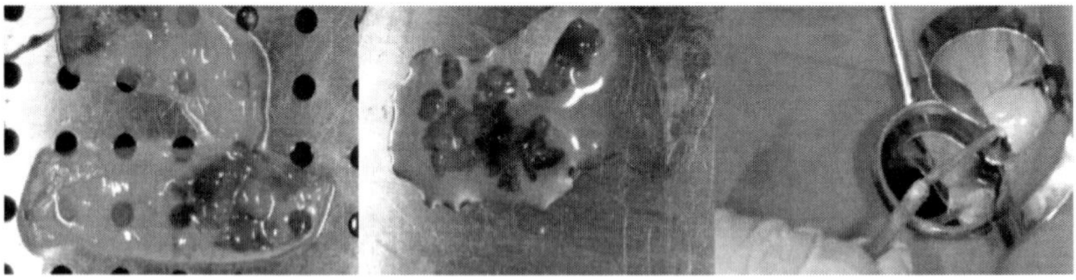

Figure 2. Placement of L-PRF into the root canal in small pieces(Author's own archive, taken by Furkan Yavaş and Serap Kaşıkcı).

Platelet Concentrations in Bone Regeneration of the Socket

Tooth extraction starts a cascade of biological processes that finally alter a previously intact alveolar bone morphology. However, in order to use the region for implantation, more research has been applied on the maintenance of future implant-bearing structures. The aim of the socket preservation procedure is to prevent progressive bone resorption after tooth extraction. This could be accomplished using different surgical techniques and bone substitutes with or without collagen membranes or the use of biological mediators. One of the most crucial factors is the ability of the biomaterial to be resorbed and replaced by newly formed hard tissue. PRF is the most investigated type of platelet concentrates in order to accelerate wound healing after tooth extraction. The application of PRF can reduce inflammation by gradually releasing autologous growth factors. To date, the bone stimulation capacity of PRF in the extraction socket is controversial; only a few randomized controlled studies have been published. The use of PRF in the socket is capable of supporting the clinician in wound closure. The regenerative effect of PRF on bone still requires more clinical studies to confirm the results (Figure 3).

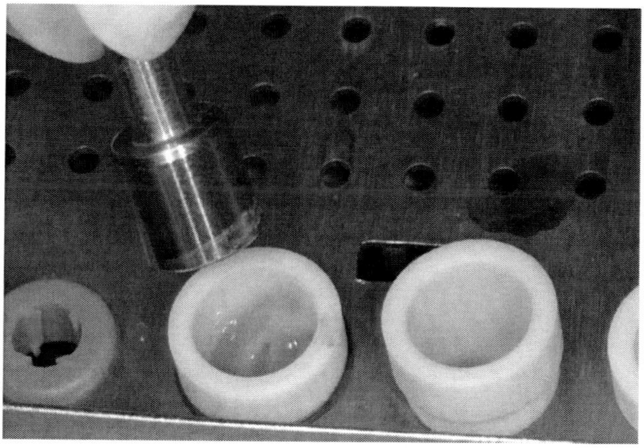

Figure 3. Preparing the PRF-plug to cover the extraction socket (Author's own archive, taken by Furkan Yavaş and Serap Kaşıkcı).

Platelet Concentrations in Periodontal Regeneration

The regenerative process of the bone and gingival tissues around the teeth has been very assuring with the PRF application. This statement is supported by various clinical studies (Choukroun et al., 2000; Choukroun et al., 2006). There is also a study that reported the success of PRF regenerative competency in cases of aggressive periodontitis. Another study has also reported the successful use of PRF as a regenerative material in cases of aggressive periodontitis (Aggour & Abd El-Hady, 2017). PRF can be utilized as a single biomaterial or in a mixture with bone grafts in terms of filling material in intrabony defects. The PRF membrane is a rigid biomaterial that is easy to adapt position in bony defects around the tooth. It can also be useful as a protection membrane on top of the graft material (Figure 4). In contrast to collagen membranes, PRF membranes experience a faster remodeling process and will promote a strong induction in the periosteum by slow release of growth factors and other matrix proteins. Current clinical evidence is not inconclusive with the root surface closure treatment of gingival recessions. The available clinical trials indicate that PRF is not successful in increasing the width of the keratinized tissue around the teeth, compared to other conventional surgical methods. However, some case reports have been published where PRF was successfully applied in single (Gupta et al., 2015; Padma et al., 2013) and multiple root coverage techniques (Aroca et al., 2009; Dixit et al., 2018). PRF membranes can also be used as a "bio-active dressing" due to reducing the morbidity related to the secondary healing site in the palate. Further corroboration is required in the form of long-term randomized control studies with larger sample sizes to confirm the mysterious potential of PRF as a biomaterial in the field of clinical periodontology.

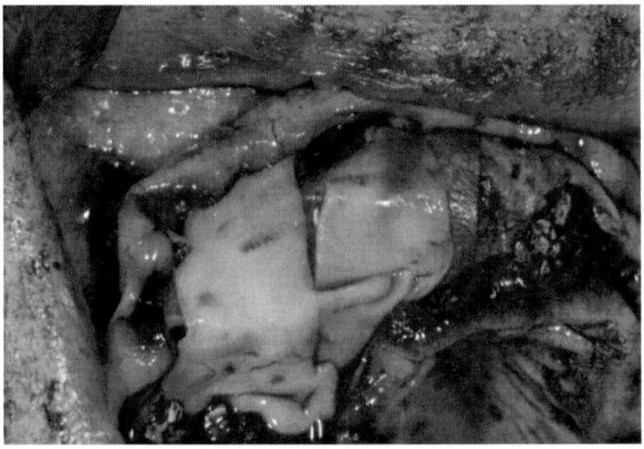

Figure 4. L-PRF membranes cover the collagen membrane before the suture (Author's own archive, taken by Furkan Yavaş and Serap Kaşıkcı).

Platelet Concentrations in Maxillary Sinus Augmentation

The posterior maxilla is a challenging region for successful dental implant installation because of its deficient bone volume caused by ridge resorption and sinus pneumatization after tooth extraction. There are different surgical approaches in order to achieve the vertical bone height required for implant placement with adequate length. Sinus augmentation surgery is considered one of the most predictable procedures that can be performed using different bone substitutes (Hallman & Thor, 2008). The final choice of grafting material has been a matter of disagreement between the authors. In terms of osteoinductive, osteogenic, and osteoconductive competencies, autogenous bone graft is still considered the gold standard for augmentation procedures (Lundgren et al., 1996; Tong et al., 1998). However, autologous bone graft has some disadvantages, the most serious being its higher morbidity after the surgery and unpredictable reabsorption of the bone (van den Bergh et al., 1998). These disadvantages have led to the spread of the use of biological and synthetic bone grafts in order to simplify the surgeries and to avoid the aforementioned complications. To avoid the aforementioned possible complications, the use of biological and synthetic bone substitutes has gained popularity. Mixing injectable platelet-rich fibrin (IPRF) with the particles of different types of bone grafts resulted in the formation of sticky bone (Mourão et al., 2015) (Figure 5). Sticky bone has been described as a structure, combination of bone graft granules and concentrated growth factors (Sohn et al., 2011). The mechanical possessions of this aggregate simplify its placement and stabilization in the maxillary sinus cavity. The clinician can mold it into the desired shape during the application. Although the addition of PRF to bone substitutes is commonly and clinically accepted standard to enhance the residual bone in the sinus cavity, resulting in high rates of success, numerous authors have established that augmentation with PRF alone could be satisfactory for promoting the bone healing process (Pichotano et al., 2019; Shreehari et al., 2022; Simonpieri et al., 2011). A second way to use PRF during sinus augmentation surgeries has been for the repair of Schneiderian membranes (Testori et al., 2019). Perforation of the Schneiderian membrane is the most common complication during sinus lift surgery (Figure 6). Usually, these perforations are covered with bioabsorbable collagen membranes during the surgery. However, it has been suggested that the solid structure of the collagen membrane may delay the osteogenic potential of the Schneiderian membrane. Furthermore, the PRF membrane contains an autologous fibrin matrix with "trapped" platelets and cytokines, which allows a slow release of growth factors. Based on these biological and mechanical features, PRF has been suggested to cover membrane perforations during sinus augmentation procedures.

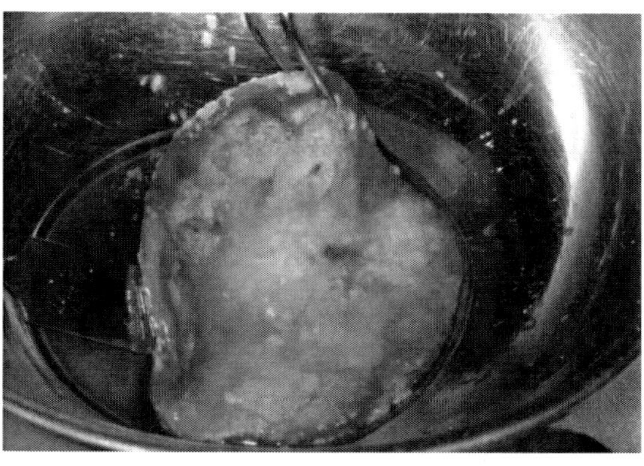

Figure 5. Xenograft after agglutination with i-PRF (Author's own archive, taken by Furkan Yavaş and Serap Kaşıkcı).

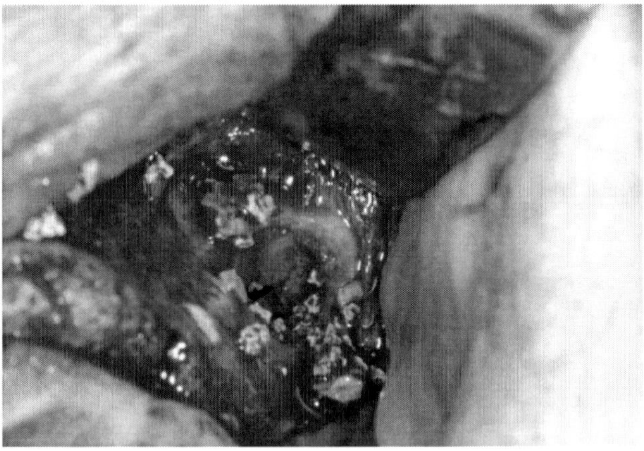

Figure 6. Schneiderian membrane perforation (Author's own archive, taken by Furkan Yavaş and Serap Kaşıkcı).

Conclusion

In summary, as a biological surgical autologous material, platelet concentrations have been successfully applied for various applications in dental regenerative medicine. Clinical studies have established safe and promising outcomes related to the use of PRF alone or in combination with other bone substitutes. Currently, platelet-rich fibrin appears to be a scientifically recognized minimally invasive technique with low risks and satisfactory clinical results. Overall, the treatments with platelet concentration materials seem to have an optimistic future in clinical regenerative dentistry.

References

Aggour, R. L., & Abd El-Hady, H. M. G. (2017). Platelet-rich fibrin for the treatment of intrabony periodontal defects in patients with generalized aggressive periodontitis: A randomized controlled clinical study. *J Int Acad Periodontol*, *19*(1), 28-34.

Anusaksathien, O., & Giannobile, W. V. (2002). Growth factor delivery to re-engineer periodontal tissues. *Current pharmaceutical biotechnology*, *3*(2), 129-139. https://doi.org/10.2174/1389201023378391.

Aroca, S., Keglevich, T., Barbieri, B., Gera, I., & Etienne, D. (2009). Clinical evaluation of a modified coronally advanced flap alone or in combination with a platelet-rich fibrin membrane for the treatment of adjacent multiple gingival recessions: A 6-month study. *Journal of periodontology*, *80*(2), 244-252. https://doi.org/10.1902/jop. 2009.080253.

Choukroun, J., Adda, F., Schoeffer, C., & Vervelle, A. (2000). PRF: an opportunity in perio-implantology. *Implantodontie*, *42*, 55-62.

Choukroun, J., Diss, A., Simonpieri, A., Girard, M.-O., Schoeffler, C., Dohan, S. L., Dohan, A. J., Mouhyi, J., & Dohan, D. M. (2006). Platelet-rich fibrin (PRF): a second-generation platelet concentrate. Part IV: clinical effects on tissue healing. *Oral Surgery, Oral Medicine, Oral Pathology, Oral Radiology, and Endodontology*, *101*(3), e56-e60. https://doi.org/10.1016/j.tripleo.2005.07.011.

Dixit, N., Lamba, A. K., Faraz, F., Tandon, S., Aggarwal, K., & Ahad, A. (2018). Root coverage by modified coronally advanced flap with and without platelet-rich fibrin: A clinical study. *Indian Journal of Dental Research*, *29*(5), 600. https://doi.org/10.4103/ ijdr.IJDR_22_17.

ElSheshtawy, A., Nazzal, H., El Shahawy, O., El Baz, A., Ismail, S., Kang, J., & Ezzat, K. (2020). The effect of platelet-rich plasma as a scaffold in regeneration/revitalization endodontics of immature permanent teeth assessed using 2-dimensional radiographs and cone beam computed tomography: a randomized controlled trial. *International endodontic journal*, *53*(7), 905-921. https://doi.org/10.1111/iej.13303.

Giannobile, W. (1996). Periodontal tissue engineering by growth factors. *Bone*, *19*(1), S23-S37. https://doi.org/10.1016/s8756-3282(96)00127-5.

Grigoratos, D., Knowles, J., Ng, Y. L., & Gulabivala, K. (2001). Effect of exposing dentine to sodium hypochlorite and calcium hydroxide on its flexural strength and elastic modulus. *International endodontic journal*, *34*(2), 113-119. https://doi.org/10.1046/ j.1365-2591.2001.00356.x.

Gupta, S., Banthia, R., Singh, P., Banthia, P., Raje, S., & Aggarwal, N. (2015). Clinical evaluation and comparison of the efficacy of coronally advanced flap alone and in combination with platelet rich fibrin membrane in the treatment of Miller Class I and II gingival recessions. *Contemporary clinical dentistry*, *6*(2), 153. https://doi.org/10.4103/0976-237X.156034.

Hallman, M., & Thor, A. (2008). Bone substitutes and growth factors as an alternative/complement to autogenous bone for grafting in implant dentistry. *Periodontology 2000*, *47*(1), 172-192. https://doi.org/10.1111/j.1600-0757.2008. 00251.x.

Hotwani, K., & Sharma, K. (2014). Platelet rich fibrin-a novel acumen into regenerative endodontic therapy. *Restorative dentistry & endodontics*, *39*(1), 1-6. https://doi.org/ 10.5395/rde.2014.39.1.1.

López-Valverde, I., Vignoletti, F., Vignoletti, G., Martin, C., & Sanz, M. (2023). Long-term tooth survival and success following primary root canal treatment: a 5-to 37-year retrospective observation. *Clinical Oral Investigations*, *27*(6), 3233-3244.. https://doi.org/10.1007/s00784-023-04938-y.

Lundgren, S., Moy, P., Johansson, C., & Nilsson, H. (1996). Augmentation of the maxillary sinus floor with particulated mandible: a histologic and histomorphometric study. *International Journal of Oral & Maxillofacial Implants*, *11*(6), 760-766.

Marx, R. E. (2004). Platelet-rich plasma: evidence to support its use. *Journal of oral and maxillofacial surgery*, *62*(4), 489-496. https://doi.org/10.1016/j.joms.2003.12.003.

Mourão, C. F. d. A. B., Valiense, H., Melo, E. R., Mourão, N. B. M. F., & Maia, M. D.-C. (2015). Obtention of injectable platelets rich-fibrin (i-PRF) and its polymerization with bone graft. *Revista do Colégio Brasileiro de Cirurgiões*, *42*, 421-423. https://doi.org/10.1590/0100-69912015006013.

Padma, R., Shilpa, A., Kumar, P. A., Nagasri, M., Kumar, C., & Sreedhar, A. (2013). A split mouth randomized controlled study to evaluate the adjunctive effect of platelet-rich fibrin to coronally advanced flap in Miller's class-I and II recession defects. *Journal of Indian Society of Periodontology*, *17*(5), 631.

Pichotano, E. C., de Molon, R. S., de Souza, R. V., Austin, R. S., Marcantonio, E., & Zandim-Barcelos, D. L. (2019). Evaluation of L-PRF combined with deproteinized bovine bone mineral for early implant placement after maxillary sinus augmentation: a randomized clinical trial. *Clinical implant dentistry and related research*, *21*(2), 253-262.

Shreehari, A., Sahoo, N., Kumar, D., & Malhi, R. (2022). Efficacy of platelet-rich fibrin in maxillary sinus augmentation and simultaneous implant placement in deficient maxillary ridges: A pilot comparative study. *Medical Journal Armed Forces India*, Early Access, 1-8. https://doi.org/10.1016/j.mjafi.2022.08.007.

Simonpieri, A., Choukroun, J., Del Corso, M., Sammartino, G., & Ehrenfest, D. M. D. (2011). Simultaneous sinus-lift and implantation using microthreaded implants and leukocyte-and platelet-rich fibrin as sole grafting material: a six-year experience. *Implant dentistry*, *20*(1), 2-12.

Sohn, D.-S., Heo, J.-U., Kwak, D.-H., Kim, D.-E., Kim, J.-M., Moon, J.-W., Lee, J.-H., & Park, I.-S. (2011). Bone regeneration in the maxillary sinus using an autologous fibrin-rich block with concentrated growth factors alone. *Implant dentistry*, *20*(5), 389-395.

Testori, T., Weinstein, T., Taschieri, S., & Wallace, S. S. (2019). Risk factors in lateral window sinus elevation surgery. *Periodontology 2000*, *81*(1), 91-123.

Tong, D. C., Rioux, K., Drangsholt, M., & Beirne, O. R. (1998). A review of survival rates for implants placed in grafted maxillary sinuses using meta-analysis. *International Journal of Oral & Maxillofacial Implants*, *13*(2), 175-182.

van den Bergh, J. P., ten Bruggenkate, C. M., Krekeler, G., & Tuinzing, D. B. (1998). Sinusfloor elevation and grafting with autogenous iliac crest bone. *Clin Oral Implants Res*, *9*(6), 429-435. https://doi.org/10.1034/j.1600-0501.1996.090608.x.

Chapter 13

PRP Treatment for Male Infertility

Tansu Güdelci*, MD

Department of Urology, Acıbadem Maslak Hospital, İstanbul, Turkiye

Abstract

The World Health Organization currently defines infertility as 'a disease of the male or female reproductive system defined by the failure to achieve a pregnancy after 12 months or more of regular unprotected sexual intercourse.' A male factor is solely responsible for about 20% of infertile couples and contributes to another 30-40%. Azoospermia, defined as the complete absence of sperm from the ejaculate, is present in about 1% of all men and in approximately 10-15% of infertile men. Azoospermia is classified into two categories in clinical practice: Obstructive azoospermia (OA) and non-obstructive azoospermia (NOA). Platelets are known for their therapeutic effects, containing many active proteins that are involved in mitogenic, chemotactic, adhesion, angiogenic, antiangiogenic, and neurotrophic processes. In recent years, the successful use of PRP in many clinical fields has led to research on its use in male infertility. Despite the limited availability of data in the literature, the use of PRP therapy is a promising new experimental method in the field of male infertility. However, further investigation with randomized controlled trials is needed to refine the technique and determine the effectiveness of this therapy.

Keywords: male infertility, azoospermia, platelet-rich plasma

* Corresponding Author's Email: drtansugudelci@gmail.com.

In: Current Clinical Recommendations ...
Editors: Nazan Yurtcu and Emel Güler
ISBN: 979-8-89113-723-3

Introduction

Infertility is a disease that affects the male or female reproductive system and is characterized by the inability to conceive a pregnancy despite engaging in unprotected sexual intercourse regularly for a period of 12 months or more. Approximately 8-15% of couples are unable to conceive after one year of unprotected intercourse (Stephan and Chandra, 2006). Approximately 20% of infertile couples can attribute their infertility solely to a male factor, while in an additional 30-40% of cases, male factors contribute to the overall infertility issue (Thonneau et al., 1991).

Azoospermia, which refers to the complete absence of sperm in the ejaculate, is found in approximately 1% of all men and affects approximately 10-15% of men with infertility. Azoospermia is classified into two categories in clinical practice: Obstructive azoospermia (OA) and non-obstructive azoospermia (NOA). NOA is characterized by the absence of sperm in the ejaculate due to failure of spermatogenesis, representing the most severe type of male infertility (Practice Committee of the American Society for Reproductive Medicine, 2018).

Presently, men with NOA depend on surgical sperm retrieval combined with assisted reproductive technology to achieve biological parenthood. However, in the past, these men had limited options and were often left with the choices of adoption or using donor sperm to start a family. The introduction of Intracytoplasmic Sperm Injection (ICSI) in 1992 revolutionized the possibilities for men with NOA to become biological fathers. This technique involves the injection of a single sperm directly into an oocyte using a micropipette, offering new hope and opportunities for men facing NOA-related challenges to start their own families with biological children. (Palermo et al., 1992).

After the description of ICSI, the first use of testicular sperm for IVF was reported by Schoysman et al. in 1993, and Devroey et al. reported a successful case of IVF-ICSI using testicular sperm extracted through the open surgical procedure known as testicular sperm extraction (TESE) in men diagnosed with NOA in 1995 (Punjani et al., 2021).

Today, there is no specific treatment available to restore spermatogenesis in the testicular tubules of patients with testicular NOA. Micro-TESE, which refers to sperm retrieval under an operating microscope, has become the primary treatment option for patients with NOA. The successful sperm retrieval rate of micro-TESE has been reported to be up to

63% in the literature (Deruyver et al., 2014). However, there is still a subset group of NOA patients with no sperm found with surgical procedures.

Platelet-rich plasma (PRP) is obtained by centrifuging whole blood, resulting in a substance abundant in growth factors and cytokines. These components play an important role in promoting healing and tissue regeneration by stimulating cell migration, differentiation, and chemotaxis. Additionally, they facilitate processes such as angiogenesis and inflammatory responses, which are vital for tissue repair and regeneration. PRP has undergone extensive research and has found its way into standard clinical practices in various medical specialties as a rejuvenating agent. It has been applied successfully in fields such as orthopedics, plastic surgery, dermatology, and dentistry (Cakiroglu et al., 2022).

The aim of this chapter is to discuss the use of PRP in the treatment of male infertility, specifically focusing on recent developments in the literature.

Male Infertility

The impact of infertility can be significant and devastating for millions of individuals and couples worldwide. According to infertility prevalence estimates published by the World Health Organization (WHO) in 2023, based on data from 1990 to 2021, it is estimated that approximately one in six people worldwide has experienced infertility at some stage in their lives, with a lifetime prevalence of 17.5% and a period prevalence of 12.6% (WHO, 2023). Approximately 20% of infertile couples can attribute their infertility solely to a male factor, while in an additional 30-40% of cases, male factors contribute to the overall infertility issue (Thonneau et al., 1991).

Normal sperm parameters were stated in 'The Sixth Edition of the WHO Manual for Human Semen Analysis' in 2021. The normal sperm parameters according to the WHO sixth edition include volume of 1.4 milliliters (ml), concentration of 15 million sperm per milliliter (mL) o, total sperm count of 39 million sperm, total motility of 42%, progressive motility of 30%, morphology of 4% with a normal shape and vitality of 54% (WHO, 2021). Deviations from these parameters can be referred to as male subfertility or infertility.

Azoospermia, which refers to the complete absence of sperm in the ejaculate, is found in approximately 1% of all men and affects approximately 10-15% of men with infertility (Practice Committee of the American Society for Reproductive Medicine, 2015). Azoospermia can be categorized into three types based on the underlying causes: pre-testicular, testicular, and post-testicular diagnoses. Azoospermia caused by pre-testicular factors involves endocrine abnormalities that negatively impact spermatogenesis. This condition is also referred to as secondary testicular failure. Azoospermia resulting from testicular factors, known as primary testicular failure, involves disorders of spermatogenesis that originate within the testes themselves. Azoospermia due to post-testicular causes is associated with issues related to ejaculatory dysfunction or ductal obstruction, leading to difficulties in sperm transit. In clinical practice, a commonly used classification system differentiates between two main types of azoospermia: obstructive azoospermia (OA) and non-obstructive azoospermia (NOA). NOA can be categorized into two types: central NOA and testicular NOA. Patients with OA usually have normal serum follicle-stimulating hormone (FSH) levels and normal-sized testes, indicating that they are more likely to have normal spermatogenesis. On the other hand, men with a notable elevation in FSH often exhibit testicular failure, indicating a diagnosis of testicular NOA. A central diagnosis of NOA is suggested when gonadotropin levels are low, and testosterone (T) levels are also low or low-normal. The determination of the underlying cause is established through a comprehensive assessment of the patient's medical history, a thorough physical examination, and an endocrine evaluation, together with additional tests (Practice Committee of the American Society for Reproductive Medicine, 2018).

In clinical practice, testicular NOA is commonly referred to as NOA. Therefore, throughout this chapter, we will use NOA to specifically refer to testicular non-obstructive azoospermia.

Milestones of Male Infertility

Before the invention of the in vitro fertilization (IVF) method in 1978, azoospermic males or couples with unexplained infertility were historically relegated to using adoption to have a family.

Steptoe and Edwards published the first successful IVF process in 1978. They defined the first successful use of ejaculated sperm from fertile men, and oocytes are fertilized outside of the body and then later implanted in the uterus, resulting in live birth. However, this method required the use of motile sperm (Steptoe and Edwards, 1978).

Temple-Smith et al. reported the first use of aspirated sperm in 1985. In this particular case, a 42-year-old man with a prior vasectomy and two unsuccessful vasoepididymostomies was involved. After a long-term epididymal massage and aspiration, a total of 0.2 mL of aspirate was obtained, which had 76% motility and an estimated 4.28 million sperm per milliliter. Using this sample, successful fertilization and clinical pregnancy were achieved through IVF (Temple-Smith et al., 1985).

In 1988, Silber et al. introduced their technique for microsurgical epididymal sperm aspiration (MESA). The article describes a method for aspirating epididymal sperm using magnification ranging from 10x to 40x. The procedure begins at the distal corpus of the epididymis and progresses towards the proximal region until motile sperm are successfully collected. In this publication, the technique was applied to two patients who had a congenital bilateral absence of the vas deferens (CBAVD). The combination of this new technique with ICSI had sparked significant excitement due to its potential to increase the likelihood that OA patients would have their own biological children. However, the fertilization and pregnancy rates have not yielded satisfactory results. A success rate of less than 10% has been reported by many centers. The use of the MESA technique has been limited due to low fertilization and pregnancy rates and the requirement for an operating microscope (Silber et al., 1988).

In 1992, intracytoplasmic sperm injection (ICSI) was introduced, which involves the injection of a single sperm into an oocyte using a micropipette (Palermo et al., 1992). This potentially provided an opportunity for men with NOA and total immotile sperm to achieve fertilization and become biological fathers of their own children.

Schoysman et al. reported the first use of testicular sperm for fertilization in 1993. They reported for the first time the achievement of pregnancy using sperm obtained by testicular biopsy in men who had previously been unable to obtain an epididymal sperm sample (Schoysman et al., 1993).

In 1995 Devroey et al. reported the first pregnancies after TESE and ICSI in NOA patients. The achievement marked a groundbreaking advancement in the treatment of men with NOA, who were previously considered to be sterile (Devroey et al., 1995). An early academic review, which included seven studies conducted between 1999 and 2013, documented that the sperm retrieval rate of TESE ranged from 16.7% to 45% (Deruyver et al., 2014).

The latest development in obtaining sperm from the testis is micro-TESE, which was described by Peter Schlegel in 1999. After observing that seminiferous tubules had different morphological characteristics under a surgical microscope, Schlegel selectively extracted the larger and more opaque tubules that were more likely to contain sperm. This technique resulted in less tissue loss from the testis and increased the percentage of successful sperm retrieval (Schlegel, 1999). Subsequent studies have shown that this technique is more effective and reliable than classic TESE in non-obstructive azoospermic men. In the same review mentioned above, which summarized seven studies conducted between 1999 and 2013, it was reported that the sperm retrieval rate of micro-TESE ranged from 42.9% to 63% (Deruyver et al., 2014). In men diagnosed with NOA, micro-TESE is widely recognized as the current gold standard procedure (Schlegel et al., 2021). However, despite all these improvements in the area of male infertility, there is still a subset group of NOA patients with no sperm found with surgical procedures who are still considered to be sterile in 2023. The search for new treatment methods for this group of patients, along with the proven effectiveness of PRP treatment in many clinical fields, has led to an investigation of whether PRP therapy is effective in the field of male infertility.

The Use of PRP in Male Infertility

In recent years, the successful use of PRP in many clinical fields has led to research on its use in male infertility. Increasing publications on the use of PRP therapy in male infertility have been seen in the literature in recent years. While animal experiments were initially more commonly seen, in vitro and in vivo human studies have recently begun to be published. The positive results obtained from the first published animal experiments provided a basis for conducting in vitro and in vivo human studies. In this section, the results obtained in light of the information obtained from animal studies will be objectively examined, followed by an examination of the results of in vitro and in vivo human studies. It should be noted that in vivo human studies are limited to only three studies in the literature as of today. The latest study is a comprehensive study conducted by me and my team, which was presented as a poster at ASRM, and detailed information on this study will be shared at the end of this section.

PRP is obtained through the centrifugation of whole blood and contains a high concentration of growth factors and cytokines. The growth factors present in PRP actively stimulate and support the processes of chemotaxis, cell proliferation, and differentiation. Apart from growth factors, platelets release a wide array of other substances, including fibronectin, vitronectin, sphingosine 1-phosphate, and various others, all of which serve crucial functions in the process of tissue repair and regeneration.

There are many studies that investigate the therapeutic potential of growth factors found in platelets, particularly in PRP, in various medical fields. These growth factors, such as vascular endothelial growth factor (VEGF), insulin-like growth factor-1 (IGF-1), fibroblast growth factor (FGF), epidermal growth factor (EGF), platelet-derived growth factor (PDGF), and nerve growth factor (NGF), play essential roles in cell proliferation, differentiation, and tissue regulation.

In the context of male fertility, these growth factors and cytokines have shown promising effects on spermatogenesis, the survival of sperm stem cells, sperm viability, motility, and DNA integrity. Notably, VEGF is crucial for the survival of sperm stem cells, while IGF-1, EGF, FGF, and PDGF contribute to spermatogenesis and steroidogenesis, impacting male hormones and fertility regulation. Additionally, NGF plays a role in maintaining sperm viability and motility, while also being involved in the development of the reproductive system (Angellee et al., 2021).

Dehghani et al. reported in 2019 that in a study in which they used 32 rats, intra-testicular injection of PRP may be able to improve the structural and functional damage caused by busulfan in the testes (Dehghani et al., 2019).

A study by Sayed and Elzainy in 2021 examined the protective effects of selenium and PRP on methotrexate-induced testicular toxicity in rats. The rats were divided into four groups and analyzed using histological, immunohistochemical, and genetic techniques. The study found that PRP improved the histological structure of the testes, increased cell regeneration, and elevated certain genetic markers. The study also found that both selenium and PRP had anti-inflammatory and anti-oxidative effects. The study suggests that PRP has a positive impact on rat testicular toxicity, as confirmed by various analyses (Sayed and Elzainy, 2021).

In 2022, Saleh et al. investigated the potential use of PRP to protect and regenerate testicular tissue against cisplatin-induced toxicity. The study used intra-testicular injection of PRP as a biomaterial to protect and regenerate testicular tissue in rats exposed to cisplatin. The results showed that PRP treatment was effective in restoring sperm counts and morphology, reproductive hormonal balance, and minimizing histological damage to testicular tissue caused by cisplatin. Furthermore, PRP treatment increased the number of spermatocytes in all stages of spermatogenesis, as well as the number of Leydig cells and the thickness of interstitial tissue. They concluded that PRP has the potential to promote tissue regeneration in addition to tissue repair, which may have promising applications in different aspects related to chemotherapy (Saleh et al., 2022).

The findings of a 2017 study by Sekerci et al., which involved 18 rats, and the 2020 study by Samy et al., which involved 40 albino rats, suggest that intra-testicular PRP application may have a protective effect against testicular ischemia/reperfusion injury (Sekerci et al., 2020).

Kutluhan et al. reported in 2020 that, in a study involving 18 rats, intra-testicular PRP had beneficial effects on spermatogenesis and hormone production in an experimental testicular torsion model (Kutluhan et al., 2020).

In 2020, Rizal et al. investigated the effect of PRP on testicular oxidative stress induced by d-galactose (d-gal) in Wistar rats. The study showed that d-gal administration increases the production of reactive oxygen species (ROS) and decreases antioxidant enzymes, leading to oxidative stress and testicular damage. The study also demonstrates that PRP has anti-inflammatory and antioxidant properties that can reduce the levels of malondialdehyde (MDA) and interleukin-6 (IL-6) in the testes of rats induced by d-gal. They concluded that intratesticular PRP injection can be an effective approach to reduce oxidative stress and inflammation in the testes (Rizal et al., 2020).

Demyashkin et al. showed the normalizing effect of PRP on the structural and functional disorders of the testis caused by electron irradiation in an animal model in 2022 (Demyashkin et al., 2022).

In a study conducted by Farhan and Al-Maathidy in 2022, the aim was to investigate the effect of PRP on the testis structure and function in rabbits. In this study, thirty male rabbits were divided into two groups: the PRP group, which received an injection of PRP, and the control group, which received normal saline. The study found that the PRP group had a higher mean of germinal layer width, Leydig cell number, and Sertoli cell number than the control group. Additionally, the PRP group exhibited a higher mean sperm concentration and normal morphology compared to the control group. Based on these results, the study concluded that PRP has the potential to improve testicular tissue histology and function and is promising as a future potential treatment for hypogonadism in different medical conditions (Farhan and Al-Maathidy, 2022).

In a study published in 2022, it was suggested that intratesticular injection of PRP can enhance the effectiveness of rabbit sperm cryopreservation (Abdulla et al., 2022).

Abduljabar et al. investigated the effects of PRP and glass wool filtration on sperm characteristics in normozoospermic and asthenozoospermic infertile men. Semen samples were collected from 60 infertile men and divided into three tubes for analysis before activation, after activation of glass wool filtration, and after activation with PRP. The results showed that both techniques improved sperm motility, but PRP was more effective in increasing sperm grade A and B motility % while decreasing sperm grade C and D motility %. These findings suggest that PRP can significantly improve sperm activity and motility, making it a promising therapeutic agent for the treatment of male infertility (Abduljabar et al., 2021).

In December 2020, Khadivi et al. published a study titled " Application of PRP improves the self-renewal of human spermatogonial stem cells in two-dimensional and three-dimensional culture systems" in the Acta Histochemica journal. In this study, it was shown that PRP application in a culture medium had a greater effect on the renewal of stem cells compared to the control group in reversing the effects of chemotherapy using testicular cells obtained from four patients who had experienced brain death (Khadivi et al., 2020).

Al-Nasser et al. evaluated the potential effectiveness of PRP therapy in 71 infertile men with NOA. They performed a fine needle aspiration (FNA) before and after intratesticular PRP injection. Each patient received ½ ml of PRP in each testicle, which was prepared by centrifuging their own blood. The patients' FSH, testosterone levels, and FNA parameters were measured before and after the procedure, and the required data were retrospectively collected. The study found that some cases of NOA developed normal spermatogenesis, and patients with spermatocytes in the initial FNA report had a lower percentage of azoospermia compared to their counterparts. The post-procedure FSH was higher than the pre-procedure FSH. The study concluded that PRP therapy has potential for the treatment of male infertility, and its potential for treatment should not be underestimated (Al-Nasser et al., 2018).

Farhan et al. conducted a study on 50 non-obstructive azoospermic infertile men to evaluate the effects of intratesticular PRP injection on spermatogenesis and hormonal levels. Autologous PRP was prepared and injected into each testicle at least three times at a one-month interval. The study found that PRP therapy can improve the structural and functional impairment of the testis in non-obstructive azoospermic infertile men, with significant differences observed in FSH and testosterone levels, as well as in sperm count (Farhan et al., 2022).

In our study, it was aimed to investigate the effect of intratesticular injection of PRP on sperm retrieval rates in men with NOA who had previously undergone at least one failed micro-TESE procedure. The study included 135 men diagnosed with NOA without genetic or anatomical abnormalities. We obtained PRP by centrifuging peripheral blood using the T-lab preparation kit. The same day, within 1 hour of preparing the PRP sample, patients were taken to the operating room and given PRP percutaneously through an 18 G butterfly needle into the seminiferous tubules or interstitial space under local anesthesia or sedation anesthesia. The amount of PRP administered was up to a maximum of 10% of each testis volume, and the injection was performed in a manner that did not cause tension in the tunica albuginea as determined by palpation. Three months after the PRP injection, micro-TESE was performed. We analyzed the outcomes based on the number of previous micro-TESE procedures. The participants were divided into two groups: Group 1, consisting of individuals who had undergone one previous unsuccessful micro-TESE procedure, and Group 2, which included those who had undergone two or more previous unsuccessful micro-TESE procedures. In Group 1, out of the 80 men who had experienced at least one unsuccessful micro-TESE operation, sperm cells were observed in 22 patients, resulting in a successful sperm retrieval rate of 27.5%. In Group 2, among the 55 men who had undergone two or more unsuccessful micro-TESE procedures, sperm cells were observed in 9 patients, resulting in a successful sperm retrieval rate of 16.4% (Gudelci et al., 2021).

Conclusion

The use of PRP therapy is a promising new experimental method in the field of male infertility. However, more research with randomized controlled trials is needed to refine the technique and determine the effectiveness of this therapy.

References

Abduljabar, W. A., Mossa, H. A. L., Abood, M. S. (2021). Beneficial role of platelet-rich plasma combined with glass wool filtration for best recovery of spermatozoa in infertile men. *European Journal of Clinical Medicine*, 2(5), 11-13. https://doi.org/10.24018/clinicmed.2021.2.5.125.

Abdulla, A. K., Rebai, T., & Al-Delemi, D. H. J. (2022). Protective Effects of Autologous Platelet-Rich Plasma (PRP) on the Outcome of Cryopreservation in Rabbit Sperm. *Cellular and Molecular Biology*, 68(4), 113-121. https://doi.org/10.14715/cmb/2022.68.4.14.

Al-Nasser, R., Khrait, Z., & Jamali, S. (2018). The Effectiveness of Autologous Platelet-Rich Plasma (PRP) in the Therapy of Infertile Men with Non-Abstractive Azoospermia. *Journal of Reproductive Medicine Gynaecology and Obstetrics*, 3(1), 100011. https://doi.org/10.24966/RMGO-2574/100011.

Angellee, J., Ginting, C. N., Chiuman, L., & Halim, B. (2021). Role of Platelet-Rich Plasma to Sperm Quality in Male Partners Undergoing Infertility Treatment. *In 2021 IEEE International Conference on Health, Instrumentation & Measurement, and Natural Sciences (InHeNce)* (pp. 1-5). IEEE. https://doi.org/10.1109/InHeNce52833.2021.9537240.

Cakiroglu Y., Yuceturk A., Karaosmanoglu O., Kopuk S. Y., Korun Z. E. U., Herlihy N., Scott R. T., Tiras B., Seli E. (2022). Ovarian reserve parameters and IVF outcomes in 510 women with poor ovarian response (POR) treated with intraovarian injection of autologous platelet-rich plasma (PRP). *Aging (Albany NY),* 14, 2513-2523. https://doi.org/10.18632/aging.203972.

Dehghani, F., Sotoude, N., Bordbar, H., Panjeshahin, M. R., & Karbalay-Doust, S. (2019). The use of platelet-rich plasma (PRP) to improve structural impairment of rat testis induced by busulfan. *Platelets*, 30(4), 513-520. https://doi.org/10.1080/09537104.2018.1478400.

Demyashkin, G. A., Borovaya, T. G., Andreeva, Y. Y., Nedorubov, A. A., Stepanova, Y. Y., Vadyukhin, M. A., Shchekin, V. I., Koryakin, S. N., Shegay, P. V., Kaprin, A. D. (2022). An experimental approach to comprehend the influence of platelet rich growth factors on spermatogenesis. *International Journal of Radiation Biology*, 98(8), 1330-1343. https://doi.org/10.1080/09553002.2022.2047820.

Deruyver, Y., Vanderschueren, D., & Van der Aa, F. (2014). Outcome of microdissection TESE compared with conventional TESE in non-obstructive azoospermia: a systematic review. *Andrology*, 2(1), 20-24. https://doi.org/10.1111/j.2047-2927.2013.00148.x.

Devroey, P., Liu, J., Nagy, Z., Goossens, A., Tournaye, H., Camus, M., Van Steirteghem, A., & Silber, S. (1995). Pregnancies after testicular sperm extraction and intracytoplasmic sperm injection in non-obstructive azoospermia. *Human Reproduction*, 10(6), 1457-1460. https://doi.org/10.1093/humrep/10.6.1457.

Farhan, R. H., Al-Temimi, M. H., Abdullah, B. J., Mohammad, M. K., Al-Dulaimi, H. A., & Al-Jebori, S. H. (2022). In Vivo Effects of PRP Intratesticle Injection on Spermatogenesis and Reproductive Hormonal Level in Non-Obstructive

Azoospermic Infertile Men. *Neuro Quantology*, 20(8), 9387-9393. https://doi.org/10.14704/nq.2022.20.8.NQ44959.

Farhan, T. M., & Al-Maathidy, A. (2022). Histo-Functional Improvement of Mammalian Testis after Platelets-Rich Plasma Treatment. *International Journal of Anatomy and Research*, 10(3), 8463-8467. https://dx.doi.org/10.16965/ijar.2022.203.

Gudelci, T., Cakiroglu, Y., Yuceturk, A., Yuksel, S. B., Karaosmanoglu, O., Kopuk, S. Y., Korun, Z. E. U., Scott Jr., R. T., Tiras, B., Kural, A. R., & Seli, E. (2021). The effect of intratesticular injection of autologous platelet-rich plasma (PRP) on sperm retrieval rates and IVF outcomes in men with non-obstructive azoospermia and history of failed testicular sperm extraction. *Fertility and Sterility*, 116(3), Supplement, E331. https://doi.org/10.1016/j.fertnstert.2021.07.893.

Khadivi, F., Koruji, M., Akbari, M., Jabari, A., Talebi, A., Ashouri Movassagh, S., Panahi Boroujeni, A., Feizollahi, N., Nikmahzar, A., Pourahmadi, M., & Abbasi, M. (2020). Application of platelet-rich plasma (PRP) improves self-renewal of human spermatogonial stem cells in two-dimensional and three-dimensional culture systems. *Acta Histochemica*, 122(8), 151627. https://doi.org/10.1016/j.acthis.2020.151627.

Kutluhan, M. A., Özsoy, E., Şahin, A., Ürkmez, A., Topaktaş, R., Toprak, T., Gümrükçü, G., & Verit, A. (2021). Effects of platelet-rich plasma on spermatogenesis and hormone production in an experimental testicular torsion model. *Andrology*, 9(1), 407-413. https://doi.org/10.1111/andr.12895.

Palermo, G., Joris, H., Devroey, P., & Van Steirteghem, A. C. (1992). Pregnancies after intracytoplasmic injection of single spermatozoon into an oocyte. *The Lancet*, 340(8810), 17-18. https://doi.org/10.1016/0140-6736(92)92425-F.

Practice Committee of the American Society for Reproductive Medicine. (2015). Diagnostic evaluation of the infertile male: A committee opinion. *Fertility and Sterility*, 103(3), e18-e25. https://doi.org/10.1016/j.fertnstert.2014.12.103.

Practice Committee of the American Society for Reproductive Medicine. (2018). Evaluation of the azoospermic male: A committee opinion. *Fertility and Sterility*, 109, 777-782. https://doi.org/10.1016/j.fertnstert.2018.01.043.

Punjani, N., Kang, C., & Schlegel, P. N. (2019). Two decades from the introduction of microdissection testicular sperm extraction: How this surgical technique has improved the management of NOA. *Journal of Clinical Medicine*, 8(10), 1593. https://doi.org/10.3390/jcm10071374.

Rizal, D. M., Puspitasari, I., & Yuliandari, A. (2020). Protective effect of PRP against testicular oxidative stress on D-galactose induced male rats. *AIP Conference Proceedings*, 2260(1), 040005. https://doi.org/10.1063/5.0015830.

Saleh, H. S., Kraidi, S. Y., & Abdulhasan, A. S. (2022). Evaluation intra-testicular injection of platelet-rich plasma in restoration male rat fertility affected by cisplatin. *Journal of Pharmaceutical Negative Results*, 13(3), 295-301. https://doi.org/10.47750/pnr.2022.13.03.047.

Sayed, W. M., & Elzainy, A. (2021). Impact of platelet-rich plasma versus selenium in ameliorating induced toxicity in rat testis: histological, immunohistochemical, and molecular study. *Cell and Tissue Research*, 385(1), 223-238. https://doi.org/10.1007/s00441-021-03439-2.

Schlegel, P. N. (1999). Testicular sperm extraction: microdissection improves sperm yield with minimal tissue excision. *Human Reproduction,* 14(1), 131-135. https://doi.org/10.1093/humrep/14.1.131.

Schlegel, P. N., Sigman, M., Collura, B., De Jonge, C. J., Eisenberg, M. L., Lamb, D. J., Mulhall, J. P., Niederberger, C., Sandlow, J. I., Sokol, R. Z., Spandorfer, S. D., Tanrikut, C., Treadwell, J. R., Oristaglio, J. T., & Zini, A. (2021). Diagnosis and Treatment of Infertility in Men: AUA/ASRM Guideline PART II. *Journal of Urology*, 205(1), 44-51. https://doi.org/10.1097/JU.0000000000001520.

Schoysman, R., Vanderzwalmen, P., Nijs, M., Segal, L., Segal-Bertin, G., Geerts, L., van Roosendaal, E., & Schoysman, D. (1993). Pregnancy after fertilisation with human testicular spermatozoa. *Lancet*, 342(8881), 1237. https://doi.org/10.1016/0140-6736(93)92217-h.

Silber, S. J., Balmaceda, J., Borrero, C., Ord, T., & Asch, R. (1988). Pregnancy with sperm aspiration from the proximal head of the epididymis: a new treatment for congenital absence of the vas deferens. *Fertility and Sterility*, 50(3), 525-528. https://doi.org/10.1016/s0015-0282(16)60147-4.

Sekerci, C. A., Tanidir, Y., Sener, T. E., Sener, G., Cevik, O., Yarat, A., Alev-Tuzuner, B., Cetinel, S., Kervancioglu, E., Sahan, A., & Akbal, C. (2017). Effects of platelet-rich plasma against experimental ischemia/reperfusion injury in rat testis. *Journal of Pediatric Urology*, 13(3), 317.e1-317.e9. https://doi.org/10.1016/j.jpurol.2016.12.016.

Stephan E. H., & Chandra A. (2006) Declining estimates of infertility in the United States:1982-2002. *Fertil Steril* 86:516-523. https://doi.org/10.1016/j.fertnstert.2006.02.129.

Steptoe, P. C., & Edwards, R. G. (1978). Birth after the reimplantation of a human embryo. *Lancet*, 2(8085), 366. https://doi.org/10.1016/s0140-6736(78)92957-4.

Temple-Smith, P. D., Southwick, G. J., Yates, C. A., Trounson, A. O., & de Kretser, D. M. (1985). Human pregnancy by in vitro fertilization (IVF) using sperm aspirated from the epididymis. *Journal of in vitro fertilization and embryo transfer,* 2(3), 119-122. https://doi.org/10.1007/BF01131497.

Thonneau P., Marchand S., Tallec a., Ferial M. L., Ducot B., Lansac J., Lopes P., Tabaste J. M., Spira A. (1991) Incidence and main causes of infertility in a resident population (1,850,000) of three French regions (1988-1989). *Hum Reprod* 6(6):811-816 https://doi.org/10.1093/oxfordjournals.humrep.a137433.

WHO (World Health Organization). (2021). *WHO laboratory manual for the examination and processing of human semen* (6th ed.). Geneva, Switzerland. CC BY-NC-SA 3.0 IGO.

WHO (World Health Organization). (2023). *Infertility prevalence estimates, 1990–2021 [Data set].* Geneva, Switzerland. CC BY-NC-SA 3.0 IGO.

Chapter 14

PRP Treatment for Genital Aesthetics

Gamze Sönmez Ünal*, **MD**
Department of Gynecology and Obstetrics, Sivas Numune Hospital, Sivas, Turkiye

Abstract

Genital aesthetics (cosmetic) is all of the procedures for the correction of genital organs that are defective or are believed to be defective. The genital aesthetic applications are as follows; labiaplasty, vaginoplasty, perineoplasty, hymenoplasty, G shot, O shot applications, genital laser applications, and PRP applications. Aesthetic concerns have been in women for centuries. With the widespread use of the Internet, access to information has become easier, so the perception of beauty has changed, and people have been searching for it. Socially, the growing importance given to appearance has increased the interest in aesthetic applications. While aesthetic applications are increasing rapidly, new alternative applications to surgical treatment have emerged. PRP is obtained by centrifuging one's blood. Genital PRP is a non-surgical, functional injection applied in the genital area. The advantages of PRP are that it can be taken from the person and injected in the same session without anesthesia, and it is not allergic. PRP is extremely effective in wound and tissue healing with its high amount of growth factors in platelets.

Keywords: platelet-rich plasma, vaginal atrophy, genital PRP

* Corresponding Author's Email: gmzsnmz@hotmail.com.

In: Current Clinical Recommendations ...
Editors: Nazan Yurtcu and Emel Güler
ISBN: 979-8-89113-723-3

Introduction

With the development of technology in our age, the perception of beauty has been reshaped. The appearance of the external genital organs of women varies due to factors such as age, weight, hormonal status, skin type, and ethnicity. Sociocultural differences between countries also make it difficult to make a universal definition of the standard appearance of the vulva (González, 2015; Hodgkinson & Hait, 1984).

Women's curiosity about their genital areas has been going on since ancient Egypt. To make the genital area look more beautiful and attract attention, painting, tattooing, ornamentation, and genital area jewelry are common in different societies (Gulia et al., 2017). The widespread use of the Internet and easy access to all kinds of information, the sharing of people on social media, and the growing importance given to external appearance as a society have increased the interest in genital aesthetics. The attribution of sexuality as the source of marital problems and is no longer a social taboo has caused women to question themselves and become more interested in their genital areas. The word aesthetic originates from French and means 'related to the sense of beauty'. Genital aesthetics are all of the surgical methods applied for the correction of defective organs. Genital aesthetic applications are also known as cosmetic gynecological applications (Eserdağ, 2021). The concept of cosmetic gynecology can be defined as surgical and non-surgical procedures applied to the vulva and vaginal area in women (Daşıkan et al., 2019). Cosmetic gynecology can also be summarized as female genital aesthetic practices and includes numerous procedures including labiaplasty, clitoral hood reduction, hymenoplasty, labia majora augmentation, vaginoplasty, and G-spot amplification (Goodman et al., 2010). These procedures are also marketed under names such as "design vagina," "vaginal rejuvenation," "laser vaginal rejuvenation," and "G shot" (Daşıkan et al., 2019).

Modern cosmetic gynecology practices have become widespread since the 2000s.

Hodgkinson and Hait, in their study in 1984, stated the ideal vulva image as the labia minora lying between the labia majora and its dimensions smaller than the labia majora (Hodgkinson & Hait, 1984). To achieve this aesthetic appearance, the labia minora must be located symmetrically and must not exceed the limits of the labia majora (Braun, 2005).

Interest in genital cosmetic applications has increased in recent years (Goodman, 2020). The growing interest of women in their bodies is the reason for this increase. Physical and psychological factors are effective in the growth of this interest. There are publications stating that post-operative body love and self-perception are improved in women who need aesthetic intervention (Daşıkan et al., 2019).

Genital aesthetic applications are divided into surgical and non-surgical applications (Eserdağ, 2021).

Surgical applications:

- Labiaplasty
- Vaginoplasty
- Perineoplasty
- Hymenoplasty
- Clitoral surgeries
- Labium majora and minora surgeries (reduction and augmentation)

Non-surgical applications:

- Radiofrequency applications
- Genital laser applications
- G-shot applications
- O shot applications
- Hyaluronic acid applications
- Regenerative applications (platelet-rich plasma (PRP), stromal vascular fraction (SVF), stem cell)
- Other non-invasive applications (mesotherapy, rope suspension applications, etc.).

Patient selection is very important in genital cosmetology. At the first application to the physician, a detailed anamnesis should be performed, the attitudes and psychological status of the patients should be evaluated in detail, and a psychiatric consultation should be requested when seemed necessary. Before the operation, the patient should be discussed in detail about her expectations and what kind of result she wants, and information should be given without setting high expectations.

Genital PRP (Platelet Rich Plasma)

Genital PRP is a non-surgical, functional injection applied in the genital area. The PRP procedure is the injection of the platelet-rich part obtained by centrifugation of the venous blood taken from the person herself. The advantages of PRP are that it can be taken from the person and injected in the same session without anesthesia, and it is not allergic. PRP is extremely effective in wound and tissue healing with its high amount of growth factors in platelets.

Platelets are the smallest of blood cells and originate from megakaryocytes (ACOG, 2020). They are of critical importance in tissue regeneration and hemostasis (George, 2000). Megakaryocyte maturation includes nuclear duplication without cell segmentation, resulting in huge cells. Cytoplasmic organelles are organized into domains representing nascent platelets, limited by a network of invaginated plasma membranes. Within the marrow, megakaryocytes located next to sinusoidal walls, which (Oneto & Etulain, 2021). Thrombotic diseases occur when platelet functions become abnormal. Platelet adhesion to damaged vessels through fibrinogen starts the secretion of granules containing serotonin, thromboxane, and adenosine to initiate the coagulation process. Platelets then secrete several growth factors from this insoluble network to the wound site, the most important of which are PDGF, TGF-ß, and IGF. PDGF is known to be characteristic of monocytes and macrophages. Besides, it also acts as an activator for collagenase, which increases the strength and durability of healing tissues. TGF-ß stimulates fibroblasts to form procollagen; then collagen begins to accumulate in the wound area (Robey et al., 1987) and thus wound healing occurs.

PRP Preparation

15-20 cc of whole blood is taken from the venous peripheral veins of the arm before the procedure. The amount of blood to be taken can be increased according to the area of PRP application. The collected blood is quickly transferred to tubes containing sodium citrate and centrifuged, avoiding hemolysis. Centrifugation of collected blood should be performed at 1200 rpm for 12 minutes or at 3000 rpm for 8 minutes. After centrifugation, 3 layers are formed in the tube. The middle layer is the part of the PRP where the white blood cells and platelets are located (Eserdağ, 2021).

Usage Areas of PRP in Cosmetic Gynecology

Functional Treatments

Sexual Pleasure Treatments

Female sexual dysfunction is defined as sexual desire, arousal, orgasm, and sexual pain disorders that result in personal problems and impair quality of life and affect intercouple relationships (Walton et al., 2003). Many factors are considered responsible for the etiology. The use of PRP in functional treatments has become widespread in recent years. Intravaginal and intraclitoral PRP applications have been reported to be used in the treatment of dyspareunia, sexual reluctance, and orgasmic disorders (Gravina et al., 2008). Before the genital PRP application, the patient should have a general gynecological examination and anamnesis. The area to be applied should be cleaned with disinfectant. Local anesthetics can be used in patients with a high sensitivity to pain. The prepared PRP fluid is injected into the 1/3 lower anterior wall of the vagina, around the clitoris, the clitoral hood, and the vestibular area with 27G or 30G needles (Eserdağ, 2021).

In a study, significant regression in sexual dysfunction and an increase in sexual satisfaction were reported after the PRP application to the anterior vaginal wall (Sukgen et al., 2019).

Genitourinary Syndrome of Menopause

The genitourinary syndrome of menopause is defined as signs and symptoms including labia majora, labia minora, clitoris, vestibule, vagina, urethra, and bladder alterations as a result of a decrease in estrogen and other sex hormones (Portman et al., 2014). Vulvar atrophy is common due to menopause. The first step in treatment is non-hormonal vaginal oils and moisturizers (NAMS, 2013). Vaginal moisturizers are designed to reduce vaginal dryness when used regularly (Levine et al., 2008).

Local low-dose estrogen preparations are considered first-line pharmacological therapy for persistent symptoms of vulvovaginal atrophy, and systemic estrogen+/-progesterone therapy is recommended (Hutchinson & Segal, 2015).

The inability to use estrogen in people who have had breast cancer or are at risk of cancer has led to the search for alternative treatment methods.

The use of PRP in the treatment of menopausal vulvovaginal atrophy and vaginal dryness has been reported to reduce vaginal dryness and dyspareunia (Saleh & Abdelghani, 2022).

Lichen Sclerosus

Lichen sclerosus is a chronic inflammatory skin disease of unknown cause that often occurs in the anogenital system. It is seen with a high incidence in women in the menopausal period (Lopez & Baptista, 2017). If left untreated, lichen sclerosus is associated with a higher degree of scarring and a higher risk of cancer in the genital area (Kirtschig, 2016).

Anogenital lichen sclerosus often causes itching and pain. The first choice for treatment is highly potent local corticosteroids (Fistarol and Itin, 2013).

In a study, 28 patients in the postmenopausal period, diagnosed by pathological examination and did not respond to corticosteroid treatment, received 3 sessions of PRP and were followed up in 6 and 12-month periods. They reported that complaints related to lichen sclerosus in patients included in the study decreased significantly and this effect continued throughout the year (Medina Garrido et al., 2023).

Another study reported that a 67-year-old patient with lichen sclerosus with postmenopausal vaginal atrophy and no response from topical estrogen treatment had a significant decrease in the patient's complaints after PRP application (Kim et al., 2017).

Use in Aesthetic Treatments

PRP can be used for the correction of age-related wrinkles, discoloration, and loss of skin tone in the labium majus and minus. In vulva rejuvenation procedures, a combination of PRP and energy-based technologies is used (Eserdağ, 2021).

PRP can also be used to correct episiotomy-related scarring.

Effect of Cosmetic Gynecology Applications on Sexual Function

Female genital aesthetic practices are applications made to the vagina and/or vulva for cosmetic or functional purposes and are also called cosmetic gynecological applications. The frequency of cosmetic gynecological practices has increased in recent years. Modern cosmetic gynecological procedures have been applied increasingly since the 2000s. While surgical procedures have been widely applied since the beginning of the 2000s, non-invasive applications have also started to become widespread since the 2010s.

According to the UK National Health Service, the number of labiaplasty procedures performed in the UK has increased fivefold in the nine years from 2001 to 2010 (Moran & Lee, 2014; Daşıkan et al., 2019).

Women tend to these applications with complaints of pain, vulvar irritation, and friction while doing sports. The rate of women going to genital plastic surgery for both aesthetic and functional reasons such as the feeling of width during sexual intercourse, not feeling the penis, increasing penile-vaginal friction, and increasing sexual pleasure by increasing penile pressure in the clitoral complex (Goodman et al., 2010; Goodman, 2011; Miklos & Moore, 2008).

Problems in the genital area can cause sexual troubles in the individual and her sexual partner. Impairment of sexual health can lead to deterioration of physical, mental, familial, and social health. The fact that women who achieve the desired appearance and function in their genitals with genital plastic surgery feel better contributes to an increase in their sexual self-confidence and sexual satisfaction (Giarenis & Cardozo, 2019; Goodman et al., 2010).

A multicenter study of 258 women undergoing genital plastic surgery stated that 64% of women had GCS due to physical discomfort, 48% for cosmetic reasons, 33% for lack of self-confidence, and 30% because of a desire to improve their sex life. 54.2% of these women had vaginoplasty or perineoplasty to increase their male partner's sexual experience, and about 5% of them had surgery, especially at the insistence of their husbands. It has been shown that 32% of women who have vaginoplasty have it performed to increase their partner's sexual pleasure. Women's attitudes and expectations, and the decision to request genital cosmetic surgery may also develop as a result of pressure from the sexual partner (Goodman et al., 2010).

Period after PRP Application

The PRP procedure is a non-invasive, non-allergic, safe, and complication-free treatment option. Therefore, it can be safely preferred in suitable patients and appropriate indications. There may be temporary redness and mild edema in the applied area after the procedure. After the procedure, the patient can easily return to her routine life and have sexual intercourse one day later. Paracetamol group painkillers should be preferred for post-procedure pain. The expected effects begin to appear after 3 weeks.

Conclusion

The PRP procedure is a non-invasive, non-allergic, safe, and complication-free treatment choice. Therefore, it can be safely preferred in suitable patients and appropriate indications. PRP can be used in treatments for sexual pleasure and lichen sclerosis, in relief of genitourinary symptoms due to menopause, and in treatments for genital aesthetic purposes.

References

ACOG. (2020). Elective Female Genital Cosmetic Surgery: ACOG Committee Opinion, Number 795. *Obstetrics and Gynecology*, 135(1), e36–e42. https://doi.org/10.1097/AOG.0000000000003616.

Braun, V. (2005). In search of (Better) Sexual Pleasure: Female Genital 'Cosmetic' Surgery. *Sage Journals*, 8(4), 407–424. https://doi.org/10.1177/1363460705056625.

Daşıkan, Z., Kıratlı, D., & Erdoğan, M. (2019). Kadınların genital görünüm memnuniyeti: Genital kozmetik cerrahi [Female genital appearance satisfaction: Genital cosmetic surgery]. *The Journal of Gynecology-Obstetrics and Neonatology*, 16(4), 238-243.

Eserdağ, S. (2021). *Kadın genital estetik & fonksiyonel cerrahisi* [Female genital aesthetic & functional surgery]. Hipokrat Bookstore.

Fistarol, S. K., & Itin, P. H. (2013). Diagnosis and treatment of lichen sclerosus: an update. *American Journal of Clinical Dermatology*, 14(1), 27–47. https://doi.org/10.1007/s40257-012-0006-4.

George, J. N. (2000). Platelets. *Lancet* (London, England), 355(9214), 1531–1539. https://doi.org/10.1016/S0140-6736(00)02175-9.

Giarenis, I., & Cardozo, L. (2014). Cosmetic genital surgery. *Obstetrics, Gynaecology and Reproductive Medicine*, 24(9), 286-288. https://doi.org/10.1016/j.ogrm.2014.06.003.

González, P. I. (2015). Classification of Hypertrophy of Labia Minora: Consideration of a Multiple Component Approach. *Surgical Technology International*, 27, 191–194.

Goodman, M. P. (2011). Female genital cosmetic and plastic surgery: a review. *The Journal of Sexual Medicine*, 8(6), 1813–1825. https://doi.org/10.1111/j.1743-6109.2011.02254.x.

Goodman, M. P. (2020). *Female Genital Plastic and Cosmetic Surgery*. Wiley Blackwell.

Goodman, M. P., Placik, O. J., Benson, R. H., 3rd, Miklos, J. R., Moore, R. D., Jason, R. A., Matlock, D. L., Simopoulos, A. F., Stern, B. H., Stanton, R. A., Kolb, S. E., & Gonzalez, F. (2010). A large multicenter outcome study of female genital plastic surgery. *The Journal of Sexual Medicine*, 7(4 Pt 1), 1565–1577. https://doi.org/10.1111/j.1743-6109.2009.01573.x.

Gravina, G. L., Brandetti, F., Martini, P., Carosa, E., Di Stasi, S. M., Morano, S., Lenzi, A., & Jannini, E. A. (2008). Measurement of the thickness of the urethrovaginal space in women with or without vaginal orgasm. *The Journal of Sexual Medicine*, 5(3), 610–618. https://doi.org/10.1111/j.1743-6109.2007.00739.x.

Gulia, C., Zangari, A., Briganti, V., Bateni, Z. H., Porrello, A., & Piergentili, R. (2017). Labia minora hypertrophy: causes, impact on women's health, and treatment options. *International Urogynecology Journal*, 28(10), 1453–1461. https://doi.org/10.1007/s00192-016-3253-8.

Hodgkinson, D. J., & Hait, G. (1984). Aesthetic vaginal labioplasty. *Plastic and Reconstructive Surgery*, 74(3), 414–416. https://doi.org/10.1097/00006534-198409000-00015.

Hutchinson-Colas, J., & Segal, S. (2015). Genitourinary syndrome of menopause and the use of laser therapy. *Maturitas*, 82(4), 342–345. https://doi.org/10.1016/j.maturitas.2015.08.001.

Kim, S. H., Park, E. S., & Kim, T. H. (2017). Rejuvenation Using Platelet-rich Plasma and Lipofilling for Vaginal Atrophy and Lichen Sclerosus. *Journal of Menopausal Medicine*, 23(1), 63–68. https://doi.org/10.6118/jmm.2017.23.1.63.

Kirtschig, G. (2016). Lichen Sclerosus-Presentation, Diagnosis and Management. *Deutsches Ärzteblatt International*, 113(19), 337–343. https://doi.org/10.3238/arztebl.2016.0337.

Levine, K. B., Williams, R. E., & Hartmann, K. E. (2008). Vulvovaginal atrophy is strongly associated with female sexual dysfunction among sexually active postmenopausal women. *Menopause* (New York, N.Y.), 15(4 Pt 1), 661–666. https://doi.org/10.1097/gme.0b013e31815a5168.

Medina Garrido, C., Cano García, A., de la Cruz Cea, L., & Oreja Cuesta, A. B. (2023). Mid-term symptomatic relief after platelet-rich plasma infiltration in vulvar lichen sclerosus. *Archives of Dermatological Research*. Advance online publication. https://doi.org/10.1007/s00403-023-02529-1.

Miklos, J. R., & Moore, R. D. (2008). Labiaplasty of the labia minora: patients' indications for pursuing surgery. *The Journal of Sexual Medicine*, 5(6), 1492–1495. https://doi.org/10.1111/j.1743-6109.2008.00813.x.

Moran, C., & Lee, C. (2014). What's normal? Influencing women's perceptions of normal genitalia: an experiment involving exposure to modified and nonmodified images. *BJOG: An International Journal of Obstetrics and Gynaecology*, 121(6), 761–766. https://doi.org/10.1111/1471-0528.12578.

NAMS. (2013). Management of symptomatic vulvovaginal atrophy: 2013 position statement of The North American Menopause Society. *Menopause* (New York, N.Y.), 20(9), 888–904. https://doi.org/10.1097/GME.0b013e3182a122c2.

Oneto, P., & Etulain, J. (2021). PRP in wound healing applications. *Platelets*, 32(2), 189–199. https://doi.org/10.1080/09537104.2020.1849605.

Pérez-López, F. R., & Vieira-Baptista, P. (2017). Lichen sclerosus in women: a review. *Climacteric: The Journal of the International Menopause Society*, 20(4), 339–347. https://doi.org/10.1080/13697137.2017.1343295.

Portman, D. J., Gass, M. L., & Vulvovaginal Atrophy Terminology Consensus Conference Panel. (2014). Genitourinary syndrome of menopause: new terminology for vulvovaginal atrophy from the International Society for the Study of Women's Sexual Health and The North American Menopause Society. *Climacteric: The Journal of the International Menopause Society*, 17(5), 557–563. https://doi.org/10.3109/13697137.2014.946279.

Robey, P. G., Young, M. F., Flanders, K. C., Roche, N. S., Kondaiah, P., Reddi, A. H., Termine, J. D., Sporn, M. B., & Roberts, A. B. (1987). Osteoblasts synthesize and respond to transforming growth factor-type beta (TGF-beta) in vitro. *The Journal of Cell Biology*, 105(1), 457–463. https://doi.org/10.1083/jcb.105.1.457.

Saleh, D. M., & Abdelghani, R. (2022). Clinical evaluation of autologous platelet rich plasma injection in postmenopausal vulvovaginal atrophy: A pilot study. *Journal of Cosmetic Dermatology*, 21(10), 4269–4275. https://doi.org/10.1111/jocd.14873.

Sukgen, G., Ellibeş Kaya, A., Karagün, E., & Çalışkan, E. (2019). Platelet-rich plasma administration to the lower anterior vaginal wall to improve female sexuality satisfaction. *Turkish Journal of Obstetrics and Gynecology*, 16(4), 228–234. https://doi.org/10.4274/tjod.galenos.2019.23356.

Walton, B., & Thornton, T. (2003). Female sexual dysfunction. *Current Women's Health Reports*, 3(4), 319–326.

Chapter 15

PRP Treatment for Erectile Dysfunction

Ali Ünal*, MD
Department of Urology, Sivas Cumhuriyet University, Sivas, Turkiye

Abstract

Erectile dysfunction is a health problem that is believed to affect millions of men around the world. It is considered a precursor of cardiovascular diseases. Due to its organic and psychological reasons, it required multidisciplinary treatment. Various protocols are applied in their treatment that range from patient education and lifestyle changes to penile prosthesis surgery. Platelet-rich plasma has been the focus of attention in recent years because it reduces the need for medical treatment and provides spontaneous erection. It provides tissue regeneration due to the growth factors, cytokines, and chemokines it contains. In preclinical studies, it has been observed to increase intracavernosal pressure and reverse the pathological process. In recent clinical studies, it has provided a noticeable change in the IIEF-5 scores of patients. However, no controlled studies have been conducted with large participation homogenized groups for PRP treatment in erectile dysfunction and no standard treatment protocol has been established. With large-scale studies and standardized treatment protocols, PRP is likely to take its place in the future in the treatment of erectile dysfunction.

Keywords: erectile dysfunction, PRP, intracavernosal injection

---

* Corresponding Author's Email: draliunal58@gmail.com.

In: Current Clinical Recommendations ...
Editors: Nazan Yurtcu and Emel Güler
ISBN: 979-8-89113-723-3

Introduction

Humanity's definition of erectile dysfunction and the search for a solution has been going on for hundreds of years. In the earliest proven written texts, Aristotle (364-322 BC) described an erection as "It seems medically proven that the air that we breathe in with the lungs reaches the penis via the heart, liver, and veins and is responsible for the erection." Leonardo Da Vinci, on the other hand, rejected Aristotle and suggested that arterial blood flow provides an erection. Researchers began to explore the anatomy and physiology of penile tissue in the 19th century. It took another century to find therapeutic agents (Hauri, 2004).

Erectile dysfunction is defined as the inability to achieve or maintain an erection sufficient for satisfactory sexual intercourse (Montorsi et al., 2010). It is a health problem that is believed to affect millions of men around the world. Due to the scarcity of studies and ethical, religious, and cultural reasons, it is difficult to accurately estimate its global incidence and prevalence.

Numerous scoring systems have been established for the diagnosis and severity of erectile dysfunction, the most widely used is IIEF. This form questions the sexual functions of the person in the last 4 weeks. It consists of a total of 15 questions under 5 sub-headings. Although its reliability is quite high, the difficulty of its use in clinical practice has led clinicians to more practical tests. The Sexual Health Inventory for Men (SHIM/IIEF-5) asks participants 5 questions from the IIEF questionnaire. Makes inquiries about ED from their sexual life in the last 6 months. Participants are evaluated from 30 points. It is classified as severe (0-10), moderate (11-16), mild-moderate (17-21), and mild (22-25) erectile dysfunction (Rosen et al., 1997).

The Massachusetts Male Aging Study is the first broad-based multidisciplinary study of erectile dysfunction. Men between the ages of 40-70 were included in the study. Many factors such as medical drug use, smoking, general health status, demographic variables, and psychological factors were evaluated. The study showed that the overall ED rate was 52%. The prevalence of mild, moderate, and severe ED was found to be 17.2%, 25.2%, and 9.6%, respectively (Feldman et al., 1994).

In a study in which 27500 people of both genders over the age of 40 from 29 countries participated, 80% of the participants stated that they had had sexual intercourse in the last year. However, 28% of the male participants and 42% of the female participants stated that they could not have satisfactory sexual intercourse for various reasons (premature ejaculation, erectile dysfunction, sexual reluctance, inability to reach orgasm, and difficulty in lubrication) (Nicolosi et al., 2004).

A recent ED study involving eight countries was conducted with 97159 participants. Patients over the age of 18 who had difficulty reaching and maintaining an erection in the last 6 months were included. It was shown that the highest prevalence in all age groups was in Italy (48.6%) and the lowest prevalence was in Brazil (37.2%). The prevalence was found to be 40.5% in all groups. The prevalence of ED in European Union countries is 42.3%, which corresponds to approximately 53.9 million men. Data show that since 2011, men with ED have increased approximately 2.5 times (Goldstein et al., 2020; Jannini et al., 2014).

Etiology

Erectile dysfunction can be classified etiologically as psychogenic, organic, and mixed type. Most cases involve both psychogenic and organic causes. Therefore, it is recommended to use the terms "primary organic" or "primary psychogenic" (Guideline). Organic causes can be classified as hormonal, vascular, neuronal, anatomical, and iatrogenic.

ED is also considered an indicator of systemic endothelial function (Virag et al., 1981). It has similar risk factors with cardiovascular diseases (age, smoking, dyslipidemia, and obesity) and progresses through similar pathophysiological mechanisms (arterial insufficiencies, endothelial dysfunction, and inflammation). Therefore, it is considered an early finding for coronary artery diseases (Grover et al., 2006).

Montorsi et al. suggested that ED is a precursor to CVD, with the idea that smaller penile arteries (1-2mm) may be affected earlier by atherosclerosis. It was predicted that larger diameters of coronary arteries (3-4mm) and carotid arteries (5-7mm) may show symptoms at later ages (Montorsi et al., 2003). Thompson et al. reported that cardiovascular disease developed at a rate of 2% in 1 year and 11% in 5 years after the first diagnosis of erectile dysfunction (Thompson et al., 2005).

The penis consists of two corpus cavernosum located laterally and a corpus spongiosum located ventrally. The corpus cavernosum, which forms most of the penis, contains erectile tissue in a dense fibroelastic sheath rich in connective tissue. The smooth muscle bundles inside give the erectile tissue a spongy appearance and form the cavernosal sinuses covered by the endothelium. The corpus spongiosum, located ventral to the corpus cavernosum, forms the urethra in the form of a median groove.

Penile erection begins with the sexual stimulus carrying the sensory impulse through the pudendal nerves. Penile tumescence and detumescence occur when the sympathetic and parasympathetic systems work in coordination. The sacral plexus (S2-S4) provides parasympathetic motor innervation. It is innervated by the inferior hypogastric plexus, by transmission of the pelvic splanchnic nerves. Under the dominance of the parasympathetic system, blood coming from the internal pudendal artery provides blood supply to the glans penis through the penile dorsal artery, and blood supply to the corpus cavernosum through the cavernous artery. The cavernous artery divides into helicine arterial branches along both corporal trunks, and penile engorgement occurs with the filling of the cavernous. With the resulting fullness, the deep dorsal vein is compressed between the tunica albuginea and an erection is achieved. At the end of the erection, the blood in the cavernous is poured into the prostatic venous plexus, and detumescence is achieved (Panchatsharam et al., 2022).

The physiology of penile erection can be explained by the mechanism of arterial dilatation and venous occlusion. After sexual stimulation, the release of nitric oxide (NO) from endothelium-derived non-adrenergic non-cholinergic nerve fibers and acetylcholine from parasympathetic cholinergic nerve endings initiate an erection. The diffusion of NO at the cellular level activates guanylate cyclase. The protein kinase-mediated cascade (phosphatidylinositol-3-kinase/protein kinase B) causes cell hyperpolarization and decreased intracellular calcium levels. With this effect, the blood flow of the sinusoids in the cavernous increases 20-40 times. The cavernosal pressure that exceeds the systolic pressure and constitutes the full erection phase. Contraction of the ischiocavernosus and bulbospongiosus muscles leads to the transition to the hard erection phase (Panchatsharam et al., 2022).

Anamnesis, Physical Examination, and Auxiliary Tests

As in all medical practices, a detailed medical and sexual history should be taken from the patient presenting with ED. If possible, the anamnesis should be performed with the partner. Anamnesis is of great importance in determining the etiology. While taking anamnesis, it should be ensured that the patient can express himself comfortably. The EAU guidelines state that symptoms often have a combination of organic and psychogenic components. It is classified as primary organic and primary psychogenic according to the time and frequency of symptoms.

At the first presentation of the patient, it should be determined whether the ED is primary or secondary. For primary reasons, the biological and sexual development process of childhood and adolescence, family and cultural structure, first sexual experience, whether or not he has a regular partner, the duration of relationship and interaction with his partner, and masturbation habit should be questioned (Porst et al., 2013). Chronic and systemic diseases related to secondary ED should be questioned. In addition, the patient's LUTS (Lower Urinary System Symptoms), (Seftel et al., 2013) ejaculation disorder (Rosen et al., 2003), history of previous trauma and abdominopelvic surgery, smoking, and drug use, and alcohol habits should also be questioned. The use of drugs that cause ED, such as non-selective beta-blockers, SSRIs, antihistamines, and opioid derivatives, should also be questioned (Francis et al., 2007).

The hardness and duration of morning erections, sexual desire, arousal, ejaculation, and orgasm status should be discussed in detail. The IIEF test may be requested from the patient for a more quantitative evaluation of anamnesis (Rosen et al., 1997). Thus, the underlying factors and treatment potential can be more objectively evaluated. Psychometric analyses support the use of EHS (Erectile Hardness Score) in the evaluation of penile hardness (Mulhall et al., 2007). Beck Depressive Index can be used in patients with mood disorders (Corona et al., 2016).

In addition to the urogenital examination, cardiological, endocrinological, and neurological examinations should also be performed in detail in patients with ED. Consultation with these departments should be requested when necessary (Shamloul & Ghanem, 2013). The examination should begin with an inspection. Due to its association with cardiovascular diseases, measurements of height, weight, and waist circumference, which are components of metabolic syndrome, should be performed. Secondary sex characteristics such as androgenetic alopecia, midline body hair, and gynecomastia should be investigated. A genital examination should be performed in the standing and supine position. In the scrotum examination, the size, consistency, and localization of the testicles should be evaluated. In the penis examination, the external urethral meatus should be seen by retracting the prepuce of the uncircumcised patient. Anatomical disorders such as hypospadias and epispadias should be defined. If there is a micropenis, its relationship with hypogonadism and secondary sexual characteristics should be evaluated. The penis shaft should be palpated along the penis. The presence of fibrous plaque, deformity, and congenital chordee in the penis should be evaluated. Anatomical disorders such as Peyronie's disease should be examined. All patients over the age of 50 and patients with LUTS should undergo a digital rectal examination.

Laboratory tests should be adjusted according to the patient's complaints and risk factors. Fasting blood glucose or HbA1C and lipid profile measurement should be performed in patients who have not been evaluated in the last 12 months. Hormone tests should be evaluated in the morning and when the patient is hungry. Erection occurs even at very low testosterone levels. If ED is associated with testosterone, the patient should be considered to have severe hypogonadism (Corona et al., 2016). In patients with specific symptoms, laboratory values of these symptoms should be studied (Figure 1).

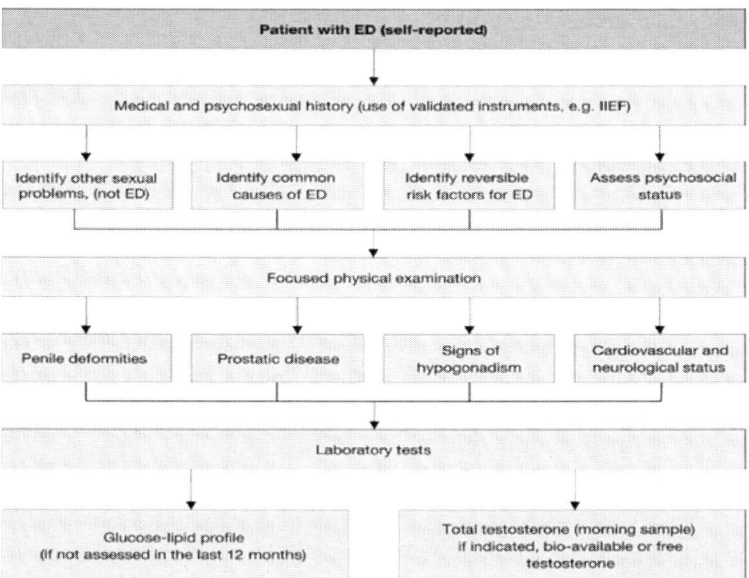

Figure 1. Minimal diagnostic evaluation in patients with ED (EAU, 2022).

Advanced Tests

The nocturnal penile tumescence and rigidity (NPTR) test is a nocturnal test that measures the number of erectile periods, its rigidity, maximum penile stiffness, and rigidity. NPTR should be administered on at least two separate nights. More than 10 minutes and at least 60% stiffness at the penile tip are considered sufficient (Zou et al., 2019). NPTR is significant in distinguishing between psychogenic and organic ED. The disadvantage is that it cannot measure axial erection when measuring radial erection, and false negatives can be seen in some neurodegenerative diseases.

The intracavernous injection test is the injection of drugs such as papaverine, phentolamine, and alprostadil into the corpus cavernosum. The hardness of the penis that cannot be bent within 10 minutes after the injection and its persistence for 30 minutes are considered significant. It is insufficient for diagnosis.

Dynamic Duplex Ultrasound of the penis examines the hemodynamic pathophysiology of erection. A Duplex-Doppler ultrasound probe producing a grayscale (continuous wave) or pulse wave should be placed at the root of the penis to display arterial flow. After the injection into the penile tissue (papaverine, phentolamine, and alprostadil), the maximum systolic blood flow >30 cm/s, end-diastolic velocity <3 cm/s, and the resistive index >0.8 are considered normal. If the patient is thought to have ED due to a vasculogenic cause and the ultrasound evaluation is normal, no additional screening methods are needed.

Arteriography or Cavernosography: Cavernosography is the application of contrast under fluoroscopy when the maximum systolic flow increases to 90 cmHg after penile Doppler USG. It is the gold standard in the investigation of vasculogenic structures. Its use is limited, as it is invasive and time-consuming.

Penile arteriography is the imaging of the pudendal artery with contrast. It is used in the investigation of penile vascular damage or secondary erectile dysfunction in young patients. Recent studies suggest the use of CT angiography before penile angiography in patients with isolated penile artery stenosis (Wang et al., 2016).

Psychiatric Evaluation

Mental health and psychological problems trigger ED (Li et al., 2021). Organic and psychological causes are intertwined in ED. Therefore, psychiatric evaluation is necessary for almost every patient. In addition, the loss of self-confidence can make the patient resistant to the treatment. Evaluations should be made with the partner, if possible, and include the factors that cause stress. Psychiatric consultation should be conducted when necessary. Brief Symptom Inventory (Derogatis & Melisaratos, 1983), Sexual Dysfunctional Blief Questionnaire (Nobre & Pinto, 2010), and Sexual Modes Questionnaire (Nobre & Pinto, 2003) can be used for detailed evaluation of patients.

Treatment

Patient Education and Lifestyle Changes: The treatment process should be carried out together with the patient, the patient's sexual partner, the physician, and the consultants. Information about diagnostic tests should be provided. The needs and expectations of the patient and sexual partner should be discussed. It should be discussed whether ED is adequately understood by the patient and his partner. Considering the diagnostic tests and patient expectations, the necessity and plan of treatment should be discussed.

Lifestyle changes show major benefits in people who lead a sedentary lifestyle and have specific comorbid diseases. In particular, metabolic syndrome is closely associated with ED. The benefits of exercise, weight loss, and a Mediterranean diet are important in the treatment of ED against potential risks, especially obesity.

Medical Treatments: Phosphodiesterase 5 inhibitors catalyze the hydrolysis of cGMP, the secondary messenger signaling molecule, in cavernous tissue. It provides relaxation in penile arteries by decreasing intracellular Ca++ levels. Increased blood flow provides compression in the subtunical venous plexus and erection.

Four drugs selected from PDE5I have been licensed by the European Medicines Agency (EMA). The mechanisms of action are similar. However, they differ from each other in their biochemical structures, pharmacokinetic properties, and clinical effects. They do not have erection-inducing effects. There must be s suitable sexual stimulus for erection. In the use of the drug, the intake of fatty foods should be reduced, it should be tested at least 6 times, and hormonal and metabolic control should be provided. The absolute contraindication is the use of drugs containing nitrates. Caution should also be exercised in its use with alpha-adrenergic agents. They should be used at least 4 hours apart. Both agents have a hypotension effect.

Sildenafil is the first PDE5I group drug that was introduced to the market in 1998. Available in 50 mg and 100 mg forms. A starting dose of 50 mg is recommended. Using after fatty meals may reduce or delay absorption.

Tadalafil was licensed in 2003. It shows activity in 30 minutes and maximal activity in about 2 hours. It has advantages such as being effective for up to 36 hours and not affected by food intake. It is available in 5 mg, 10 mg, and 20 mg forms. The recommended form is 5 mg in daily intake and 10 mg in optional intake. It has been shown that 40% of men over 45 years of age respond to ED/BPH symptoms with daily use of 5 mg of tadalafil, and symptoms improve after 12 weeks.

Vardenafil shows activity for about 30 minutes. It is available in 5 mg, 10 mg, and 20 mg forms. Drug absorption decreases with food intake. It has given successful results even in difficult-to-treat subgroups, such as diabetes mellitus. Orodispersible tablet forms offered ease of use and eliminated the association of absorption with food absorption.

Avanafil was licensed in 2013. It is a selective PDE5I and highly inhibits. It is available in 50 mg, 100 mg, and 200 mg forms. The recommended dose for ED is 100 mg. There is limited absorption with food.

The most common side effects of PDE5I agents are headache, dyspepsia, hot flashes, nasal congestion, back pain, and visual disturbances. Hot flashes and visual disturbances are more common in sildenafil and vardenafil. Back pain/myalgia is more common in tadalafil. The PDE5I drugs should be chosen according to the frequency of sexual intercourse, the patient's personal experiences, the duration of the drug action, side effects, and the way of use, by deciding with the patient. It should not be used together with drugs containing organic nitrates, and care should be taken when using it with alpha-adrenergic and other antihypertensives.

Topical/Intraurethral Alprostadil: Alprostadil is a Prostaglandin E1 analog. It binds to the G protein by binding to the PGE1 receptor on the surface of smooth muscle cells and activates the cAMP pathway. Thus, it provides relaxation of the vascular smooth muscle.

Topical Alprostadil: Available in 200 µg and 300 µg forms. It is applied from the external meatus with the help of a permeation-enhancing cream. Systemic side effects are minimal. Penile erythema, pain, and burning are its side effects that can develop within 2 hours.

Intraurethral Alprostadil: It is used by placing it intraurethral with the help of a pellet (125-1000 µg). The recommended dose is 500 µg. Penile pain, dizziness, and urethral bleeding may occur.

Medical Devices

ESWT: It has been applied as an alternative treatment for vasculogenic ED in recent years. It has been reported to give effective results in studies. However, there is no consensus on standardization such as shock wave generating devices (electrohydraulic, electromagnetic, piezoelectric, and electro-pneumatic), the type of shock waves (focused, semi-focused, linear, and unfocused), the application time, the number of applications, and the region to be applied (Sokolakis et al., 2019). Data limitations require larger randomized controlled studies.

Vacuum Pump Devices: It works based on the principle of passive blood supply of the corpus cavernosum by exposing the penis to negative pressure in a bell jar and compressing the root of the penis with tape and trapping the blood in the penis. Regardless of the cause of ED, it provides more than 90% satisfactory erection. Patients usually stop using within 3 months due to penile pain, bruising, numbness, and time-consuming. It is contraindicated in patients with bleeding disorders and using anticoagulants.

Intracavernosal Treatments

Alprostadil is the first and only drug used in the intracavernosal treatment of ED. It is used as monotherapy at a dose of 5-40 µg. Erection occurs within 5-15 minutes. The patient should be trained for the injection technique and, if he does not have sufficient skills, should be taught to his partner. The most common side effect is penile pain. Long-term pain and priapism are less common side effects. Its systemic side effect is mild hypertension due to high-dose use.

Bimix, Trimix: Papaverine (7.5-45 mg) + phentolamine (0.25-1.5 mg) (also known as Bimix) and papaverine (8-16 mg) + phentolamine (0.2-0.4 mg) + alprostadil (10-20 µg) (also known as Trimix). Although they were never licensed for ED, they are widely used with improved efficacy rates.

Invicorp is a combination of vasoactive intestinal peptide (25 µg) and phentolamine mesylate (1-2 mg) licensed in Scandinavia.

Surgical Treatments

Penile prosthesis implantation is the most frequently performed surgery today in the treatment of organically caused ED. It is generally preferred in patients with vascular disease, diabetes, and previous pelvic surgery/trauma. There are two types of penile prostheses.

Inflatable Dentures: It has two or three parts. It is preferred because it provides a more natural appearance. It is used with the help of a pump placed in the scrotum. It is more difficult to use and more costly.

Flexible Prostheses: It is easier to implant. It is easier to use and less expensive. The disadvantage is that the penis is permanently semirigid.

The satisfaction rate is 92-100% in patients and 91-95% in partners. The most important complications of penile prosthesis implantation are mechanical failure and infection. Mechanical failure is often seen in 3-piece prostheses. In recent years, this rate has decreased below 5% in a 5-year follow-up. Penile prosthesis infection was reduced to 2-3% with antibiotic prophylaxis and compliance with hygiene. In case of infection, the prosthesis should be removed and antibiotic therapy should be administered. Alternatively, removal of the prosthesis, washing the cavernous with antibiotics, and insertion of a new prosthesis have been reported to provide 80% success (Mulcahy, 2000).

PRP

PRP is the centrifugation of whole blood and the separation of the platelet-rich layer. In this layer, which is separated from whole blood, there is a platelet concentration that exceeds physiological limits by 3-7 times. It shows its therapeutic effect when the platelet count in the final product reaches 1,000,000 U/μl. Platelet-rich plasma is rich in cytokines and growth factors that will reverse the pathophysiology of ED through both angiogenesis and stem cell activation. Current medical treatments, ESWT, and vacuum devices provide symptomatic treatment rather than treating the pathophysiology of the disease. The application of intracavernosal PRP both provides spontaneous erection and reduces the need for medical treatment (Khodamoradi et al., 2022).

PRP contains many growth factors, chemokines, and cytokines. PF-4 (Platelet-factor 4) attracts neutrophils and eosinophils to the site of inflammation. PDGF (Platelet-derived growth factor) and TGF-β (transforming growth factor beta) synthesize collagen. VEGF (vascular endothelial growth factor) and EGF (epidermal growth factor) provide new blood vessel formation (Figure 2).

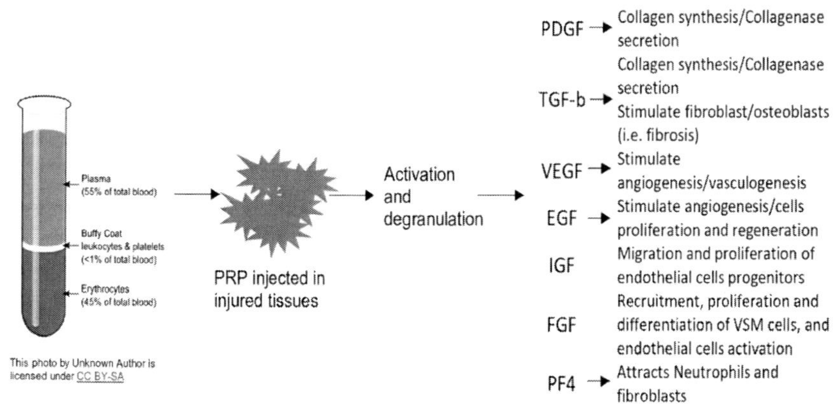

Figure 2. PRP mechanism of action (Alkandari et al., 2022).

The release of chemokine factors at the time of inflammation, stabilization of the extracellular matrix with collagen synthesis, and increased blood flow are expected responses for tissue regeneration. Local application of PRP allows the increase of various growth factors and rapid regeneration in the damaged area (Alkandari et al., 2022).

In animal models in preclinical studies, investigators frequently used intracavernous pressure measurement and histopathological evaluations (Ding et al., 2009; Wu et al., 2012). In a recent animal study, erectile dysfunction parameters were examined for a total of 18 weeks after streptozocin was loaded onto rats for 12 weeks. In the study, in which intracavernous pressure and systemic blood pressure were closely followed, a regression was observed in ED parameters with PRP treatment. Histologically, increased regeneration of myelinated nerve fibers and decreased corporal smooth muscle atrophy were observed (Liao et al., 2022).

Poulios et al. administered 10 ml of PRP and placebo intracavernosal injection to 30 patients with mild to moderate ED. Applications made at one-month intervals were evaluated in the 1st, 3rd, and 6th months. It was determined that there was an improvement of 2.7, 2.8, and 3.9 points in the IIEF scores, respectively (Poulios et al., 2021).

Ruffo et al. conducted a study of 60 patients with mild to severe ED. In the study, they gave ESWT (1500 shock/session) treatment for 6 weeks to one group, and ESWT (1500 shock/session) + PRP injection (every 2 weeks) to the other group for 6 weeks. At 6-months of follow-up, the mean IIEF-5 score increased from 11 to 18 in the ESWT group, while it increased from 10 to 22 in the ESWT+PRP group (Ruffo et al., 2018).

In the study by Alkhayal et al., PRP was administered to 61 patients who applied with the complaint of organic ED. After 11 weeks of follow-up, mean IIEF-5 scores increased from 12.5 to 17.7 (Alkhayal et al., 2019) (method not clear).

In the study by Taş et al., 3 PRP injections were administered to ED patients with metabolic syndrome at 15-day intervals. Control IIEF-5 scores increased moderately from 18 to 20 in the 1st, 3rd, and 6th months (Taş et al., 2021).

The most commonly reported side effects in human-based studies are pain at the injection site, bruising, palpable penile stiffness, and plaque formation. In the current studies, no systemic side effects have been reported.

The recent popularity of PRP has led academic studies to focus on the subject. Both animal experiments and studies on human volunteers enable us to obtain more quantitative results.

Studies have shown that intracavernosal PRP leads to significant increases in IIEF-5 scores. The scarcity and heterogeneity of the patient groups participating in clinical studies show the need to study larger and homogeneous groups. Clinical physicians, especially urologists, need both studies with larger patient groups and standardized treatment protocols for the use of PRP in the treatment of ED. In studies conducted in different centers, different techniques are used to obtain PRP. In addition, there are non-standardized data on the treatment dose to be administered, the number of doses to be administered, the interval between doses, and the total treatment time. The limited data that the researchers reported on the method is another problem. In particular, the area where PRP will be applied on the penis and the use of the penile clamp should be detailed.

Conclusion

The American Urological Association (AUA) and the European Association of Urology (EAU) recommended that PRP be considered only experimentally due to the lack of evidence on the potential benefits and risks of ED treatment.

- PRP should not be recommended to men with ED unless administered in the context of an IRB-approved experimental clinical research protocol. At this time, no peer-reviewed full-text publications are available to constitute an evidence base. Therefore, reliable information about the potential benefits and risks/costs of PRP therapy is not available. Because of the absence of evidence and given the availability of multiple other proven treatment options, the Panel's expert opinion is that PRP therapy is not appropriate for men with ED except as part of an IRB-approved research trial (AUA, 2022).
- Do not use PRP to treat ED outside the confines of a clinical trial (EAU, 2022).

According to current literature studies and guidelines, there is insufficient evidence for the use of PRP in the clinical treatment of ED. In addition, the treatment protocol is not standardized. According to the successful results obtained in the experimental studies, due to its potential benefits, PRP is a strong candidate to be one of the main treatment modalities for ED in the future.

References

Alkandari, M. H., Touma, N., & Carrier, S. (2022). Platelet-Rich Plasma Injections for Erectile Dysfunction and Peyronie's Disease: A Systematic Review of Evidence. *Sexual Medicine Reviews*, 10(2), 341–352. https://doi.org/10.1016/j.sxmr.2020.12.004.

Alkhayal, M., & Lourdes, M. (2019). Platelet Rich Plasma Penile Rejuvenation as a Treatment for Erectile Dysfunction: An Update. *The Journal of Sexual Medicine*, 16(2), 71. https://doi.org/10.1016/j.jsxm.2019.03.228.

AUA. (2022). Erectile Dysfunction: AUA Guideline. Retrieved 2 March 2023 from https://www.auanet.org/guidelines-and-quality/guidelines/erectile-dysfunction-(ed)-guideline.

Corona, G., Isidori, A. M., Aversa, A., Burnett, A. L., & Maggi, M. (2016). Endocrinologic Control of Men's Sexual Desire and Arousal/Erection. *The Journal of Sexual Medicine*, 13(3), 317–337. https://doi.org/10.1016/j.jsxm.2016.01.007.

Derogatis, L. R., & Melisaratos, N. (1983). The Brief Symptom Inventory: An introductory report. *Psychological Medicine*, 13(3), 595–605.

Ding, X. G., Li, S. W., Zheng, X. M., Hu, L. Q., Hu, W. L., & Luo, Y. (2009). The effect of platelet-rich plasma on cavernous nerve regeneration in a rat model. *Asian Journal of Andrology*, 11(2), 215–221. https://doi.org/10.1038/aja.2008.37.

EAU. (2022). Sexual and Reproductive Health: EAU Guideline. Retrieved 2 March 2023 from https://uroweb.org/guidelines/sexual-and-reproductive-health/chapter/management-of-erectile-dysfunction.

Feldman, H. A., Goldstein, I., Hatzichristou, D. G., Krane, R. J., & McKinlay, J. B. (1994). Impotence and its medical and psychosocial correlates: Results of the Massachusetts Male Aging Study. *The Journal of Urology*, 151(1), 54–61. https://doi.org/10.1016/s0022-5347(17)34871-1.

Francis, M. E., Kusek, J. W., Nyberg, L. M., & Eggers, P. W. (2007). The contribution of common medical conditions and drug exposures to erectile dysfunction in adult males. *The Journal of Urology,* 178(2), 591–596. https://doi.org/10.1016/j.juro.2007.03.127.

Goldstein, I., Goren, A., Li, V. W., Tang, W. Y., & Hassan, T. A. (2020). Epidemiology Update of Erectile Dysfunction in Eight Countries with High Burden. *Sexual Medicine Reviews*, 8(1), 48–58. https://doi.org/10.1016/j.sxmr.2019.06.008.

Grover, S. A., Lowensteyn, I., Kaouache, M., Marchand, S., Coupal, L., DeCarolis, E., Zoccoli, J., & Defoy, I. (2006). The prevalence of erectile dysfunction in the primary care setting: Importance of risk factors for diabetes and vascular disease. *Archives of Internal Medicine*, 166(2), 213–219. https://doi.org/10.1001/archinte.166.2.213.

Hauri, D. (2004). Physiologie und Pathophysiologie der erektilen Dysfunktion. Eine Erfindung von heute? [Physiology and pathophysiology of erectile dysfunction. A modern contrivance?]. *Der Urologe. Ausg. A*, 43(11), 1423–1429. https://doi.org/10.1007/s00120-004-0674-7.

Jannini, E. A., Sternbach, N., Limoncin, E., Ciocca, G., Gravina, G. L., Tripodi, F., Petruccelli, I., Keijzer, S., Isherwood, G., Wiedemann, B., & Simonelli, C. (2014). Health-related characteristics and unmet needs of men with erectile dysfunction: A survey in five European countries. *The Journal of Sexual Medicine*, 11(1), 40–50. https://doi.org/10.1111/jsm.12344.

Khodamoradi, K., Dullea, A., Golan, R., Molina, M., Arora, H., Masterson, T. A., & Ramasamy, R. (2022). Platelet Rich Plasma (PRP) Growth Factor Concentration Varies in Men With Erectile Dysfunction. *The Journal of Sexual Medicine*, 19(9), 1488–1493. https://doi.org/10.1016/j.jsxm.2022.06.003.

Li, K., Liang, S., Shi, Y., Zhou, Y., Xie, L., Feng, J., Chen, Z., Li, Q., & Gan, Z. (2021). The Relationships of Dehydroepiandrosterone Sulfate, Erectile Function and General Psychological Health. *Sexual Medicine*, 9(4), 100386. https://doi.org/10.1016/j.esxm.2021.100386.

Liao, C. H., Lee, K. H., Chung, S. D., Chen, K. C., Praveen Rajneesh, C., Chen, B. H., Cheng, J. H., Lin, W. Y., Chiang, H. S., & Wu, Y. N. (2022). Intracavernous Injection of Platelet-Rich Plasma Therapy Enhances Erectile Function and Decreases the Mortality Rate in Streptozotocin-Induced Diabetic Rats. *International Journal of Molecular Sciences*, 23(6), 3017. https://doi.org/10.3390/ijms23063017.

Montorsi, F., Adaikan, G., Becher, E., Giuliano, F., Khoury, S., Lue, T. F., Sharlip, I., Althof, S. E., Andersson, K. E., Brock, G., Broderick, G., Burnett, A., Buvat, J., Dean, J., Donatucci, C., Eardley, I., Fugl-Meyer, K. S., Goldstein, I., Hackett, G., Hatzichristou, D., Hellstrom, W., Incrocci, L., Jackson, G., Kadioglu, A., Levine, L., Lewis, R. W., Maggi, M., McCabe, M., McMahon, C. G., Montague, D., Montorsi, P., Mulhall, J., Pfaus, J., Porst, H., Ralph, D., Rosen, R., Rowland, D., Sadeghi-Nejad, H., Shabsigh, R., Stief, C., Vardi, Y., Wallen, K., & Wasserman, M. (2010). Summary of the recommendations on sexual dysfunctions in men. *The Journal of Sexual Medicine*, 7(11), 3572–3588. https://doi.org/10.1111/j.1743-6109.2010.02062.x.

Montorsi, F., Briganti, A., Salonia, A., Rigatti, P., Margonato, A., Macchi, A., Galli, S., Ravagnani, P. M., & Montorsi, P. (2003). Erectile dysfunction prevalence, time of onset and association with risk factors in 300 consecutive patients with acute chest pain and angiographically documented coronary artery disease. *European Urology*, 44(3), 360–365. https://doi.org/10.1016/s0302-2838(03)00305-1.

Mulcahy, J. J. (2000). Long-term experience with salvage of infected penile implants. *The Journal of Urology*, 163(2), 481–482.

Mulhall, J. P., Goldstein, I., Bushmakin, A. G., Cappelleri, J. C., & Hvidsten, K. (2007). Validation of the erection hardness score. *The Journal of Sexual Medicine*, 4(6), 1626–1634. https://doi.org/10.1111/j.1743-6109.2007.00600.x.

Nicolosi, A., Laumann, E. O., Glasser, D. B., Moreira, E. D., Jr, Paik, A., & Gingell, C., & Global Study of Sexual Attitudes and Behaviors Investigators' Group. (2004). Sexual behavior and sexual dysfunctions after age 40: the global study of sexual attitudes and behaviors. *Urology*, 64(5), 991–997. https://doi.org/10.1016/j.urology.2004.06.055.

Nobre, P. J., & Pinto-Gouveia, J. (2003). Sexual modes questionnaire: measure to assess the interaction among cognitions, emotions, and sexual response. *Journal of Sex Research*, 40(4), 368–382. https://doi.org/10.1080/00224490209552203.

Nobre, P. J., & Pinto-Gouveia, J. (2006). Dysfunctional sexual beliefs as vulnerability factors to sexual dysfunction. *Journal of Sex Research*, 43(1), 68–75. https://doi.org/10.1080/00224490609552300.

Panchatsharam, P. K., Durland, J., & Zito, P. M. (2022). Physiology, Erection. In *StatPearls*. StatPearls Publishing.

Porst, H., Burnett, A., Brock, G., Ghanem, H., Giuliano, F., Glina, S., Hellstrom, W., Martin-Morales, A., Salonia, A., Sharlip, I., & ISSM Standards Committee for Sexual Medicine. (2013). SOP conservative (medical and mechanical) treatment of erectile dysfunction. *The Journal of Sexual Medicine*, 10(1), 130–171. https://doi.org/
10.1111/jsm.12023.

Poulios, E., Mykoniatis, I., Pyrgidis, N., Zilotis, F., Kapoteli, P., Kotsiris, D., Kalyvianakis, D., & Hatzichristou, D. (2021). Platelet-Rich Plasma (PRP) Improves Erectile Function: A Double-Blind, Randomized, Placebo-Controlled Clinical Trial. *The Journal of Sexual Medicine*, 18(5), 926–935. https://doi.org/10.1016/j.jsxm.2021.03.008.

Richter, P., Werner, J., Heerlein, A., Kraus, A., & Sauer, H. (1998). On the validity of the Beck Depression Inventory: A review. *Psychopathology*, 31(3), 160–168. https://doi.org/10.1159/000066239.

Roehrborn, C. G., Egan, K. B., Miner, M. M., Ni, X., Wong, D. G., & Rosen, R. C. (2016). Erectile dysfunction and lower urinary tract symptoms associated with benign prostatic hyperplasia (LUTS/BPH) combined responders to tadalafil after 12 weeks of treatment. *BJU International*, 118(1), 153–160. https://doi.org/10.1111/bju.13406.

Rosen, R., Altwein, J., Boyle, P., Kirby, R. S., Lukacs, B., Meuleman, E., O'Leary, M. P., Puppo, P., Robertson, C., & Giuliano, F. (2003). Lower urinary tract symptoms and male sexual dysfunction: the multinational survey of the aging male (MSAM-7). *European Urology*, 44(6), 637–649. https://doi.org/10.1016/j.eururo.2003.08.015.

Rosen, R. C., Riley, A., Wagner, G., Osterloh, I. H., Kirkpatrick, J., & Mishra, A. (1997). The international index of erectile function (IIEF): a multidimensional scale for assessment of erectile dysfunction. *Urology*, 49(6), 822–830. https://doi.org/ 10.1016/s0090-4295(97)00238-0.

Ruffo, N., Stanojevic, F., Iacono, L., Romis, G., Romeo, G., & Di Lauro, G. (2018). Treating erectile dysfunction with a combination of low-intensity shock waves (LISW) and platelet-rich plasma (PRP) injections. *The Journal of Sexual Medicine*, 15(3), 318–319. https://doi.org/10.1016/j.jsxm.2018.04.435.

Seftel, A. D., de la Rosette, J., Birt, J., Porter, V., Zarotsky, V., & Viktrup, L. (2013). Coexisting lower urinary tract symptoms and erectile dysfunction: a systematic review of epidemiological data. *International Journal of Clinical Practice*, 67(1), 32–45. https://doi.org/10.1111/ijcp.12044.

Shamloul, R., & Ghanem, H. (2013). Erectile dysfunction. *Lancet (London, England)*, 381(9861), 153–165. https://doi.org/10.1016/S0140-6736(12)60520-0.

Sokolakis, I., & Hatzichristodoulou, G. (2019). Clinical studies on low-intensity extracorporeal shockwave therapy for erectile dysfunction: a systematic review and meta-analysis of randomised controlled trials. *International Journal of Impotence Research*, 31(3), 177–194. https://doi.org/10.1038/s41443-019-011.

Taş, T., Çakıroğlu, B., Arda, E., Onuk, Ö., & Nuhoğlu, B. (2021). Early clinical results of the tolerability, safety, and efficacy of autologous platelet-rich plasma administration in erectile dysfunction. *Sexual Medicine, 9(2),* 100313. https://doi.org/ 10.1016/j.esxm.2020.100313.

Thompson, I. M., Tangen, C. M., Goodman, P. J., Probstfield, J. L., Moinpour, C. M., & Coltman, C. A. (2005). Erectile dysfunction and subsequent cardiovascular disease. *JAMA, 294(23),* 2996–3002. https://doi.org/10.1001/jama.294.23.2996.

Virag, R., Zwang, G., Dermange, H., & Legman, M. (1981). Vasculogenic impotence: A review of 92 cases with 54 surgical operations. *Vascular Surgery, 15(1),* 9-17. https://doi.org/10.1177/153857448101500102.

Wang, T. D., Lee, W. J., Yang, S. C., Lin, P. C., Tai, H. C., Liu, S. P., Huang, C. H., Chen, W. J., Chen, M. F., & Hsieh, J. T. (2016). Clinical and imaging outcomes up to 1 year following balloon angioplasty for isolated penile artery stenoses in patients with erectile dysfunction: The PERFECT-2 study. *Journal of Endovascular*

Therapy: An Official Journal of the International Society of Endovascular Specialists, 23(6), 867–877. https://doi.org/10.1177/1526602816669337.
Wu, C. C., Wu, Y. N., Ho, H. O., Chen, K. C., Sheu, M. T., & Chiang, H. S. (2012). The neuroprotective effect of platelet-rich plasma on erectile function in bilateral cavernous nerve injury rat model. *The Journal of Sexual Medicine, 9(11),* 2838–2848. https://doi.org/10.1111/j.1743-6109.2012.02881.x.
Zou, Z., Lin, H., Zhang, Y., & Wang, R. (2019). The role of nocturnal penile tumescence and rigidity (NPTR) monitoring in the diagnosis of psychogenic erectile dysfunction: A review. *Sexual Medicine Reviews, 7(3),* 442–454. https://doi.org/10.1016/j.sxmr.2018.10.005.

Chapter 16

PRP Treatment for Sexual Dysfunction

Hayri Bozkurt*, **MD**
Department of Family Medicine, Heykel Family Health Center, Bursa, Turkiye

Abstract

Sexual dysfunction occurs in men and women, and the prevalence increases with age. Dysfunction can occur in one or more areas of the normal sexual response cycle: desire, arousal, or orgasm. It can also be due to pain. In addition to medical and surgical treatments, PRP has recently been tested in patients with sexual dysfunction. Platelet-rich plasma (PRP) found its use in the treatment of different conditions and diseases because concentrated plasma PRP consists of many growth factors. Their interaction with surrounding cells, intracellular matrix, and mediators at the site of injection leads to tissue regeneration. Due to the angiogenic, vasculogenic, and regenerative effects of PRP, it has recently been widely used in the treatment of male and female sexual dysfunctions. Platelet-rich plasma (PRP) treatments, which seem to offer hope here, have given satisfactory results in the treatment of patients with this dysfunction. PRP is an innovative therapeutic modality, as it is affordable, simple, easily performed, and effective. It is also a non-invasive modality with promising results and no side effects. For this treatment to become widespread, it needs trials in larger populations and a timeline of proven literature.

Keywords: platelet-rich plasma, female sexual dysfunction, male sexual dysfunction, ınjection, current treatment approaches

---

* Corresponding Author's Email: bozkurt_hayri19@hotmail.com.

In: Current Clinical Recommendations ...
Editors: Nazan Yurtcu and Emel Güler
ISBN: 979-8-89113-723-3

Introduction

Sexual dysfunction is a condition that is seen in both sexes and also increases with advancing age (Anderson et al., 2022). Dysfunction can occur during all three phases of the sexual cycle: desire, arousal, or orgasm. Human sexual function has a very complex structure consisting of physiological and psychological components. A detailed sexual history and a focused physical examination are very important in diagnosis because it is based on clinical findings (Anderson et al., 2022).

Impaired sexual function has a very important place in human quality of life as it has detrimental effects on self-esteem, sense of integrity, and interpersonal relationships in both sexes. It is often emotionally distressing and stressful. Especially if female sexuality is disrupted, this can lead to family conflicts and divorces (Gaber & Shaltout, 2021).

Platelet-rich plasma (PRP) was discovered to be useful in the treatment of various conditions and diseases, on the grounds that concentrated plasma PRP comprises of numerous growth factors. The angiogenic, vasculogenic, and regenerative effects of PRP are now being used in the treatment of patients diagnosed with sexual dysfunction.

Platelet-rich plasma (PRP), which is considered a new non-surgical outpatient treatment; It helps patients with sexual dysfunction recover using one's own growth factors (Gaber & Shaltout, 2021).

PRP has no known contraindications as it is completely autologous and technically offers the advantage of injection into the tissue as a non-viscous liquid rather than a gel as in hyaluronic acid fillers. The unique aqueous structure of PRP provides an even distribution throughout the tissue surrounding the injection site (Dhillon et al., 2012).

Sexual Function

People's understanding of sexuality has a very complex structure and can also act in different ways. The main elements of the understanding of sexuality in people; to enjoy and ensure the continuation of the generation. In studies, it is stated that there are many factors in the structure of sexuality, and this structure is very complex (Meston & Buss, 2007).

Buss (2003) stated that sexuality is experienced within certain limits within the cultural environment. The most impressive ones in the experience of sexuality are status, roles, and prestige in society. In the realization of sexual intercourse, it is stated that sexual intercourse is experienced for reasons such as reducing sexual tension, getting pleasure, emotional togetherness, being happy, experience, and curiosity, and there may be more than 200 reasons like these (Meston & Buss, 2007).

The sexual response process stages of people (Keçe, 2013):

1. Arousal: It is a physiological state that allows people to have sexual intercourse to prepare their bodies for intercourse (Kaplan, 2014). While arousal in women is manifested by wetting the vagina and filling the lips with blood, it is seen as an erection in men (Özdel, 2001).
2. Plateau: This phase is both a continuation and a part of arousal. This phase begins with the continuation of sexual stimuli and increased sexual excitement. In the plateau phase, the individual's pleasure and sexual tension increase. The plateau phase continues until the couples reach orgasm, and this phase is the orgasm entry phase (İncesu, 2004).
   The plateau phase lasts from 30 seconds to several minutes. At this stage, while there is growth in the testicles in men, in women, contractions are observed. As women's breasts enlarge, enlargement and color changes appear in the vagina and penis. While contractions seen in women affect large muscles, heartbeat and breathing accelerate and blood pressure increases (Bozkurt et al., 2013).
3. Orgasm: The orgasm phase is very short in terms of duration and very satisfying in terms of pleasure. Orgasm increases intensity in the clitoral region and vagina in women, and in the penis and prostate in men. In this phase, ejaculation is observed in men and contractions in women (İncesu, 2004).
4. Dissolution: In this phase, the physical changes that occur after orgasm occurs or when orgasm is not achieved gradually disappear. Men enter a period of numbness after orgasm. During this period, nerves, heart, and skeletal muscles are not affected by stimuli. In women, orgasm can be seen again with the re-activation of sexual stimulation.

Sexual Dysfunction

Sexual dysfunction is a condition that is affected by psychophysiological changes seen in men and women, manifested by deterioration in sexual responsiveness and sexual desire (Aydin, 2012).

Sexual disorders consist of three main groups (DSM-IV 1994).

1) Paraphilias 2) Sexual identity disorders (Transsexuality) 3) Sexual dysfunctions

Paraphilia is characterized by recurrent sexual urges and fantasies involving various objects, abnormal actions, or situations for sexual arousal and orgasm. In order to be called paraphilia, the person must be able to orgasm depending on some compulsory and repetitive conditions.

Exhibitism (exhibitionism, showing off), Frottorism (frictionism), Pedophilia: Engaging in sexual activity with a child or children who have not reached puberty, Fetishism: Sexual interest in inanimate objects, zoophilia (animal sexual act), necrophilia (corpses).

Gender identity disorders (Transsexuality): It is characterized by a persistent feeling of discomfort with one's own biological sex. The person rejects his/her own sexual organs since childhood, adopts attitudes, behaviors, and roles appropriate to the sexual identity of the opposite sex. Wants to dress, play, act like the opposite sex.

Sexual dysfunctions in women; It consists of low sexual desire, arousal and orgasm disorder, vaginismus, and painful sexual intercourse. In men, it consists of low sexual desire, sexual aversion disorder, erectile dysfunction (erectile dysfunction), premature ejaculation and other ejaculation disorders, and painful sexual intercourse problems.

Etiology in Sexual Dysfunction

Predisposing factors in sexual dysfunctions: Inadequate sexual education, Sexual myths, Growing up in a conservative environment, Inadequate sexual experience, Lifestyle, Broken family relationships, Personality traits, Traumatic sexual experiences, and Insecurity in the psychosexual role.

Initiating factors in sexual dysfunctions; Physical illnesses, Depression and other psychiatric disorders, Side effects of drugs, Alcohol and substance use, Exaggerated performance expectations, Pregnancy, Birth and lactation, Relationship problems, Aging, Infidelity, Spouse loss, and Sexual dysfunction in partner.

Sustaining factors in sexual dysfunctions; Performance anxiety, Relationship problems, Sexual myths, Psychiatric disorders, Physical illnesses, Side effects of drugs, Alcohol and substance use, Feeling of guilt and sinfulness, and Loss of attraction between partners.

Incidence of Sexual Dysfunctions

Female: In a UK study, Burri and Spector found that 15.5% of women report lifetime FSD. In this study hypoactive sexual desire is the most common sexual complaint with 17.3%-21.4%, followed by 11.4% new arousal, 8.7% slipperiness, 8.8% orgasm, and 6.0% sexual pain (Burri & Spector, 2011).

An Australian study found that 36% of women reported at least one new symptom of sexual dysfunction in the last year of their life. These symptoms were 11% indifference to sex, inability to orgasm (10%), vaginal dryness problem (9%), inability to enjoy sexual intercourse (8%), anxiety about having sexual intercourse (6%), experiencing physical pain during sexual intercourse (5%), and very fast orgasm (2%). Lack of interest in sex and lack of sexual pleasure, interestingly younger women were more likely to develop new sexual difficulties compared to older women (Martin et al., 2014).

Male: Premature ejaculation and erectile dysfunction are the most common sexual dysfunctions (Johannes et al., 2000; Martin et al., 2014). Studying premature ejaculation (PE) has been difficult as there are inconsistencies and difficulties in defining the condition. The literature on the prevalence of interest and desire disorders in men is limited (Martin et al., 2014). In studies conducted (for varying age ranges and geographic locations), a decreased in the prevalence of interest and desire has been reported in the 15% to 25% range. There is little literature on the prevalence of dyspareunia in men. Nickel et al. reported that the prevalence of painful ejaculation was 16.8% in a world study (Moreira Jr et al., 2003).

Platelet-Rich Plasma (PRP) Treatment for Female Sexual Dysfunction

Platelet-rich plasma (PRP) is effective; In addition, studies in areas such as wound care, orthopedics, dental surgery, and the cosmetic sector have also shown that it does not have significant side effects (Kakudo et al., 2008; Kon et al., 2011; Sclafani, 2011). The main mechanism of action of PRP is to activate pluripotent stem cells, to rejuvenate the tissue in that area and to help its development (Azzena et al., 2008; Carroll et al., 2005). Many articles, such as the absence of granuloma after PRP injection and the absence of infection-like side effects, show the reliability of this treatment method (Dhillon et al., 2012).

In some women who describe sexual dysfunction, it is also known that PRP injections into the periurethral region of the Skenes glands and clitoris reduce the symptoms they describe (in all three stages of the sex cycle) and respond well to treatment.

Due to the effect of PRP to increase angiogenesis and neovascularization, it is also used in the treatment of diseases such as vaginal lichen sclerosis, stress urinary incontinence, episiotomy scars, vaginal wetting disorders due to increased collagen in the wall as a result of intermittent applications to the anterior vaginal wall (Neto, 2017).

Improvement in sexual functions has been reported with the application of PRP to the G-spot (Puppo, 2013). Its first use for female sexual dysfunction was made by Charles Runels under the name O-Shot (Runels et al., 2014). Gynecologists use PRP in treatments such as vaginal rejuvenation and O-shot therapy, since 35 growth factors that were found to be released from platelets provide tissue healing, regeneration, and growth (Ramos et al., 2013).

O-Shot therapy: As a result of the injection of PRP into certain parts of the vagina with the help of local anesthetic drugs and the effect mechanism of PRP. The regression symptoms of sexual dysfunction such as increased sexual response, increased arousal, strong orgasm, and decreased dyspareunia in women is called "O-shot" treatment (Jain et al., 2015). In another study, they applied PRP to the clitoris and vagina of 11 women who had sexual dysfunction. As a result, it has been observed that PRP is an effective and reliable method in the treatment of sexual dysfunctions, especially because of the increase and improvement in desire, arousal, lubrication, and orgasms (Runels et al., 2014).

In addition, vaginal PRP was applied 4 times a month to 52 female patients who applied to a private clinic due to sexual dysfunction. As a result of this application, a significant increase was found in the sexual satisfaction of all patients who applied (Sukgen et al., 2019).

Platelet-Rich Plasma (PRP) Treatment for Male Sexual Dysfunction

Erectile dysfunction (ED) and Peyronie's disease (PD) are the most common sexual dysfunctions in men. Erectile dysfunction is the inability of a man's penis to become as erect as it should be, or to maintain it for a long time, during sexual intercourse. Peyronie's disease is a deformity that occurs with the abnormal development of the connective tissue in the body of the male genitalia. All deformations of the penis at the moment of erection, except the right angle of 90 degrees left, right, up or down. Penile curvature is an important problem in erection and quality of sexual intercourse. It also negatively affects the quality of life in the future of both women and men (Hellstrom & Bivalacqua, 2000).

In the treatment of ED, a wide range of treatment methods have been used, from minimally invasive procedures to more invasive procedures such as penile implants. Even intracavernosal injections (ICI), intracavernous stem cell therapy (SCT), and platelet-rich plasma (PRP) injections have been tried (Scott et al., 2019). Although the use of PRP in urology is new, it is increasing day by day due to positive results.

As we mentioned above, ED is a problem in which an erection is absent or cannot be achieved in sufficient time. Furthermore, its frequency increases with age; while the prevalence is 22% under the age of 40, it has been shown to be 49% between the ages of 40-70. It has been shown that the prevalence of ED increases with age and is also directly proportional to the loss of body smooth muscle mass (Moreland, 1998).

In a study conducted in 2013-2015 to evaluate the safety and efficacy of PRP in the treatment of ED, promising microscopic and macroscopic results were obtained. PRP also significantly improved intracavernosal peak systolic velocity (PSV), IIEF-5, and sexual encounter profile (SEP) scores (Chalyj et al., 2015; Epifanova et al., 2019; Epifanova et al., 2020).

PRP therapy is a profoundly powerful technique for treating and fixing erectile dysfunction among all age groups. It is exceptionally protected and does not cause any incidental effects. The impacts of PRP on harmed tissues and their regenerative capacities are very much reported. In this way, in case for a non-obtrusive, nonsurgical answer for performance issues, PRP therapy may be a decent decision for you.

Peyronie's disease (PD) is defined as a painful penile deformity resulting from tunica albuginea fibrosis (Nehra et al., 2015). The exact pathogenesis of

PD is unknown. It is considered a complex disease characterized by a genetic predisposition in its etiology and a traumatic event that occurs as a result of inflammation of the penile tissue (Bivalacqua et al., 2000).

In a case of prp method treatment in Peyronie's disease made and published by Marcovici; penile curvature angle decreased significantly after 2 months (Marcovici, 2018).

Conclusion

PRP is simple, easy to apply, cost-effective, non-invasive, and effective which are some of the benefits it provides. Due to the benefits we have mentioned, PRP has recently become a frequently used treatment method that provides orgasm, desire, satisfaction, arousal, and lubricity in women; in the treatment of erectile dysfunction and Peyronie's disease in men. Although PRP is a reliable treatment method, it is still in the trial phase for ED and PH, and it is also not included in the routine treatment algorithm. Although the exact mechanism of action of PRP is not known, it is strongly believed that it acts by regeneration of the endothelium, smooth muscle cells, and connective tissue. The available data are currently insufficient to conduct a systematic review and meta-analysis. Therefore, very large, placebo-controlled, and multicenter studies are needed to confirm or not confirm the efficacy and safety of PRP.

References

Anderson, D., Laforge, J., Ross, M. M., Vanlangendonck, R., Hasoon, J., Viswanath, O., Kaye, A. D., & Urits, I. (2022). Male sexual dysfunction. *Health Psychol Res, 10*(3), 37533. https://doi.org/10.52965/001c.37533.

Aydin, D. (2012). Sağlık çalışanı evli kadınlarda cinsel mitlere inanma durumu ve cinsel işlev bozuklukları [Belief in sexual myths and sexual dysfunctions in married women of healthcare professionals]. *Health Sciences Institute, Ankara.*

Azzena, B., Mazzoleni, F., Abatangelo, G., Zavan, B., & Vindigni, V. (2008). Autologous platelet-rich plasma as an adipocyte in vivo delivery system: Case report. *Aesthetic Plast Surg, 32*(1), 155-158. https://doi.org/10.1007/s00266-007-9022-9.

Bivalacqua, T. J., Diner, E. K., Novak, T. E., Vohra, Y., Sikka, S. C., Champion, H. C., Kadowitz, P. J., & Hellstrom, W. J. G. (2000). A rat model of Peyronie's disease associated with a decrease in erectile activity and an increase in inducible nitric oxide synthase protein expression. *The Journal of Urology, 163*(6), 1992-1998. https://doi.org/10.1016/S0022-5347(05)67616-1.

Bozkurt, A., Özmenler, K. N., Karlıdere, T., Işıklı, H., Gülsün, M., Ak, M., Yetkin, S., Özgen, F., Özşahin, A., & Aydın, H. İ. (2013). Characteristics of male sexual dysfunction subjects from a sociocultural perspective: Analysis of 18 years. *New/Yeni Symposium Journal, 51*,1.

Burnett, A. L., Nehra, A., Breau, R. H., Culkin, D. J., Faraday, M. M., Hakim, L. S., Heidelbaugh, J., Khera, M., McVary, K. T., Miner, M. M., Nelson, C. J., Sadeghi-Nejad, H., Seftel, A. D., & Shindel, A. W. (2018). Erectile Dysfunction: AUA Guideline. *The Journal of Urology, 200*(3), 633-641. https://doi.org/10.1016/j.juro.2018.05.004.

Burri, A., & Spector, T. (2011). Recent and lifelong sexual dysfunction in a female UK population sample: Prevalence and risk factors. *The Journal of Sexual Medicine, 8*(9), 2420-2430.

Carroll, R. J., Arnoczky, S. P., Graham, S., & O'Connell, S. M. (2005). Characterization of autologous growth factors in Cascade platelet rich fibrin matrix (PRFM). *Edison, NJ: Musculoskeletal Transplant Foundation*.

Chalyj, M., Grigorjan, V., Epifanova, M., & Krasnov, A. (2015). The effectiveness of intracavernous autologous platelet-rich plasma in the treatment of erectile dysfunction. *Urologiia*, 4, 76-79.

Dhillon, R. S., Schwarz, E. M., & Maloney, M. D. (2012). Platelet-rich plasma therapy-future or trend? *Arthritis Research & Therapy, 14*(4), 1-10.

EAU. (2009). European Association of Urology Guidelines 2009 Edition. Retrieved from https://uroweb.org/eau-guidelines/male-sexual-dysfunction/2009.

Epifanova, M., Gvasalia, B., Chaliy, M., & Artemenko, S. (2019, April). Combined therapy for treating erectile dysfunction: First results on the use of low-intensity extracorporeal shock wave therapy and platelet-rich plasma. *Bju International, 123*, 25-25.

Epifanova, M. V., Gvasalia, B. R., Durashov, M. A., & Artemenko, S. A. (2020). Platelet-rich plasma therapy for male sexual dysfunction: Myth or reality? *Sexual Medicine Reviews, 8*(1), 106-113.

Gaber, M. A., & Shaltout, S. A. (2021). Assessment of autologous platelet-rich plasma as a local therapy for female sexual dysfunction. *Menoufia Medical Journal, 34*(1), 61.

Hellstrom, W. J., & Bivalacqua, T. J. (2000). Peyronie's disease: etiology, medical, and surgical therapy. *J Androl, 21*(3), 347-354.

İncesu, C. (2004). Cinsel işlevler ve cinsel işlev bozuklukları [Sexual functions and sexual dysfunctions]. *Journal of Clinical Psychiatry, 7*(Suppl 3), 3-13.

Jain, A., Bedi, R. K., & Mittal, K. (2015). Platelet-rich plasma therapy: A novel application in regenerative medicine. *Asian J Transfus Sci, 9*(2), 113-114. https://doi.org/10.4103/0973-6247.162679.

Johannes, C. B., Araujo, A. B., Feldman, H. A., Derby, C. A., Kleinman, K. P., & McKINLAY, J. B. (2000). Incidence of erectile dysfunction in men 40 to 69 years old: longitudinal results from the Massachusetts male aging study. *The Journal of Urology, 163*(2), 460-463.

Kakudo, N., Minakata, T., Mitsui, T., Kushida, S., Notodihardjo, F. Z., & Kusumoto, K. (2008). Proliferation-promoting effect of platelet-rich plasma on human adipose-derived stem cells and human dermal fibroblasts. *Plast Reconstr Surg, 122*(5), 1352-1360. https://doi.org/10.1097/PRS.0b013e3181882046.

Kaplan, H. S. (2014). *Yeni cinsel terapi: Cinsel işlev bozukluklarının etkin tedavisi* [New sex therapy: effective treatment of sexual dysfunctions]. Ankara: Ck Publishing House.

Keçe, C. (2013). *Cinselliğin Dayanılmaz Ağırlığı Sağlıklı ve Mutlu Bir Cinsel Yaşama Yardımcı Olan Teknikler* [The Unbearable Weight of Sexuality Techniques That Help A Healthy And Happy Sexual Life] (2nd Edition). Ankara: Compass Publishing House.

Kon, E., Mandelbaum, B., Buda, R., Filardo, G., Delcogliano, M., Timoncini, A., Fornasari, P. M., Giannini, S., & Marcacci, M. (2011). Platelet-rich plasma intra-articular injection versus hyaluronic acid viscosupplementation as treatments for cartilage pathology: from early degeneration to osteoarthritis. *Arthroscopy, 27*(11), 1490-1501. https://doi.org/10.1016/j.arthro.2011.05.011.

Marcovici, I. (2018). PRP and correction of penile curvature (Peyronie's Disease). *The American Journal of Cosmetic Surgery, 36*(3), 117-120. https://doi.org/10.1177/0748806818798280.

Martin, S. A., Atlantis, E., Lange, K., Taylor, A. W., O'Loughlin, P., & Wittert, G. A. (2014). Predictors of sexual dysfunction incidence and remission in men. *The Journal of Sexual Medicine, 11*(5), 1136-1147.

Martínez-Zapata, M. J., Martí-Carvajal, A., Solà, I., Bolibar, I., Angel Expósito, J., Rodriguez, L., & García, J. (2009). Efficacy and safety of the use of autologous plasma rich in platelets for tissue regeneration: A systematic review. *Transfusion, 49*(1), 44-56. https://doi.org/10.1111/j.1537-2995.2008.01945.x

Meston, C. M., & Buss, D. M. (2007). Why humans have sex. *Archives of Sexual Behavior, 36*, 477-507.

Moreira Jr, E. D., Lbo, C. F. L., Diament, A., Nicolosi, A., & Glasser, D. B. (2003). Incidence of erectile dysfunction in men 40 to 69 years old: results from a population-based cohort study in Brazil. *Urology, 61*(2), 431-436.

Moreland, R. B. (1998). Is there a role of hypoxemia in penile fibrosis: a viewpoint presented to the Society for the Study of Impotence. *International Journal of Impotence Research, 10*(2), 113-120. https://doi.org/10.1038/sj.ijir.3900328.

Nehra, A., Alterowitz, R., Culkin, D. J., Faraday, M. M., Hakim, L. S., Heidelbaugh, J. J., Khera, M., Kirkby, E., McVary, K. T., Miner, M. M., Nelson, C. J., Sadeghi-Nejad, H., Seftel, A. D., Shindel, A. W., & Burnett, A. L. (2015). Peyronie's Disease: AUA Guideline. *The Journal of Urology, 194*(3), 745-753. https://doi.org/10.1016/j.juro.2015.05.098.

Neto, J. (2017). O-Shot: Platelet rich plasma in intimate female treatment. *J Women's Health Care, 6*, 395.

Özdel, O. (2001). Cinsel İşlev Bozukluklarının Anksiyete ve Depresyonla İlişkisi ile Organisite Ayırımında Nörofizyolojik İnceleme Yöntemlerinin Rolü [The Role of Neurophysiological Examination Methods in the Relation of Sexual Dysfunctions with Anxiety and Depression and Organism Distinction] Unpublished Specialization

Thesis. Pamukkale University Faculty of Medicine, Department of Psychiatry, Denizli.

Puppo, V. (2013). Anatomy and physiology of the clitoris, vestibular bulbs, and labia minora with a review of the female orgasm and the prevention of female sexual dysfunction. *Clinical Anatomy, 26*(1), 134-152.

Ramos, E. S. M., Fonteles, L. A., Lagalhard, C. S., & Fucci-da-Costa, A. P. (2013). STYLAGE®: a range of hyaluronic acid dermal fillers containing mannitol. Physical properties and review of the literature. *Clin Cosmet Investig Dermatol, 6*, 257-261. https://doi.org/10.2147/ccid.S35251.

Runels, C., Melnick, H., Debourbon, E., & Roy, L. (2014). A pilot study of the effect of localized injections of autologous platelet rich plasma (PRP) for the treatment of female sexual dysfunction. *J Women's Health Care, 3*(169), 2167-0420. https://doi.org/10.4172/2167-0420.1000169.

Sclafani, A. P. (2011). Safety, efficacy, and utility of platelet-rich fibrin matrix in facial plastic surgery. *Arch Facial Plast Surg, 13*(4), 247-251. https://doi.org/10.1001/archfacial.2011.3.

Scott, S., Roberts, M., & Chung, E. (2019). Platelet-rich plasma and treatment of erectile dysfunction: Critical review of literature and global trends in platelet-rich plasma clinics. *Sex Med Rev, 7*(2), 306-312. https://doi.org/10.1016/j.sxmr.2018.12.006.

Sukgen, G., Ellibeş Kaya, A., Karagün, E., & Çalışkan, E. (2019). Platelet-rich plasma administration to the lower anterior vaginal wall to improve female sexuality satisfaction. *Turk J Obstet Gynecol, 16*(4), 228-234. https://doi.org/10.4274/tjod.galenos.2019.23356.

Chapter 17

PRP Treatment for Anal Fistula

Zumrud Aliyeva[1,*], MD
and Aykhan Abbasov[2], MD
[1]Department of General Surgery, Central Neftchilar Hospital, Baku, Azerbaijan
[2]Department of General Surgery, EGE Hospital, Baku, Azerbaijan

Abstract

An anal fistula is one of the common benign illnesses of the anorectum seen by coloproctologists. The main goal of surgery is to eradicate the fistula and preserve anal continence. However, anal fistula treatment, especially in complex fistulas, still had a high risk of recurrences ranging to %50 despite these surgical techniques. Local application of platelet-rich plasma PRP can be a new era in the treatment of anal fistula, both alone and in order to increase surgical success. Having been defined as a treatment in selected complex cryptogenic fistula –in-ano, autologous PRP is regarded safe and equivalent to commercial fibrin glue, which is less expensive. The combined the Lift-Prp technique in a high perianal fistula increases healing results from 59% to 77% compared to the alone LIFT technique. The combined use of PRP with other surgical techniques accelerates the range of cure rate to 83%. Another difficult problem to overcome is the anal fistulas that develop due to inflammatory bowel diseases. Combining the mucosal advancement flap with platelet-rich plasma in patients suffering from Crohn's disease–related high perianal fistulas enables moderate consequences such as the healing rate accounting for 70% of the total figure. In conclusion, the use of PRP for the closure of the perianal fistula is a novel alternative method that may offer significant benefits.

* Corresponding Author's Email: dr.zumrudaliyeva@gmail.com.

In: Current Clinical Recommendations ...
Editors: Nazan Yurtcu and Emel Güler
ISBN: 979-8-89113-723-3

Platelet-rich plasma can be considered a safe, effective, alternative, and additional treatment to surgery in the anal fistula.

Keywords: platelet-rich plasma, anal fistula, cryptoglandular fistulas

Introduction

Having been one of the common benign illnesses of the anorectum observed by coloproctologists, anal fistula subjected 12.3 and 5.6 per 100,000 men and women to suffer this trouble, respectively (Sainio, 1984). Along with complaints such as involuntary smelly discharge, itching, and pain in the anal region, it can also cause serious social and psychological disorders in patients. The main goal of surgery is to eradicate the fistula and preserve anal continence (Irel, 2002). The treatment of a simple fistula is usually completed with a fistulotomy, which is healing for approximately 90% of patients and has a low risk of incontinence (Van Onkelen et al., 2014). But the discussed problem lies in the management of complex fistulas, with a risk of incontinence and recurrence. There are two main classes of surgical techniques in examining the disease, each of which includes partial sphincter–preserving procedure (cutting seton, fistulectomy, fistulotomy), while the other is sphincter– conserving procedure (mucosal advancement flap, video-assisted anal fistula treatment, over the scope clip, the ligation of intersphincteric fistula tract, fibrins, and plugs)– undergone long-term development, which still is. However, anal fistula treatment especially in complex fistulas still had a high risk of recurrences ranging to %50 despite these surgical techniques (Dudukgian et al., 2011, Soew-Choen et al., 1991). Not only does Fistula recurrence leave its advertising impact on the surgeon–patient relationship, but also the patient's life base (Di Cristofaro et al., 2014). The postoperative scars and tissue fibrosis, which require the anal sphincter, trigger some difficulties while treating recurrent anal fistulas. Due to the dense and poorly vascularized canal tissue, the healing process deteriorates. Despite the fact that in case the surgery is limited, it would induce recurrence, and aggressive management would be mainly caused by fecal incontinence (Whiteford et al., 2005).

Local application of platelet-rich plasma PRP can be a new era in the treatment of anal fistula, both alone and in order to increase surgical success. PRP is easy to obtain and apply and since it is an autologous liquid, it does not have any allergic or other side effects. In most studies, the preparation of autologous PRP was based on the method previously described by Anitua, collected in a sterilized container composed of 3.8% sodium citrate, 40 ml peripheral venous blood sample was prepared by PRP (Anitua, 2000). In general, we can explain the usefulness of PRP in anal fistula with a few factors, the first of which is that a fibrin clot, plays the role of scaffolding for granulocytes, endothelial cells, and fibroblasts following the formation of well-vascularized fresh granulation tissue and eventually in the healing process of the fistula, is formed by a range of cytokines, which have been released from platelet granularities-PDGF, TGF-B, FGF, VEGF, and IGF. Besides that, the internal orifice could be subjected to mechanical compression by locally injecting PRP fluid and the fistulas canal by edematous tissue. However, the growth factors accelerate the concentration of platelet, which enable fistula healing to accelerate considerably (Dhurat et al., 2014; Lacci et al., 2010). Due to a wide range of applications, PRP depends on the surgeon, which would be basically used alone or after surgery, around the fistula tract and inside of it.

Especially, we see that the surgical results of high complex fistulas and the recurrence rates are so high that they cannot be ignored. There are some studies that compared autologous platelet to commercial ones, featuring a lower amount of cost, autologous PRP could be equivalent to commercial fibrin glue, defined as treatment in selected complex cryptogenic fistula –in-ano, and is noted as the safest (de la Portilla et al., 2019).

At present, considered one of the most favorable techniques in high trans sphincter fistula –in-ano, LIFT, and Mucosal advancement flap have a favorable healing rate, without having any adverse effect on the continence. However, it is yet uncertain to the one why this witnesses failure in one-third of patients (Madbouly et al., 2014). Going ahead of the alone LIFT technique, the figures showing the healing rate of the patients through the method of combined LIFT-PRP in high perianal fistula changes between 59% and 77% respectively. Consequently, LIFT-PRP for the treatment of high transsphinctrecic fistula in ano could be referred to as the safe modality, featuring with significantly successful healing rate during a shorter time, subjecting the patient to comparatively less pain contrasting to LIFT alone (Khaled et al., 2021). Meanwhile, the PRP-MAF (mucosal advancement flap) technique, as well as, prove favorable results, thus the fistulous tracks with below 4 mm diameter contributed to the healing process, by exerting a considerable impact up to 87% after PRP application (Yajie et al., 2023; Qinghua et al., 2022).

The combined technique of Lift (ligation of the intersphincteric fistula tract)-PRP in a high perianal fistula increases healing results from 59% to 77% compared to the alone LIFT technique. Overall, LIFT-PRP for the treatment of high transsphincteric fistula-in-ano is a safe modality with a significantly higher successful healing rate, shorter healing time, and less postoperative pain compared to LIFT alone (Khaled et al., 2021). Similarly, combined PRP-MAF (a technique also shows good results, so the diameter of the fistulous tracts below 4 mm exerted a significant impact of up to 87% on the healing process after PRP application (Jacek et al., 2022b).

Analyzed the systematic review and meta-analysis, it can be seen that the overall cure rate of fistulas ranged from 65% to 72.11%. So, the cure rate of PRP alone composes of 62.39% of the total number. However, when PRP is combined with other applications using different surgical techniques, and it triggers acceleration in the range of cure rates up to 83%. Meanwhile, all studies experienced 12% increase in the amount of the pooled recurrence rate. As a result, according to 4 studies randomly controlled, the surgery method without PRP witnessed a significantly lower rate of cure compared to the cure rate of interventions that required the involvement of PRP (Yajie et al., 2023; Qinghua et al., 2022).

Another problem which is difficult to overcome is anal fistulas that develop due to inflammatory bowel diseases. 25% of patients with known Crohn's disease, in their life, suffer from a perianal fistula which develops usually within the first two decades after initial diagnosis (Schwartz et al., 2022). From this point of view, there is a continuous range of medical and surgical challenges represented by the management of fistulizing perianal Crohn's disease. Despite the fact that multidisciplinary care has improved considerably recently, recurrence rates still continue to show high figures, negatively impacting the life quality of young patients (Molendijk et al., 2022; Zwintscher et al., 2015). The development rate of the fistula is going through the course of IBD (inflammatory bowel disease) or after restorative proctocolectomy (IPAA), performed more frequently for ulcerative colitis (Jacek et al., 2022a). The patients suffering from Crohn's disease experience far more disappointing results in the healing rate after surgical closure due to high perianal fistula compared to those (patients) with cryptoglandular fistula. Combining the mucosal advancement flap with platelet-rich plasma in patients with Crohn's disease-related high perianal fistulas enable a moderate healing rate composing 70% of the total figure (Gottgens et al., 2015).

Conclusion

In conclusion, the application of PRP in the closure of the perianal fistula is a novel alternative method that may offer significant benefits. It gives 62% of the cure rate in criptoglandular fistula in use alone and 83% of the cure with combined techniques without impairing continence. On the other hand, complex fistulas and IBD-related fistulas have difficulties with healing rates, recurrent rates, and continence. And there are also favorable results in PRP injections combined with surgery. When you use a combined technique of application PRP, it is important to choose the right time of surgery, so the surgical area should be clean at the time of surgery for favorable results. If there is an abscess or purulent fluid leaking, it would be better not to place the cutting seton and in the second round of surgery do the combined technique with PRP injection. Furthermore, as this is an autologous product, there is no rejection risk and minimizes infection risk. Platelet-rich plasma can be considered a safe, effective, alternative, and additional treatment to surgery in the anal fistula. Notwithstanding this, to achieve adequate results, we need further studies in clinical practice.

References

Anitua, E. (2000). Plasma rich in growth factors: Preliminary results of use in the preparation of future sites for implants. *International Journal of Oral and Maxillofacial Implants, 14*, 529–535. PMID: 10453668.

de la Portilla, F., Muñoz-Cruzado, M. V. D., Maestre, M. V., García-Cabrera, A. M., Reyes, M. L., Vázquez-Monchul, J. M., Jimenez-Rodríguez, R. M., Díaz-Pavón, J. M., & Padillo, F. J. (2019). Platelet-rich plasma (PRP) versus fibrin glue in cryptogenic fistula-in-ano: A phase III single-center, randomized, double-blind trial. *International Journal of Colorectal Disease, 34*, 1113-1119. https://doi.org/10.1007/s00384-019-03290-6.

Dhurat, R., & Sukesh, M. (2014). Principles and methods of preparation of platelet-rich plasma: A review and author's perspective. *Journal of Cutaneous and Aesthetic Surgery, 7*, 189-197. https://doi.org/10.4103/0974-2077.150734.

Di Cristofaro, L., Ruffolo, C., Pinto, E., Massa, M., Antoniutti, M., Cagol, M., Massani, M., Alfieri, R., Costa, A., Bassi, N., Castoro, C., & Scarpa, M. (2014). Complications after surgery for colorectal cancer affect quality of life and surgeon-patient relationship. *Colorectal Disease: Official Journal of the Association of Coloproctology, 16*, 407-419. https://doi.org/10.1111/codi.12752.

Dudukgian, H., & Abcarian, H. (2011). Why do we have so much trouble treating anal fistula? *World Journal of Gastroenterology, 17*, 3292-3296. https://doi.org/10.3748/wjg.v17.i28.3292.

Gottgens, K. W. A., Smeets, R. R., Stassen, L. P. S., Beets, G. L., Pierik, M., & Breukink, S. O. (2015). Treatment of Crohn's disease-related high perianal fistulas combining the mucosa advancement flap with platelet-rich plasma: A pilot study. *Techniques in Coloproctology, 19*, 455–459. https://doi.org/10.1007/s10151-015-1311-8.

Irel, G. B. (2002). The outcome of surgery for complex anal fistula. *Colorectal Disease: Official Journal of the Association of Coloproctology, 4*, 254-261. https://doi.org/10.1016/j.ijsu.2019.08.003.

Jacek, H., Jarosław, C., & Tomasz, B. (2022a). Application of platelet-rich plasma in rectovaginal fistulas in patients with ulcerative colitis. *Langenbeck's Archives of Surgery, 407*(1), 429-433. https://doi.org/10.1007/s00423-021-02232-7.

Jacek, H., Jarosław, C., Tomasz, B., & Barbara, K. (2022b). Comparison between the application of platelet-rich plasma and mucosal advancement flap in patients with high transsphincteric anal fistulas: a randomized control trial. *ANZ Journal of Surgery, 92*(5), 1137-1141. https://doi.org/10.1111/ans.17656.

Khaled, M. M., Sameh, H. E., Yasmine, A. I., & Waleed, O. (2021). Ligation of intersphincteric fistula tract (LIFT) with or without injection of platelet-rich plasma (PRP) in the management of high trans-sphincteric fistula-in-ano: Short-term outcomes of a prospective, randomized trial. *Surgery, 170*(1), 61-66. https://doi.org/10.1016/j.surg.2020.12.025.

Lacci, K. M., & Dardik, A. (2010). Platelet-rich plasma: Support for its use in wound healing. *Yale Journal of Biology and Medicine, 83*, 1-9. PMC2844688.

Madbouly, K. M., El Shazly, W., Abbas, K. S., & Hussein, A. M. (2014). Ligation of intersphincteric fistula tract versus mucosal advancement flap in patients with high transsphincteric fistula-in-ano: a prospective randomized trial. *Diseases of the Colon & Rectum, 57*, 1202-1208. https://doi.org/10.1097/DCR.0000000000000194.

Molendijk, I., Nuij, V. J., van der Meulen-de Jong, A. E., & van der Woude, C. J. (2014). Disappointing durable remission rates in complex Crohn's disease fistula. *Inflammatory Bowel Diseases, 20*, 2022–2028. https://doi.org/10.1097/MIB.0000000000000148.

Qinghua, L., Ping, Z., & Shuangqing, C. (2022). Meta-analysis of platelet-rich plasma therapy for anal fistula. *Journal of Cosmetic Dermatology, 21*(10), 4559-4566. https://doi.org/10.1111/jocd.14760.

Sainio, P. (1984). Fistula-in-ano in a defined population: Incidence and epidemiological aspects. *Annals of Chirurgiae et Gynaecologiae, 73*, 219-224.

Schwartz, D. A., Loftus, E. V., Tremaine, W. J., Panaccione, R., Harmsen, W. S., Zinsmeister, A. R., & Sandborn, W. J. (2022). The natural history of fistulizing Crohn's disease in Olmsted County, Minnesota. *Gastroenterology, 122*, 875–880. https://doi.org/10.1053/gast.2002.32362.

Soew-Choen, F., Burnett, S., Bartram, C. I., & Nicholls, R. J. (1991). Comparison between anal endosonography and digital examination in the evaluation of anal fistulas. *British Journal of Surgery, 78*, 445-447. https://doi.org/10.1002/bjs.1800780418.

Van Onkelen, R. S., Gosselink, M. P., Van Rosmalen, J., Thijsse, S., & Schouten, W. R. (2014). Different characteristics of high and low transsphincteric fistulae. *Colorectal Disease, 16*, 471-475. https://doi.org/10.1111/codi.12578.

Whiteford, M. H., Kilkenny, J. 3rd, Hyman, N., Buie, W. D., Cohen, J., Orsay, C., Dunn, G., Perry, W. B., Ellis, C. N., Rakinic, J., Gregorcyk, S., Shellito, P., Nelson, R., Tjandra, J. J., Newstead, G., & The Standards Practice Task Force. (2005). Practice parameters for the treatment of perianal abscess and fistula-in-ano (revised). *Diseases of the Colon & Rectum, 48*, 1337–1342. https://doi.org/10.1007/s10350-004-0921-4.

Yajie, W., Quan, R., Yiming, M., & Xiaofei, L. (2023). Platelet-rich plasma in the treatment of anal fistula: A systematic review and meta-analysis. *International Journal of Colorectal Disease, 38*(1), 70. https://doi.org/10.1007/s00384-023-04367-z.

Zwintscher, N. P., Shah, P. M., Argawal, A., Chesley, P. M., Johnson, E. K., Newton, C. R., Maykel, J. A., & Steele, S. R. (2015). The impact of perianal disease in young patients with inflammatory bowel disease. *International Journal of Colorectal Disease, 30*, 1275-1279. https://doi.org/10.1007/s00384-015-2251-5.

Chapter 18

PRP in Wound Healing Applications

Canberk Tomruk*, MD

Department of Histology and Embryology, Samsun University Samsun Education and Research Hospital, Samsun, Turkiye

Abstract

Platelets are involved in different stages of wound healing through the growth factors and cytokines they contain. Different platelet-rich plasma products containing higher platelets than normal blood have been applied in experimental and clinical studies in different areas of regenerative medicine to use these effects of platelets. Wound healing is one of these areas, and these products show their effects by increasing angiogenesis and re-epithelialization, stimulating migration, proliferation, and differentiation of cells involved in wound healing. These effects are variable due to the variety of platelet-derived products, preparation, and application methods. Factors such as wound location, wound type, and comorbidities of the patient also contribute to this variability. With the development of more effective products with innovative methods and comprehensive studies to ensure the standardization of application doses and routes, platelet-rich plasma applications, which have been observed to have positive effects, have the potential to be used frequently in the healing process of different wounds in the future.

Keywords: PRP, wound healing, growth factors

---

* Corresponding Author's Email: canberktomruk@hotmail.com.

In: Current Clinical Recommendations ...
Editors: Nazan Yurtcu and Emel Güler
ISBN: 979-8-89113-723-3

Introduction

In addition to their critical role in hemostasis and thrombosis, platelets also participate in inflammation, tissue regeneration, and initiation and regulation of wound healing through growth factors, cytokines, and other bioactive molecules (Fréchette et al., 2005). Through these molecules, they take part in tissue repair by contributing to fibroblast migration and proliferation, angiogenesis, and mesenchymal stem cell proliferation and differentiation processes (Etulain, 2018). Based on these effects, platelet-rich plasma (PRP), a plasma component obtained by centrifugation of whole blood, has been frequently used in clinical and experimental studies in the field of regenerative medicine in recent years with the advantages of being economical, autologous origin, and easy to apply (Dhurat & Sukesh, 2014; Etulain, 2018).

PRP has a platelet concentration about 3-7 times higher than normal blood. The clinically useful concentration of PRP is thought to be 1 million/microliter (Hesseler & Shyam, 2019; Smith et al., 2019). Platelets contain mitogenic and chemotactic growth factors such as platelet-derived growth factor (PDGF), vascular endothelial growth factor (VEGF), transforming growth factor β (TGF-β), insulin-like growth factor (IGF), fibroblast growth factor (FGF), and epithelial growth factor (EGF), which are released from α-granules when they are activated. In addition, cytokines secreted from granules are involved in cell migration, and serotonin and histamine are involved in the inflammation phase of wound healing (Foster et al., 2009; Maisel-Campbell et al., 2020; Pallua et al., 2009). Platelets that release growth factors with PRP application increase the healing effect by synthesizing and releasing growth factors for the rest of their life span (Marx, 2001). Platelets are also thought to have antimicrobial and immune modulatory properties that help reduce wound infection and facilitate healing (Smith et al., 2019).

The use of platelet-derived products in regenerative medicine has started since the 1990s, and its use has been increasing with *in vivo* and *in vitro* studies in many different fields such as orthopedics, ophthalmology, and dermatology (Etulain, 2018). Studies have shown that PRP applications facilitate wound remodeling by reducing dermal scarring while increasing recollagenation, angiogenesis, wound strength, hemostasis, and tissue regeneration (Cieślik-Bielecka et al., 2018).

PRP Types

In PRP production, in general, 10-60 mL of whole blood is collected, anticoagulants are added, and centrifugation is applied to separate cell types (Hesseler & Shyam, 2019). However, there are PRP-derived products with different preparation protocols and different platelet and growth factor content. The PRP types are classified according to their leukocyte and fibrin content.

Pure-platelet-rich plasma (P-PRP) is a pure platelet concentration without leukocytes, prepared with cell separators and collecting the most superficial buffy coat sub-plasma portion. Leukocyte-platelet-rich plasma (L-PRP) does not require special cell separators, and the entire buffy coat is collected. Pure-platelet-rich fibrin (P-PRF) is prepared by adding calcium chloride to form a platelet-fibrin clot. Leukocyte-platelet-rich fibrin (L-PRF) is prepared by slow centrifugation without the addition of an anticoagulant (Cieślik-Bielecka et al., 2018; Hesseler & Shyam, 2019). PRF may have advantages over PRP due to the absence of an anticoagulant, longer growth factor release from the fibrin gel, and antimicrobial effects of leukocytes trapped in the gel (Gentile et al., 2021). PRP has also been shown to have antibacterial activity, but these effects are limited because they are short-term and weak (Shao et al., 2020). When preparing 'plasma-rich in growth factors' or 'preparations rich in growth factors' (PRGF), a single centrifugation is performed, sodium citrate is used as an anticoagulant, and calcium chloride is used as an activator. The absence of leukocytes in PRGF prevents increased inflammation in inflammatory disorders (Anitua et al., 2007; 2021). There are also types of PRP that differ from PRP and PRGF, such as platelet-rich eye plasma (E-PRP) used in ophthalmology. E-PRP, which is inexpensive and easy to prepare in the form of eye drops and clots, can be used as an effective treatment method in ophthalmologic pathologies such as corneal ulcers, dry eye syndrome, and ocular surface syndrome after Laser In Situ Keratomileusis (LASIK), as it contains growth factors and cell adhesion molecules (L. Alio et al., 2012).

Although it is theoretically conceivable that the administration of products containing only a single growth factor, such as recombinant human platelet-derived growth factor-BB (rhPDGF-BB), can be more effective, their short life span and bolus administration are disadvantages compared to PRP. In addition, the fact that studies show that PDGF-BB expression is associated with malignant transformation and that PRP is autologous, contains multiple growth factors similar to natural wound healing and can act by slow release rather than bolus through platelet plug makes PRP more advantageous (Govindarajan et al., 2005; Lacci & Dardik, 2010).

In PRP preparation, variables such as patient age, platelet count, and medication history affect the product obtained. Studies showing that cytokines such as interleukin (IL)-1β and tumor necrosis factor (TNF) are higher in PRPs prepared from men compared to PRPs prepared from women show that gender is another factor. While a low platelet concentration of the resulting product prevents a sufficient effect, high concentrations can also have an inhibitory effect and impair wound healing (Shao et al., 2020; Weibrich et al., 2004; Xiong et al., 2018).

The effect of all these different PRP products is variable in the treatment of different pathologies, and there is no standardized procedure.

Wound Healing

Wounds that develop due to disruption of the body's tissue integrity and functioning heal through physiological processes that develop to restore normal structure and function. Hemostasis, inflammation, proliferation, and remodeling constitute the four phases of wound healing (Rittié, 2016). The proper progression of these processes plays an important role in effective and proper wound healing.

Immediately after tissue damage, the coagulation process begins rapidly, hemostasis occurs, and the platelet plug adheres to the damaged endothelium of the vessels. Fibrin strands reinforce this plug. In the inflammatory phase, neutrophils and monocytes, which transform into macrophages and remove damaged structures and pathogens, arrive at the wound site. The vessels dilate to facilitate the migration of cells and allow wound-healing substances such as growth factors, nutrients, and antibodies to reach the site, leading to an increase in interstitial fluid and edema. The proliferation phase begins approximately one week later, during which the migration, differentiation, and proliferation of healing cells are at the forefront. With type 3 collagen secreted from fibroblasts, the hemostatic clot transforms into granulation tissue. As a result of the remodeling of this tissue over time, a scar develops. Systemic and local factors such as infection, burns, steroids, radiotherapy, ischemia, and diabetes delay wound healing and may lead to chronic wounds or hypertrophic scarring (Gökkaya et al., 2022; Smith et al., 2019; Zhou et al., 2021).

Growth Factors Involved in Wound Healing

After tissue damage, platelets are involved in hemostasis, and the growth factors released from activated platelets contribute to wound healing (Gökkaya et al., 2022).

Many studies have shown that growth factors such as PDGF, EGF, FGF, VEGF, IGF, and TGF-β are effective in healing. Increasing the concentration of these growth factors released from activated platelets in the fibrin clot with PRP applications is thought to have a therapeutic effect (Bijl et al., 2019; Ebrahim et al., 2021; Roubelakis et al., 2014). These growth factors bind to the transmembrane receptors of cells and induce the expression of genes associated with collagen synthesis, angiogenesis, macrophage chemotaxis, cell division, and proliferation. Platelet concentrates containing leukocytes also contribute to the resistance of wounds to infection (Bijl et al., 2019; He et al., 2022; Shi et al., 2021). Studies have shown that wound healing is impaired in *Nbeal2*-knockout mice lacking α-granules (Deppermann et al., 2013). The Notch signaling pathway, which is involved in determining cell fate, has also been shown to play a role in the regulation of impaired proliferation, angiogenesis, and apoptosis/survival processes in diabetic wounds (Siebel & Lendahl, 2017). Studies are showing that PRP is effective in wound healing by modulation of this pathway. In the study by Ebrahim et al., the combined efficacy of the application of PRP and adipose-derived mesenchymal stem cell (ADSC) was examined in a diabetic wound model developed in rats. It was observed that epidermal thickness and angiogenesis increased more in the combined application group compared to their individual applications, and Notch signaling pathway-related expressions, which increased in the non-application diabetic group, were down-regulated in the treatment groups, more in the combined application group (Ebrahim et al., 2021).

The mechanisms of action of the growth factors contained in platelets and the stage of wound healing in which they are effective are different from each other. PDGF promotes angiogenesis and stimulates the migration, proliferation, and differentiation of cells involved in wound healing. It promotes wound contraction and granulation tissue formation (Barrientos et al., 2008; Smith et al., 2019). In the study by Rees et al., topically applied PDGF gel was shown to promote wound healing in pressure ulcers (Rees et al., 1999). VEGF contributes to epithelialization, as well as increasing angiogenesis and vascular permeability (Hsu & Chang, 2004; Smith et al., 2019; Sun et al., 2020). In diabetic foot ulcers, the administration of recombinant VEGF has been shown to promote wound healing (Hanft et al., 2008). FGF, another effective growth factor in epithelialization and angiogenesis, is found in high concentrations in PRP and is thought to be more effective in the early stages of wound healing because it is rapidly released (Smith et al., 2019; Xie et al., 2008). Ortega et al. showed that wound healing was impaired in FGF2(-/-) mice (Ortega et al., 1998). TGF-β is an important growth factor involved in all phases of wound healing and is effective in collagen synthesis and deposition in addition to its effects on angiogenesis and cell differentiation (Smith et al., 2019). IGF is also one of the growth factors found in PRP and its topical application has been shown to increase re-epithelialization in experimental animal studies (Ghiasi et al., 2018). Hepatocyte growth factor (HGF) and EGF are also known to have roles in angiogenesis and epithelialization (Conway et al., 2006; Girdler et al., 1995).

Zhou et al. tried to prevent the disadvantage caused by the short half-life of these growth factors, which are effective in wound healing, with an experimental model in which they applied PRP loaded in gelatin microspheres and obtained positive results (Zhou et al., 2021). Such applications instead of direct PRP application alone may lead to the development of more effective treatment protocols in the future.

PRP Applications in Wound Healing in Experimental and Clinical Studies

Considering that PRP exerts its effects on wound healing through growth factors, prolonging the release time of these factors may lead to more effective PRP applications. In a study in mice, the effects of PRP-loaded gelatin microspheres (GMs) on wound healing were examined in full-thickness wounds. It was observed that wound healing was accelerated, inflammatory cytokines were upregulated, and macrophage infiltration and angiogenesis increased in the PRP and GM+PRP groups. As a result of inhibition of the collective activation of platelets bound in layers in GM, it was determined that the GM+PRP group prolonged the cytokine release profile compared to the PRP-only group. This suggests that these carriers can be used as more effective therapeutic models; however, the time-consuming application and the risk of gelatin-induced immune rejection limit the widespread use of these applications for now (Zhou et al., 2021).

Hyaluronic acid, an extracellular matrix component found in tissues such as cartilage, bone, and skin, prevents dry skin and gives elasticity to the tissue. Increased production of hyaluronic acid allows it to act as a scaffold during the remodeling phase. The combination of PRP and hyaluronic acid may be an effective approach in chronic ulcers (Gentile et al., 2021; He et al., 2022). In a study by Cho et al. in mice, it was shown that the collagen and hyaluronic acid-enhancing effect of PRP was efficient on photoaging-related wrinkles (Cho et al., 2011).

Specialized wound dressings can also play an important role in the treatment of chronic infected wounds. Shi et al. showed that the application of wound dressing obtained by loading gentamicin sulfate and PRP into gelatin microspheres covalently bound to carboxymethyl chitosan was effective in both reducing infection and wound healing in infected wounds (Shi et al., 2021). The use of innovative methods such as wound-on-a-chip as in the study by Biglari et al. may provide a better understanding of the effects of different variations of PRP on the complex processes of wound healing (Biglari et al., 2019; Bijl et al., 2021).

Li et al. combined artificial dermal scaffolds with PRP and examined their effects on wounds in Bama pigs. Although artificial dermal scaffolds have good biocompatibility and mechanical strength and allow cell metabolism to progress due to their porous structure, their use in the clinic is open to improvement due to insufficient vascular regeneration. Based on the assumption that combined application would increase vascular regeneration due to the abundant VEGF content of PRP, they showed that the wound healing rate was significantly higher compared to the control in their experiment. The finding that CD31 immunopositivity, which is used to evaluate angiogenesis, was also high in the PRP+artificial dermal scaffold group shows that such products have the potential for use in diabetes-induced wounds where wound healing is impaired due to insufficient vascular regeneration (Li et al., 2022).

In a study comparing the effects of PRP with ozone and hyperbaric oxygen (HBO) treatments, which are alternative methods used in wound healing, these treatments were applied experimentally to wounds created in the oral cavity of rats. As a result of histopathological and biochemical examinations, it was determined that the PRP group had the lowest inflammation rate and the highest proliferation, vessel density, and collagenization (Uslu et al., 2020).

The increase in obesity and diabetes every day is a factor that should not be ignored regarding chronic wounds. One of the most common complications caused by diabetes is skin ulcerations. These wounds increase morbidity, and their treatment requires a long and challenging process. This is an important public health problem and can lead to prolonged hospitalizations, thus burdening health expenditures (Cialdai et al., 2020; Ebrahim et al., 2021; Roubelakis et al., 2014). In diabetic foot ulcers, one of the most common causes of lower extremity amputations, chronic inflammation, and decreased growth factor production impairs wound healing. It is thought that adjuvant PRP treatments containing these factors may contribute to the wound healing process (Nolan et al., 2021). In such wounds, the application of L-PRF can be a more effective and economical adjuvant treatment method due to the prolonged release of growth factor from the fibrin network of L-PRF compared to PRP and the effect of leukocytes (Shao et al., 2020). Different studies using L-PRP and L-PRF in patients with chronic lower extremity ulcers have shown that these applications are significantly effective in closing the ulcer area compared to the control. It has also been reported that symptoms such as pain, burning, and itching decreased in patient groups where these treatments were applied (Hesseler & Shyam, 2019; Moneib et al., 2018; Pinto et al., 2018).

In patients with comorbidities, cell proliferation is reduced and impaired proliferation and migration of keratinocytes disrupt epidermalization, leading to slow and poor wound healing. Wound site infections also negatively affect this process and scars that develop differently from surrounding tissues create an undesirable aesthetic appearance, especially in the maxillofacial regions. In the study by Menchisheva et al., 100 patients who underwent maxillofacial surgery were divided into two groups, 50 in the control group and 50 in the group with treated PRP. Ultrasound examination showed that edema and infiltration around the wound were less in the PRP-treated group compared to the control group. Fibroblasts, macrophages, and collagen fibers were also found to appear earlier in this group (Menchisheva et al., 2019).

Another approach to maximize the benefits of PRP applications is the use of PRP-derived exosomes (PRP-Exos), which are cheap and easy to produce. In the study by Xu et al., the effects of PRP-Exos and Curcuma zedoaria on the chitosan/silk hydrogel were examined wound dressing in a diabetic wound model in rats, and it was found that both separate and combination applications increased collagen synthesis and deposition, dermal angiogenesis, wound contraction, and re-epithelialization. The fact that PRP-Exos can be injected as a liquid and applied as a hydrogel sponge dressing increases its potential to be used as one of the methods that accelerate diabetic wound healing (Xu et al., 2018).

In a study conducted by Monteiro et al. in horses, it was found that TGF-β1 expression was higher in the group treated with PRP compared to the untreated control group in wounds formed in the metacarpal regions, although no histological and biomechanical differences were observed. The authors suggested that autologous topical application of PRP may be more appropriate in wounds with chronic/massive tissue loss rather than small granulation wounds (Monteiro et al., 2009). Another experimental study with autologous PRP application showed that PRP application accelerated re-epithelialization in deep partial-thickness burns in Bama pigs. The observation that Ki67 (+) cells and α-SMA (+) vessels accompanying the increase in EGF, bFGF, and VEGF levels were also higher in the PRP group showed that PRP application was effective in the treatment of deep partial-thickness wounds, which are wounds with difficult healing processes compared to simple wounds, where severe scars can develop due to burn-induced dermal damage (Sun et al., 2020).

ADSCs have angiogenic and anti-inflammatory effects and the potential to differentiate into various cells. Due to the growth factors they secrete, autologous free fat transfer containing ADSCs is thought to be beneficial in wound healing and these effects have been investigated in various studies (Marangi et al., 2014; Previnaire et al., 2016; Rigotti et al., 2007; Smith et al., 2018). The synergistic effects of PRP have also been examined in many studies such as the one reviewed by Smith et al. (Smith et al., 2019). In the case study of Salemi et al. in which autologous adipose tissue and a combination of PRP were applied, it was observed that wound healing was completed, and limb function was regained at 15 months in a 65-year-old male patient with a three-year lower extremity ulcer (Salemi et al., 2008). With the synergistic effect of PRP, which acts as a scaffold for adipocytes and stem cells, allowing these cells to remain in the graft area for a long time, it was concluded that ADSCs secreted higher VEGF and FGF, thus increasing graft vascularization, decreasing necrosis, and increasing graft survival. The combined application with PRP may become an even more effective method if standardization is achieved in future studies due to both the increase in graft survival and the effect of growth factors that both have (Smith et al., 2019).

Otolaryngology is one of the clinical areas where PRP applications are used. In a study by Yildirim et al. that examined the effects of submucosal PRP injection in a model of endoscopic sinus surgery in rabbits, it was observed that PRP application had anti-inflammatory and mucus viscosity-reducing effects by reducing neutrophil and goblet cell counts and decreasing collagen density (Yildirim et al., 2020). In another study, after the application of nasal packings with saline and PRP to half of 50 patients in the postoperative period after endonasal surgery, it was observed that PRP accelerated the healing of septal and conchal mucosa and reduced the complaints of the patients (Kuzucu et al., 2017).

Finally, as a glance to the future, manned space missions to the Moon and Mars, which are planned to be carried out in the near future, will create situations where the 'treatment after stabilization and emergency return to Earth' approach applied to injuries so far will not be possible. Under these conditions, it is important to examine differences in wound healing mechanisms and plan treatment methods. For this reason, Cialdai et al. created a sutured wound model in leeches (Hirudo Medicalis) and investigated the effects of microgravity and the role of PRP application in preventing microgravity-induced changes and found that PRP was particularly effective in preventing microgravity-induced impairment of fibroblast migration to the wound site (Cialdai et al., 2020).

Conclusion

Factors such as the variety of PRP preparation methods, the timing, dose, and frequency of application, the patient's comorbidities, and the location, area, and depth of the wound lead to different clinical results. In order to prevent the variability in platelet count and function caused by autologous blood collection from patients, the use of PRP products produced from blood taken from healthy donors can ensure that standard products are given to patients.

In conclusion, PRP applications are frequently used in the treatment of acute and chronic wounds, and there are many studies showing positive effects. More in vitro and in vivo studies are needed to better understand these effects and develop standard application doses and methods. As multicenter randomized trials and systematic evaluations of the results of clinical use are conducted, qualified clinical evidence will be obtained and it will be possible to apply PRP products with optimal composition in both wound healing and other regenerative medicine fields.

References

Anitua, E., Pino, A., Aspe, L., Martínez, M., García, A., Goñi, F., & Troya, M. (2021). Anti-inflammatory effect of different PRGF formulations on cutaneous surface. *Journal of Tissue Viability, 30*(2), 183–189. https://doi.org/10.1016/j.jtv.2021.02.011.

Anitua, E., Sánchez, M., Orive, G., & Andía, I. (2007). The potential impact of the preparation rich in growth factors (PRGF) in different medical fields. *Biomaterials, 28*(31), 4551–4560. https://doi.org/10.1016/j.biomaterials.2007.06.037.

Barrientos, S., Stojadinovic, O., Golinko, M. S., Brem, H., & Tomic-Canic, M. (2008). Growth factors and cytokines in wound healing. *Wound Repair and Regeneration, 16*(5), 585–601. https://doi.org/10.1111/j.1524-475X.2008.00410.x.

Biglari, S., Le, T. Y. L., Tan, R. P., Wise, S. G., Zambon, A., Codolo, G., De Bernard, M., Warkiani, M., Schindeler, A., Naficy, S., Valtchev, P., Khademhosseini, A., & Dehghani, F. (2019). Simulating inflammation in a wound microenvironment using a dermal wound-on-a-chip model. *Advanced Healthcare Materials, 8*(1), 1801307. https://doi.org/10.1002/adhm.201801307.

Bijl, I., Korte, D., & Middelkoop, E. (2021). Variation in platelet-rich plasma compositions used for wound healing indications. *Wound Repair and Regeneration, 29*(2), 284–287. https://doi.org/10.1111/wrr.12886.

Bijl, I., Vlig, M., Middelkoop, E., & Korte, D. (2019). Allogeneic platelet-rich plasma (PRP) is superior to platelets or plasma alone in stimulating fibroblast proliferation and migration, angiogenesis, and chemotaxis as relevant processes for wound healing. *Transfusion, 59*(11), 3492–3500. https://doi.org/10.1111/trf.15535.

Cho, J. M., Lee, Y. H., Baek, R.-M., & Lee, S. W. (2011). Effect of platelet-rich plasma on ultraviolet B-induced skin wrinkles in nude mice. *Journal of Plastic, Reconstructive & Aesthetic Surgery, 64*(2), e31–e39. https://doi.org/10.1016/j.bjps.2010.08.014.

Cialdai, F., Colciago, A., Pantalone, D., Rizzo, A. M., Zava, S., Morbidelli, L., Celotti, F., Bani, D., & Monici, M. (2020). Effect of unloading condition on the healing process and effectiveness of platelet rich plasma as a countermeasure: Study on in vivo and in vitro wound healing models. *International Journal of Molecular Sciences, 21*(2), 407. https://doi.org/10.3390/ijms21020407.

Cieślik-Bielecka, A., Pierchała, M., Królikowska, A., & Reichert, P. (2018). Effect of L-PRP treatment on wound healing after surgical skin incision in an experimental animal model. *Connective Tissue Research, 59*(6), 550–560. https://doi.org/10.1080/03008207.2018.1424148.

Conway, K., Price, P., Harding, K. G., & Jiang, W. G. (2006). The molecular and clinical impact of hepatocyte growth factor, its receptor, activators, and inhibitors in wound healing. *Wound Repair and Regeneration, 14*(1), 2–10. https://doi.org/10.1111/j.1743-6109.2005.00081.x.

Deppermann, C., Cherpokova, D., Nurden, P., Schulz, J.-N., Thielmann, I., Kraft, P., Vögtle, T., Kleinschnitz, C., Dütting, S., Krohne, G., Eming, S. A., Nurden, A. T., Eckes, B., Stoll, G., Stegner, D., & Nieswandt, B. (2013). Gray platelet syndrome and defective thrombo-inflammation in Nbeal2-deficient mice. *Journal of Clinical Investigation, 123*(8), 3331–3342. https://doi.org/10.1172/JCI69210.

Dhurat, R., & Sukesh, M. (2014). Principles and methods of preparation of platelet-rich plasma: A review and author's perspective. *Journal of Cutaneous and Aesthetic Surgery, 7*(4), 189. https://doi.org/10.4103/0974-2077.150734.

Ebrahim, N., Dessouky, A. A., Mostafa, O., Hassouna, A., Yousef, M. M., Seleem, Y., El Gebaly, E. A. E. A. M., Allam, M. M., Farid, A. S., Saffaf, B. A., Sabry, D., Nawar, A., Shoulah, A. A., Khalil, A. H., Abdalla, S. F., El-Sherbiny, M., Elsherbiny, N. M., & Salim, R. F. (2021). Adipose mesenchymal stem cells combined with platelet-rich plasma accelerate diabetic wound healing by modulating the Notch pathway. *Stem Cell Research & Therapy, 12*(1), 392. https://doi.org/10.1186/s13287-021-02454-y.

Etulain, J. (2018). Platelets in wound healing and regenerative medicine. *Platelets, 29*(6), 556–568. https://doi.org/10.1080/09537104.2018.1430357.

Foster, T. E., Puskas, B. L., Mandelbaum, B. R., Gerhardt, M. B., & Rodeo, S. A. (2009). Platelet-rich plasma. *The American Journal of Sports Medicine, 37*(11), 2259–2272. https://doi.org/10.1177/0363546509349921.

Fréchette, J.-P., Martineau, I., & Gagnon, G. (2005). Platelet-rich plasmas: Growth factor content and roles in wound healing. *Journal of Dental Research, 84*(5), 434–439. https://doi.org/10.1177/154405910508400507.

Gentile, P., Alves, R., Cole, J. P., Andjelkov, K., Van Helmelryck, T., Fernandez, J., Trivisonno, A., Guillaume, L., Verpaele, A., Tonnard, P., Magalon, J., Magalon, G., & Menkes, S. (2021). AIRMESS – Academy of International Regenerative Medicine & Surgery Societies: Recommendations in the use of platelet-rich plasma (PRP), autologous stem cell-based therapy (ASC-BT) in androgenetic alopecia and wound healing. *Expert Opinion on Biological Therapy, 21*(11), 1443–1449. https://doi.org/10.1080/14712598.2021.1908995.

Ghiasi, Z., Gray, T., Tran, P., Dubielzig, R., Murphy, C., McCartney, D. L., & Reid, T. W. (2018). The effect of topical Substance-P plus insulin-like growth factor-1 (IGF-1) on epithelial healing after photorefractive keratectomy in rabbits. *Translational Vision Science & Technology, 7*(1), 12. https://doi.org/10.1167/tvst.7.1.12.

Girdler, N. M., McGurk, M., Aqual, S., & Prince, M. (1995). The effect of epidermal growth factor mouthwash on cytotoxic-induced oral ulceration. *American Journal of Clinical Oncology, 18*(5), 403–406. https://doi.org/10.1097/00000421-199510000-00009.

Gökkaya, A., Görgü, M., Kızılkan, J., Karanfil, E., & Doğan, A. (2022). The measurement of wound tensile strength and the effect of PRP on wound tensile force: an experimental investigation on rabbits. *Journal of Plastic Surgery and Hand Surgery, 56*(1), 38–46. https://doi.org/10.1080/2000656X.2021.1914637.

Govindarajan, B., Shah, A., Cohen, C., Arnold, R. S., Schechner, J., Chung, J., Mercurio, A. M., Alani, R., Ryu, B., Fan, C.-Y., Cuezva, J. M., Martinez, M., & Arbiser, J. L. (2005). Malignant transformation of human cells by constitutive expression of platelet-derived growth factor-BB. *Journal of Biological Chemistry, 280*(14), 13936–13943. https://doi.org/10.1074/jbc.M500411200.

Hanft, J. R., Pollak, R. A., Barbul, A., Van Gils, C., Kwon, P. S., Gray, S. M., Lynch, C. J., Semba, C. P., & Breen, T. J. (2008). Phase I trial on the safety of topical rhVEGF on chronic neuropathic diabetic foot ulcers. *Journal of Wound Care, 17*(1), 30–37. https://doi.org/10.12968/jowc.2008.17.1.27917.

He, Z., Liu, A., Yu, J., & Chen, X. (2022). Role of platelet-rich plasma gel in promoting wound healing based on medical images of wounds. *Contrast Media & Molecular Imaging, 2022*, 1–9. https://doi.org/10.1155/2022/1543604.

Hesseler, M. J., & Shyam, N. (2019). Platelet-rich plasma and its utility in medical dermatology: A systematic review. *Journal of the American Academy of Dermatology, 81*(3), 834–846. https://doi.org/10.1016/j.jaad.2019.04.037.

Hsu, C., & Chang, J. (2004). Clinical implications of growth factors in flexor tendon wound healing. *The Journal of Hand Surgery, 29*(4), 551–563. https://doi.org/10.1016/
j.jhsa.2004.04.020.

Kuzucu, I., Beriat, G. K., Ezerarslan, H., Ozdemir, S., & Kocaturk, S. (2017). Effects of the autologous platelet-rich plasma in nasal pack on postoperative quality of life. *Journal of Craniofacial Surgery, 28*(3), e299–e302. https://doi.org/10.1097/SCS.0000000000003664.

Alio, J. L., Arnalich-Montiel, F., & Rodriguez, A. E. (2012). The role of "eye platelet rich plasma" (E-Prp) for wound healing in ophthalmology. *Current Pharmaceutical Biotechnology, 13*(7), 1257–1265. https://doi.org/10.2174/138920112800624355.

Lacci, K. M., & Dardik, A. (2010). Platelet-rich plasma: Support for its use in wound healing. *The Yale Journal of Biology and Medicine, 83*(1), 1–9. http://www.ncbi.nlm.nih.gov/pubmed/20351977.

Li, Z.-H., Wu, G.-F., Song, H.-Q., Huang, K., Wu, B., Xu, X.-L., & Zhu, L.-X. (2022). Artificial dermal scaffold loaded with platelet-rich plasma promotes wound healing in pigs by favoring angiogenesis. *Medical Science Monitor, 28*, e936186. https://doi.org/10.12659/MSM.936186.

Maisel-Campbell, A. L., Ismail, A., Reynolds, K. A., Poon, E., Serrano, L., Grushchak, S., Farid, C., West, D. P., & Alam, M. (2020). A systematic review of the safety and effectiveness of platelet-rich plasma (PRP) for skin aging. *Archives of Dermatological Research, 312*(5), 301–315. https://doi.org/10.1007/s00403-019-01999-6.

Marangi, G. F., Pallara, T., Cagli, B., Schena, E., Giurazza, F., Faiella, E., Zobel, B. B., & Persichetti, P. (2014). Treatment of early-stage pressure ulcers by using autologous adipose tissue grafts. _Plastic Surgery International, 2014_, 1–6. https://doi.org/10.1155/2014/817283.

Marx, R. E. (2001). Platelet-rich plasma (PRP): What is PRP and what is not PRP? *Implant Dentistry, 10*(4), 225–228. https://doi.org/10.1097/00008505-200110000-00002.

Menchisheva, Y., Mirzakulova, U., & Yui, R. (2019). Use of platelet-rich plasma to facilitate wound healing. *International Wound Journal, 16*(2), 343–353. https://doi.org/10.1111/iwj.13034.

Moneib, H. A., Youssef, S. S., Aly, D. G., Rizk, M. A., & Abdelhakeem, Y. I. (2018). Autologous platelet-rich plasma versus conventional therapy for the treatment of chronic venous leg ulcers: A comparative study. *Journal of Cosmetic Dermatology, 17*(3), 495–501. https://doi.org/10.1111/jocd.12401.

Monteiro, S. O., Lepage, O. M., & Theoret, C. L. (2009). Effects of platelet-rich plasma on the repair of wounds on the distal aspect of the forelimb in horses. *American Journal of Veterinary Research, 70*(2), 277–282. https://doi.org/10.2460/ajvr.70.2.277.

Nolan, G. S., Smith, O. J., Jell, G., & Mosahebi, A. (2021). Fat grafting and platelet-rich plasma in wound healing: a review of histology from animal studies. *Adipocyte, 10*(1), 80–90. https://doi.org/10.1080/21623945.2021.1876374.

Ortega, S., Ittmann, M., Tsang, S. H., Ehrlich, M., & Basilico, C. (1998). Neuronal defects and delayed wound healing in mice lacking fibroblast growth factor 2. *Proceedings of the National Academy of Sciences, 95*(10), 5672–5677. https://doi.org/10.1073/pnas.95.10.5672.

Pallua, N., Pulsfort, A. K., Suschek, C., & Wolter, T. P. (2009). Content of the growth factors bFGF, IGF-1, VEGF, and PDGF-BB in freshly harvested lipoaspirate after centrifugation and incubation. *Plastic and Reconstructive Surgery, 123*(3), 826–833. https://doi.org/10.1097/PRS.0b013e318199ef31.

Pinto, N. R., Ubilla, M., Zamora, Y., Del Rio, V., Dohan Ehrenfest, D. M., & Quirynen, M. (2018). Leucocyte- and platelet-rich fibrin (L-PRF) as a regenerative medicine strategy for the treatment of refractory leg ulcers: a prospective cohort study. *Platelets, 29*(5), 468–475. https://doi.org/10.1080/09537104.2017.1327654.

Previnaire, J. G., Fontet, P., Opsomer, C., Simon, M., & Ducrocq, T. (2016). Lipofilling (fat grafting) in the secondary prevention of ischial tuberosity and pelvic pressure ulcers. *Spinal Cord, 54*(1), 39–45. https://doi.org/10.1038/sc.2015.184.

Rees, R. S., Robson, M. C., Smiell, J. M., & Perry, B. H. (1999). Becaplermin gel in the treatment of pressure ulcers: A phase II randomized, double-blind, placebo-controlled study. *Wound Repair and Regeneration, 7*(3), 141–147. https://doi.org/10.1046/j.1524-475X.1999.00141.x.

Rigotti, G., Marchi, A., Galiè, M., Baroni, G., Benati, D., Krampera, M., Pasini, A., & Sbarbati, A. (2007). Clinical treatment of radiotherapy tissue damage by lipoaspirate transplant: A healing process mediated by adipose-derived adult stem cells. *Plastic and Reconstructive Surgery, 119*(5), 1409–1422. https://doi.org/10.1097/01.prs.0000256047.47909.71.

Rittié, L. (2016). Cellular mechanisms of skin repair in humans and other mammals. *Journal of Cell Communication and Signaling, 10*(2), 103–120. https://doi.org/10.1007/s12079-016-0330-1.

Roubelakis, M. G., Trohatou, O., Roubelakis, A., Mili, E., Kalaitzopoulos, I., Papazoglou, G., Pappa, K. I., & Anagnou, N. P. (2014). Platelet-rich plasma (PRP) promotes fetal mesenchymal stem/stromal cell migration and wound healing process. *Stem Cell Reviews and Reports, 10*(3), 417–428. https://doi.org/10.1007/s12015-013-9494-8.

Salemi, S., Rinaldi, C., Manna, F., Guarneri, G. F., & Parodi, P. C. (2008). Reconstruction of lower leg skin ulcer with autologous adipose tissue and platelet-rich plasma. *Journal of Plastic, Reconstructive & Aesthetic Surgery, 61*(12), 1565–1567. https://doi.org/10.1016/j.bjps.2008.04.048.

Shao, S., Pan, R., & Chen, Y. (2020). Autologous platelet-rich plasma for diabetic foot ulcer. *Trends in Endocrinology & Metabolism, 31*(12), 885–890. https://doi.org/10.1016/j.tem.2020.10.003.

Shi, L., Lin, F., Zhou, M., Li, Y., Li, W., Shan, G., Xu, Y., Xu, J., & Yang, J. (2021). Preparation of biocompatible wound dressings with dual release of antibiotic and platelet-rich plasma for enhancing infected wound healing. *Journal of Biomaterials Applications, 36*(2), 219–236. https://doi.org/10.1177/0885328221996013.

Siebel, C., & Lendahl, U. (2017). Notch signaling in development, tissue homeostasis, and disease. *Physiological Reviews, 97*(4), 1235–1294. https://doi.org/10.1152/physrev.00005.2017.

Smith, O. J., Jell, G., & Mosahebi, A. (2019). The use of fat grafting and platelet-rich plasma for wound healing: A review. *International Wound Journal, 16*(1), 275–285. https://doi.org/10.1111/iwj.13029.

Smith, O. J., Kanapathy, M., Khajuria, A., Prokopenko, M., Hachach-Haram, N., Mann, H., & Mosahebi, A. (2018). Systematic review of the efficacy of fat grafting and platelet-rich plasma for wound healing. *International Wound Journal, 15*(4), 519–526. https://doi.org/10.1111/iwj.12892.

Sun, Y., Cao, Y., Zhao, R., Xu, F., Wu, D., & Wang, Y. (2020). The role of autologous PRP on deep partial-thickness burn wound healing in Bama pigs. *Journal of Burn Care & Research, 41*(3), 657–662. https://doi.org/10.1093/jbcr/iraa012.

Uslu, K., Tansuker, H. D., Tabaru, A., Egeren, S. E., Kulahci, K. K., Bulut, P., Emre, F., & Oktay, M. F. (2020). Investigation of the effects of thrombocyte-rich plasma, systemic ozone and hyperbaric oxygen treatment on intraoral wound healing in rats: Experimental study. *European Archives of Oto-Rhino-Laryngology, 277*(6), 1771–1777. https://doi.org/10.1007/s00405-020-05872-5.

Weibrich, G., Hansen, T., Kleis, W., Buch, R., & Hitzler, W. E. (2004). Effect of platelet concentration in platelet-rich plasma on peri-implant bone regeneration. *Bone, 34*(4), 665–671. https://doi.org/10.1016/j.bone.2003.12.010.

Xie, J., Bian, H., Qi, S., Xu, Y., Tang, J., Li, T., & Liu, X. (2008). Effects of basic fibroblast growth factor on the expression of extracellular matrix and matrix metalloproteinase-1 in wound healing. *Clinical and Experimental Dermatology, 33*(2), 176–182. https://doi.org/10.1111/j.1365-2230.2007.02573.x.

Xiong, G., Lingampalli, N., Koltsov, J. C. B., Leung, L. L., Bhutani, N., Robinson, W. H., & Chu, C. R. (2018). Men and women differ in the biochemical composition of platelet-rich plasma. *The American Journal of Sports Medicine, 46*(2), 409–419. https://doi.org/10.1177/0363546517740845.

Xu, N., Wang, L., Guan, J., Tang, C., He, N., Zhang, W., & Fu, S. (2018). Wound healing effects of a Curcuma zedoaria polysaccharide with platelet-rich plasma exosomes assembled on chitosan/silk hydrogel sponge in a diabetic rat model. *International Journal of Biological Macromolecules, 117*, 102–107. https://doi.org/10.1016/j.ijbiomac.2018.05.066.

Yildirim, U., Kemal, O., Aksoy, A., Karaca, E., Terzi, O., & Atmaca, S. (2020). Effects of submucosal PRP injection on wound healing in endonasal surgeries: An experimental study. *European Archives of Oto-Rhino-Laryngology, 277*(6), 1681–1689. https://doi.org/10.1007/s00405-020-05884-1.

Zhou, S., Li, L., Chen, C., Chen, Y., Zhou, L., Zhou, F. H., Dong, J., & Wang, L. (2021). Injectable gelatin microspheres loaded with platelet rich plasma improve wound healing by regulating early inflammation. *International Journal of Medical Sciences, 18*(9), 1910–1920. https://doi.org/10.7150/ijms.51060.

Chapter 19

PRP Treatment in Bone Fracture

M. Fatih Uzun*, PhD

Department of Orthopedy and Traumatology, Erciyes University Faculty of Medicine, Kayseri, Turkiye

Abstract

Although bone tissue has the potential to heal after trauma, the healing capacity of bone tissue depends on many factors, such as fracture type, age, and genetic bone disorders. The risk of non-union or delayed union varies worldwide but ranges from 1.9% to 4.9%. In elderly patients with lower extremity fractures, long-term immobilization after non-union, thromboembolism, pulmonary infection, and bed sores may increase the risk of death. Today, the basic treatment principle for fractures is surgery for a stable fixation or a plaster or splint. Platelet-rich plasma (PRP) can be used alone or in combination to increase bone regeneration. PRP is produced by the centrifugation of peripheral blood. Containing high levels of bioactive substances, PRP plays a role in neovascularization, tissue remodeling, and the regulation of inflammation. In recent years, the use of PRP has gained popularity for accelerating fracture healing and treating non-union fractures.

Keywords: platelet-rich plasma, bone healing, non-union, callus, bone fracture

* Corresponding Author's Email: drmehfatih@gmail.com.

In: Current Clinical Recommendations ...
Editors: Nazan Yurtcu and Emel Güler
ISBN: 979-8-89113-723-3

Introduction

Bone is a tissue that acts as a structural scaffold for our body by providing support and protection to soft tissues and internal organs (Kolar et al., 2010). Bone tissue has a significant capacity to repair and regenerate in response to injury and fracture. Fracture healing is a unique process that heals very similarly to its original form and does not heal with scar tissue, unlike other repair processes in the body (McKibbin, 1978). There are many studies on fracture healing and its acceleration day by day. New surgical methods are being developed with orthopedic interventions and rapid advances in medical technology. However, despite these, the healing of some fractures is not as desired; prolongation of the healing time and sometimes non-union can be observed. Platelet-rich plasma (PRP) is an autologous blood-derived biological agent that provides cytokines, growth factors, and bio-micromolecules at supraphysiological concentrations at the site of tissue damage, thereby enhancing the healing potential of tissues.

Many studies have proven that PRP has osteogenic activity (Ranjan et al., 2023).

Healing of Fractures and PRP

A fracture is a form of injury that involves disruption of the structural integrity of the bone cortex and varying degrees of damage to the surrounding soft tissues. Fracture healing is divided into primary (direct) and secondary (indirect) healing, depending on the fixation method (Müller et al., 1992). Fracture healing is mostly in the form of secondary healing. In this healing, the fibrocartilaginous callus transforms into mineralized cartilage and then endochondral bone formation occurs (Braun & Rüter, 1996; Remedios, 1999). Fracture healing phases consist of intertwined phases. These include the formation of hematomas, inflammation, the formation of new vessels, the formation of granulation tissue, the formation of fibrous tissue, the fibrocartilage, hyaline cartilage (soft callus), cartilage mineralization, woven bone (hard callus), and finally remodeling (Kolar et al., 2010). Although bone tissue has excellent healing potential after trauma, recovery depends on many factors, such as age, fracture type, and genetic bone disorders (Zhang et al., 2021). Up to 13% of tibial shaft fractures are associated with non-union or delayed union (Audigé et al., 2005). In elderly patients, the risk of lung infection, thrombosis, and bed sores increases as a result of lower extremity fractures and prolonged immobility, and deaths may occur (Colais et al., 2015).

PRP produced by centrifugation of peripheral blood is low-cost and minimally invasive. The aim here is to remove elements that are considered unusable (mostly heavy and easily separable red blood cells) from peripheral blood and to collect elements that can be used for therapeutic applications (fibrinogen/fibrin, platelets, growth factors, leukocytes, and other circulating cell forms, in solution in liquid plasma) and to concentrate (Dohan Ehrenfes et al., 2009) . Bioactive substances released from PRP can play a role in tissue remodeling, neovascularization, and the regulation of inflammation (Mazzocca et al., 2012). PRP contains high concentrations of autologous bioactive factors, including platelet-derived growth factor (PDGF), transforming growth factor beta (TGF-ß), and interleukin (Boesen et al., 2017). Growth factors released from activated platelets play an important role in intracellular signaling pathways that induce the production of proteins necessary for regenerative processes such as matrix production, cellular proliferation, collagen synthesis, and osteoid production, which are essential for fracture healing (Malhotra et al., 2015). In addition, these growth factors provide osteoprogenitor cell stimulation (Gianakos et al., 2015).

The definition of PRP refers to the volume of autologous plasma with a platelet concentration of 1,000,000 platelets/l in a plasma volume of 5 ml (Wilkins & Kelly, 2003). Platelet products obtained from peripheral blood in 2009 were classified into four groups (Dohan Ehrenfest et al., 2009).

1. P-PRP (pure platelet-rich plasma): injectable, it can be used in orthopedics, traumatology, and sports medicine
2. L-PRP (leukocytes and platelet-rich plasma): injectable, can be used in orthopedics and traumatology, sports medicine
3. P-PRF (Pure Platelet-Rich Fibrin)
4. L-PRF (leukocytes and platelet-rich fibrin)
5. This classification system is largely endorsed by the consensus published in 2012 (Dohan Ehrenfest et al., 2012).

PRP in Preclinical Studies

PRP has been shown to provide numerous potential benefits as a result of histological, radiographic, and biomechanical analysis in most studies of animal bone models. Parizi et al., in their study on an experimental bone healing model, reported that histological bone healing was superior in animals treated with PRP. Furthermore, in this study, fracture healing was faster in the PRP group (Parizi et al., 2012). Platelets have also been used in oral and maxillofacial surgery to enhance bone and soft tissue healing. In their mandibular bone graft regeneration model, Marx et al. reported that the rate of bone healing in the treated group was 2.3 times faster than in the group without PRP (Marx et al., 1998). The growth factors released from alpha granules of platelets affect cell differentiation, fracture healing, and matrix production in cell and organ culture. These growth factors modulate bone regeneration: PDGF is an insulin-like growth factor (IGF), and TGF-ß (Marx et al., 1998). TGF-ß1 and bone morphogenic proteins (BMPs), also from the TGF-ß superfamily, stimulate osteoblastic differentiation and the production of a new bone matrix (Roldán et al., 2004). These components, which make up the structure of PRP, increase bone healing and regeneration, increasing osteid bridging and fracture union (Gianakos et al., 2015). Bone proliferation and the amount of callus were radiographically evaluated in the study by Sauza et al. In this study, radiographic bone healing was found to be significantly different in the PRP group compared to the control group on the 6th and 60th days (Souza et al., 2012). These positive effects may be due to the chemotactic and mitogenic effects of PRP on fibroblasts and osteoblasts (Kurikchy et al., 2013).

PDGF has been shown to stimulate bone formation and accelerate wound healing, resulting in bone regeneration (Gianakos et al., 2015). The role of Prp in bone healing may be due to TGF-ß's increase in mesenchymal stem cell (MSC) proliferation and stimulation of osteogenic differentiation (Watabe & Miyazono, 2009). These growth factors stimulate cell mitosis by affecting collagenous and non-collagenous protein synthesis. As a result, it modulates cells in the callus as they progress through the healing stages (Cornell & Lane, 1992).

There are also studies showing that PRP increases bone healing when used with a scaffold. Kasten et al. reported that the addition of PRP to hyaluronic acid with calcium phosphate improved bone defects in rabbits with large bone defects (Kasten et al., 2008). Many other studies have reported similar results. This may be related to the fact that the scaffold facilitates the deployment of cell signaling molecules released by platelets in PRP, which can promote osteogenesis (Jungbluth et al., 2010). Type II collagen is incorporated into the cartilage structure and plays an important role in the formation of long bones through endochondral ossification

(Gianakos et al., 2015). Van Buul et al. reported that PRP reduces the IL-1ß-mediated inhibition of type II collagen and aggrecan gene expression. Interleukin-1ß is a catabolic cytokine. It has been reported to decrease the expression of PRP IL-1ß (van Buul et al., 2011). There are also studies showing that Prp also increases the biomechanical durability of bones. With biomechanically strong bones, early mobilization, an earlier return to social life, a greater postoperative range of motion, and greater patient satisfaction will be possible (Baksh et al., 2013).

PRP in the Treatment of Non-Union

The risk of non-union or delayed union varies worldwide but ranges from 1.9% to 4.9% (Wildemann et al., 2021). Non-union is defined as a fracture that does not heal for nine months or shows no signs of healing for three consecutive months (Andersen et al., 2021). The gold standard treatment in boiling is autologous bone graft. However, the limitations of this method include potential damage to the arteries, nerves, and tissues around the donor bone and pain at the donor site (Kikuchi et al., 2020). For the treatment of non-union fractures, inexpensive, non-invasive, and less-complicated adjuvant treatments are needed. Percutaneous injection of PRP in the treatment of non-union has been reported to be effective in small-scale clinical studies. However, controversial results have been obtained in randomized controlled studies (Duramaz et al., 2018). Seijas et al. applied growth factor-rich plasma to clavicle fractures with delayed union and stimulated the consolidation of the fracture (Seijas et al., 2010). Bielecki et al. reported that the platelet- and leukocyte-rich fibrin they applied percutaneously was an adequate treatment for the delay of union (Bielecki et al., 2008).

In the study conducted by PRP, a total of 94 patients without long bone union were treated with PRP, and complete union was achieved in 82 patients. They reported that percutaneous PRP injection can be performed in bone fractures without union (Malhotra et al., 2015). PRP can also be used with other forms of non-union fracture treatment, including autografts and/or fixation devices (Andersen et al., 2021). Some studies have reported that the combination of autograft and PRP is effective in the treatment of non-union (Sanchez et al., 2009; Tarallo et al., 2012). In a study investigating the effect of PRP on the healing rate of non-union fractures treated with autologous bone graft and internal fixation, the union rate was significantly higher in the

PRP group (Ghaffarpasand et al., 2016). There are also studies investigating whether the combination of PRP and mesenchymal stem cells can facilitate the healing of non-unions. In one of these studies, it was reported that PRP could be used for the union of non-union fractures using an autograft. This result highlights that PRP is effective in improving bone regeneration in difficult cases of no union (Labibzadeh et al., 2016). However, there are studies reporting that the use of PRP alone without bone grafting is not beneficial for bone regeneration.

Conclusion

Despite advances in the treatment of long bone fractures, disturbances in healing processes remain a problem. Autologous bone grafts are the gold standard of treatment for non-unions or delayed unions. However, donor site morbidity is the limitation of this treatment. Adjuvant treatments are needed for groups at risk of non-union. PRP is an inexpensive, reliable, and minimally invasive method for the treatment of non-union and the acceleration of union. However, there is a need for randomized, controlled clinical studies showing that PRP accelerates bone regeneration and its use in the treatment of non-union. In addition, preparation and application should be standardized for the further development of PRP in fractures.

References

Andersen, C., Wragg, N. M., Shariatzadeh, M., & Wilson, S. L. (2021). The use of platelet-rich plasma (PRP) for the management of non-union fractures. *Current Osteoporosis Reports, 19*(1), 1–14. https://doi.org/10.1007/s11914-020-00643-x.

Audigé, L., Griffin, D., Bhandari, M., Kellam, J., & Rüedi, T. P. (2005). Path analysis of factors for delayed healing and nonunion in 416 operatively treated tibial shaft fractures. *Clinical Orthopaedics and Related Research, 438*, 221–232. https://doi.org/10.1097/01.blo.0000163836.66906.74.

Baksh, N., Hannon, C. P., Murawski, C. D., Smyth, N. A., & Kennedy, J. G. (2013). Platelet-rich plasma in tendon models: A systematic review of basic science literature. *Arthroscopy: The Journal of Arthroscopic & Related Surgery, 29*(3), 596–607. https://doi.org/10.1016/j.arthro.2012.10.025.

Bielecki, T., Gazdzik, T. S., & Szczepanski, T. (2008). Benefit of percutaneous injection of autologous platelet-leukocyte-rich gel in patients with delayed union and nonunion. *European Surgical Research. Europaische Chirurgische Forschung.*

Recherches Chirurgicales Europeennes, 40(3), 289–296. https://doi.org/10.1159/000114967.

Braun, W., & Rüter, A. (1996). Fracture healing: Morphologic and physiologic aspects. *Der Unfallchirurg, 99*(1), 59–67.

Colais, P., Di Martino, M., Fusco, D., Perucci, C. A., & Davoli, M. (2015). The effect of early surgery after hip fracture on 1-year mortality. *BMC Geriatrics, 15*, 141. https://doi.org/10.1186/s12877-015-0140-y.

Cornell, C. N., & Lane, J. M. (1992). Newest factors in fracture healing. *Clinical Orthopaedics and Related Research, 277*, 297–311.

Dohan Ehrenfest, D. M., Bielecki, T., Mishra, A., Borzini, P., Inchingolo, F., Sammartino, G., Rasmusson, L., & Everts, P. A. (2012). In search of a consensus terminology in the field of platelet concentrates for surgical use: Platelet-rich plasma (PRP), platelet-rich fibrin (PRF), fibrin gel polymerization and leukocytes. *Current Pharmaceutical Biotechnology, 13*(7), 1131–1137. https://doi.org/10.2174/138920112800624328.

Dohan Ehrenfest, D. M., Rasmusson, L., & Albrektsson, T. (2009). Classification of platelet concentrates: From pure platelet-rich plasma (P-PRP) to leucocyte- and platelet-rich fibrin (L-PRF). *Trends in Biotechnology, 27*(3), 158–167. https://doi.org/10.1016/j.tibtech.2008.11.009.

Duramaz, A., Ursavaş, H. T., Bilgili, M. G., Bayrak, A., Bayram, B., & Avkan, M. C. (2018). Platelet-rich plasma versus exchange intramedullary nailing in treatment of long bone oligotrophic nonunions. *European Journal of Orthopaedic Surgery & Traumatology: Orthopedie Traumatologie, 28*(1), 131–137. https://doi.org/10.1007/s00590-017-2024-7.

Ghaffarpasand, F., Shahrezaei, M., & Dehghankhalili, M. (2016). Effects of platelet-rich plasma on healing rate of long bone non-union fractures: A randomized double-blind placebo-controlled clinical trial. *Bulletin of Emergency and Trauma, 4*(3), 134–140.

Gianakos, A., Zambrana, L., Savage-Elliott, I., Lane, J. M., & Kennedy, J. G. (2015). Platelet-rich plasma in the animal long-bone model: An analysis of basic science evidence. *Orthopedics, 38*(12), e1079-90. https://doi.org/10.3928/01477447-20151120-04.

Jungbluth, P., Wild, M., Grassmann, J.-P., Ar, E., Sager, M., Herten, M., Jäger, M., Becker, J., Windolf, J., & Hakimi, M. (2010). Platelet-rich plasma on calcium phosphate granules promotes metaphyseal bone healing in mini-pigs. *Journal of Orthopaedic Research: Official Publication of the Orthopaedic Research Society, 28*(11), 1448–1455. https://doi.org/10.1002/jor.21152.

Kasten, P., Vogel, J., Geiger, F., Niemeyer, P., Luginbühl, R., & Szalay, K. (2008). The effect of platelet-rich plasma on healing in critical-size long-bone defects. *Biomaterials, 29*(29), 3983–3992. https://doi.org/10.1016/j.biomaterials.2008.06.014.

Kikuchi, N., Yoshioka, T., Arai, N., Hyodo, K., Kanamori, A., & Yamazaki, M. (2020). A radiological study of bone remodeling with two different types of porous β-tricalcium phosphate in humans. *Scientific Reports, 10*(1), 19886. https://doi.org/10.1038/s41598-020-77011-3.

Kolar, P., Schmidt-Bleek, K., Schell, H., Gaber, T., Toben, D., Schmidmaier, G., Perka, C., Buttgereit, F., & Duda, G. N. (2010). The early fracture hematoma and its potential role in fracture healing. *Tissue Engineering. Part B, Reviews, 16*(4), 427–434. https://doi.org/10.1089/ten.TEB.2009.0687.

Kurikchy, M. Q., Al-Rawi, N. H., Ayoub, R. S., & Mohammed, S. S. (2013). Histological evaluation of bone healing using organic bovine bone in combination with platelet-rich plasma (an experimental study on rabbits). *Clinical Oral Investigations, 17*(3), 897–904. https://doi.org/10.1007/s00784-012-0751-z.

Labibzadeh, N., Emadedin, M., Fazeli, R., Mohseni, F., Hosseini, S. E., Moghadasali, R., Mardpour, S., Azimian, V., Ghorbani Liastani, M., Mirazimi Bafghi, A., Baghaban Eslaminejad, M., & Aghdami, N. (2016). Mesenchymal stromal cells implantation in combination with platelet lysate product is safe for reconstruction of human long bone nonunion. *Cell Journal, 18*(3), 302–309. https://doi.org/10.22074/cellj.2016.4557.

Malhotra, R., Kumar, V., Garg, B., Singh, R., Jain, V., Coshic, P., & Chatterjee, K. (2015). Role of autologous platelet-rich plasma in treatment of long-bone nonunions: a prospective study. *Musculoskeletal Surgery, 99*(3), 243–248. https://doi.org/10.1007/ s12306-015-0378-8.

Marx, R. E., Carlson, E. R., Eichstaedt, R. M., Schimmele, S. R., Strauss, J. E., & Georgeff, K. R. (1998). Platelet-rich plasma: Growth factor enhancement for bone grafts. *Oral Surgery, Oral Medicine, Oral Pathology, Oral Radiology, and Endodontics, 85*(6), 638–646. https://doi.org/10.1016/s1079-2104(98)90029-4.

Mazzocca, A. D., McCarthy, M. B. R., Chowaniec, D. M., Dugdale, E. M., Hansen, D., Cote, M. P., Bradley, J. P., Romeo, A. A., Arciero, R. A., & Beitzel, K. (2012). The positive effects of different platelet-rich plasma methods on human muscle, bone, and tendon cells. *The American Journal of Sports Medicine, 40*(8), 1742–1749. https://doi.org/10.1177/0363546512452713.

McKibbin, B. (1978). The biology of fracture healing in long bones. *The Journal of Bone and Joint Surgery. British Volume, 60-B*(2), 150–162. https://doi.org/10.1302/0301-620X.60B2.350882.

Müller, M. E., Allgöwer, M., Schneider, R., & Willenegger, H. (1992). Manual der Osteosynthese. In *Manual der Osteosynthese* (3rd ed.). Springer.

Parizi, A. M., Oryan, A., Shafiei-Sarvestani, Z., & Bigham, A. S. (2012). Human platelet rich plasma plus Persian Gulf coral effects on experimental bone healing in rabbit model: Radiological, histological, macroscopical and biomechanical evaluation. *Journal of Materials Science: Materials in Medicine, 23*(2), 473–483. https://doi.org/10.1007/s10856-011-4478-1.

Ranjan, R., Kumar, R., Jeyaraman, M., Arora, A., Kumar, S., & Nallakumarasamy, A. (2023). Autologous platelet-rich plasma in the delayed union of long bone fractures - A quasi experimental study. *Journal of Orthopaedics, 36*, 76–81. https://doi.org/10.1016/j.jor.2022.12.013.

Remedios, A. (1999). Bone and bone healing. *Veterinary Clinics of North America: Small Animal Practice, 29*(5), 1029–1044. https://doi.org/10.1016/S0195-5616(99)50101-0.

Roldán, J. C., Jepsen, S., Miller, J., Freitag, S., Rueger, D. C., Açil, Y., & Terheyden, H. (2004). Bone formation in the presence of platelet-rich plasma vs. bone morphogenetic protein-7. *Bone, 34*(1), 80–90. https://doi.org/10.1016/j.bone.2003.09.011.

Sanchez, M., Anitua, E., Cugat, R., Azofra, J., Guadilla, J., Seijas, R., & Andia, I. (2009). Nonunions treated with autologous preparation rich in growth factors. *Journal of Orthopaedic Trauma, 23*(1), 52–59. https://doi.org/10.1097/BOT.0b013e31818faded.

Seijas, R., Santana-Suarez, R. Y., Garcia-Balletbo, M., Cuscó, X., Ares, O., & Cugat, R. (2010). Delayed union of the clavicle treated with plasma rich in growth factors. *Acta Orthopaedica Belgica, 76*(5), 689–693.

Souza, T. F. B., Andrade, A. L., Ferreira, G. T. N. M., Sakamoto, S. S., Albuquerque, V. B., Bonfim, S. R. M., Luvizotto, M. C. R., & Louzada, M. J. Q. (2012). Healing and expression of growth factors (TGF-β and PDGF) in canine radial ostectomy gap containing platelet-rich plasma. *Veterinary and Comparative Orthopaedics and Traumatology: V.C.O.T, 25*(6), 445–452. https://doi.org/10.3415/VCOT-10-10-0146.

Tarallo, L., Mugnai, R., Adani, R., & Catani, F. (2012). Treatment of the ulna non-unions using dynamic compression plate fixation, iliac bone grafting and autologous platelet-rich plasma. *European Journal of Orthopaedic Surgery & Traumatology: Orthopedie Traumatologie, 22*(8), 681–687. https://doi.org/10.1007/s00590-011-0902-y.

van Buul, G. M., Koevoet, W. L. M., Kops, N., Bos, P. K., Verhaar, J. A. N., Weinans, H., Bernsen, M. R., & van Osch, G. J. V. M. (2011). Platelet-rich plasma releasate inhibits inflammatory processes in osteoarthritic chondrocytes. *The American Journal of Sports Medicine, 39*(11), 2362–2370. https://doi.org/10.1177/0363546511419278.

Watabe, T., & Miyazono, K. (2009). Roles of TGF-beta family signaling in stem cell renewal and differentiation. *Cell Research, 19*(1), 103–115. https://doi.org/10.1038/cr.2008.323.

Wildemann, B., Ignatius, A., Leung, F., Taitsman, L. A., Smith, R. M., Pesántez, R., Stoddart, M. J., Richards, R. G., & Jupiter, J. B. (2021). Non-union bone fractures. *Nature Reviews. Disease Primers, 7*(1), 57. https://doi.org/10.1038/s41572-021-00289-8.

Zhang, Y., Xing, F., Luo, R., & Duan, X. (2021). Platelet-rich plasma for bone fracture treatment: A systematic review of current evidence in preclinical and clinical studies. In *Frontiers in Medicine* (Vol. 8, p. 676033). https://doi.org/10.3389/fmed.2021.676033.

Chapter 20

PRP Treatment for Skin Disorders

Derya Bostan Ağırdıcı*, **MD**
Department of Dermatology, İzmir Tınaztepe University, İzmir, Turkiye

Abstract

Platelet-rich plasma therapy is an autologous blood product that is obtained by centrifugation of blood and contains high concentrations of platelets. Platelets contain many growth factors with regenerative properties that are involved in cell proliferation and differentiation, angiogenesis, and extracellular matrix production. Because of these unique properties, PRP has been used in many different fields such as dermatology, plastic surgery, orthopedics, urology, and obstetrics. Recently, PRP applications in skin diseases have become more and more prevalent. PRP will be used in dermatology for skin diseases, mainly alopecia, acne scars, skin rejuvenation, striae, and vitiligo. The results obtained from the studies are promising and point to a new indication every day. Although promising results have been obtained with the use of PRP, larger studies are needed to prove its effectiveness.

Keywords: platelet-rich plasma, skin, dermatology

Introduction

Platelet-rich plasma (PRP) is an autologous blood product obtained by centrifuging the patient's own venous blood (Leo et al., 2015). Homologous was used for the first time in 1987 after cardiac surgery. It has been used to

* Corresponding Author's Email: drybstn@yahoo.com.tr.

In: Current Clinical Recommendations ...
Editors: Nazan Yurtcu and Emel Güler
ISBN: 979-8-89113-723-3

reduce the transfusion of blood products. Today, in addition to dermatology and plastic surgery, orthopedics, cardiovascular surgery, maxillofacial surgery, urology, ophthalmology, etc. It is used in many branches (Dhillon et al., 2012). It is used because of its healing-accelerating effect in sports medicine and orthopedics, tendon, ligament, muscle, and bone tissue (Foster et al., 2009). The use of PRP in dermatology has ranged from chronic ulcer treatment to cosmetic procedures (Dhurat & Sukesh, 2014). In recent years, it has been used in many different indications with increasing frequency in cosmetic dermatology (Leo et al., 2015).

Acne Scars

PRP activates TGF-β fibroblasts in connective tissue cells. It causes an increase in the number and production of collagen. It contributes to the reduction of scar tissue by increasing dermal regeneration with its growth factors. In a study of 23 cases whose use of PRP was not controlled, it was reported to show significant efficacy in acne scars (Redaelli et al., 2010). In a study in which the micro-needling system and PRP were combined, it was shown that the combination was better than micro-needling alone (Asif et al., 2016). In a meta-analysis conducted in 2018, it was shown that PRP contributes significantly to acne scars and is suitable for combined treatments (Alser & Goutos, 2018).

After ablative application of CO2 laser to 14 patients, intradermal PRP on one half of the face and on the other side placebo was administered. The combination of the two treatments has been shown to be synergistic in the treatment of acne scars and ablative laser erythema and edema due to the application of PRP. It was found that it took a shorter time in the group (Lee et al., 2011). In another study, it was shown that the combination of fractional ablative CO2 laser applied to atrophic acne scars with intradermal or topical PRP application gave significantly better results than laser application alone. Among the success of topical and intradermal PRP applications, no significant difference was found (Gawdat et al., 2014).

Melasma

Melasma is a chronic inflammatory disease characterized by melanocyte hyperfunction and increased melanin deposition on the skin (Pixley et al., 2023).

It was thought that PRP could be used in melasma because of the melanogenesis inhibitory property of TGF-β1 (D.-S. Kim et al., 2004). It is a matter of debate whether increasing the vascular plexus with high levels of VEGF and PDGF, which also have angiogenic potential, will increase the vascular structure of the melasma (Chatterjee & Vasudevan, 2014). In a clinical study conducted with 33 patients in 2018, the efficacy of PRP in melasma was demonstrated (Hofny et al., 2019).

Psoriasis Vulgaris

Psoriasis is a chronic disease characterized by erythematous scaly plaques (*Psoriasis: epidemiology, clinical features, and quality of life | Annals of the Rheumatic Diseases*, t.y.). PRP reduces chemotaxis by inhibiting chemokine transactivation and CXCR4-receptor expression, thereby possibly controlling local inflammation. The combination of methotrexate and PRP in psoriasis vulgaris was compared with methotrexate monotherapy, and it was found to be effective (Chakravdhanula et al., 2016).

Nail Disorders

Inflammatory nail disorders are a group of conditions that can be isolated from the nail or associated with systemic diseases. These disorders include lichen planus, lichen striatus, and idiopathic trachyonychia. Topical tacrolimus, intralesional or systemic steroids, azathioprine and etretinate have been tried in the treatment (*Treatment of inflammatory nail disorders - Dehesa - 2012 - Dermatologic Therapy - Wiley Online Library*, t.y.).

PRP has been proposed as a treatment for inflammatory nail disorders based on its anti-inflammatory properties and growth factors. The literature that evaluates the treatment of these disorders with PRP is limited to a comparable intra-individual study and two case reports. In these studies, it was reported that nail changes improved with PRP treatment. It has been reported that the combination of PRP and triamcinolone provides more improvement than triamcinolone alone (Kaur & Jakhar, 2019; Pixley et al., 2023).

Pemfigus Vulgaris

In a study conducted in 2015, PRP was shown to be effective in resistant pemphigus vulgaris oral lesions. PRP has shown that in pemphigus lesions, TGF-β prevents inflammation and autoimmunity by affecting T regulator and other T helper cells (EL-Komy et al., 2015).

Vitiligo

Vitiligo is an acquired idiopathic disease that is clinically characterized by amelanotic lesions on the skin and causes significant deterioration in the quality of life of patients. In recent years, the use of platelet-rich plasma (PRP) has received increasing attention as a new treatment modality in the treatment of various dermatological diseases, including vitiligo (Mercuri et al., 2020).

It has been shown that growth factors secreted from alpha granules of platelets increase the release of adhesion molecules and chemokines that allow the migration of melanocytes (Domaszewska-Szostek et al., 2023).

It has been shown that PRP application increases the efficacy and reduces the cumulative dose when used with dbUVB (Z. A. Ibrahim et al., 2016). In another study, it was shown that PRP increases the efficacy by combining it with fractional laser therapy in vitiligo (Kadry et al., 2018). PRP in the treatment of vitiligo is a very new view, its clinical studies are very few, and therefore there is no consensus yet.

Skin Rejuvenation

It has been thought that PRP can be used in skin rejuvenation through the increase in fibroblastic activity and the synthesis of other matrix proteins, especially collagen (Yuksel et al., 2014).

In one study, positive results were found when PRP was applied to the head and neck region of 23 patients three times with an interval of one month and evaluated with dermoscopic and digital photography one month after the last application. Improvement was found in nasolabial grooves, neck lines, skin tone, and periocular wrinkles (Redaelli et al., 2010).

In the evaluation of PRP application three months after treatment in 10 patients with periorbital hyperpigmentation and crow's feet wrinkles, only an improvement in infraorbital color homogeneity showed a significant difference. No change was found in the amount of melanin, stratum corneum hydration, wrinkle volume, and visibility (Mehryan et al., 2014).

On the other hand, in another study, it was shown that PRP provided a significant improvement in tone and wrinkles on infraorbital skin (Kang et al., 2014).

In a prospective study conducted on 20 female patients, it was emphasized that the growth factors contained in PRP application is a reliable method that can be used in skin rejuvenation with the effect of the micro-needling method (Abuaf et al., 2016).

In one study, it was reported that the combination of fractional laser and topically applied PRP provided an increase in skin elasticity and reduced erythema compared to patients treated with laser alone. Histological findings in the combined therapy group increased dermoepidermal junction length significantly more. It is known that PRP increases the production of hyaluronic acid, thereby increasing skin elasticity (Shin et al., 2012).

Successful autologous fat transfer with PRP has been reported in the literature. There are studies reporting combinations. PRP has been used as a support to reduce the rejection of the fat graft and increase its stability (Park et al., 2012; Willemsen et al., 2013).

Stria

In striae with dermal scar tissue accompanied by epidermal atrophy, current treatments are generally not successful enough (I. S. Kim et al., 2012).

PRP stimulates fibroblast growth and induces the expression of type I collagen and metalloproteinase proteins (MMP) in fibroblasts. On the other hand, metalloproteinase proteins provide cleaning of old and damaged collagen. Therefore, PRP induces the remodeling of the extracellular matrix and the formation of collagen and elastic fibers (Suh et al., 2012).

In a study conducted in 68 patients, the efficacy of PRP alone, microdermabrasion alone, and combined treatment applied a maximum of 6 times with an interval of 2 weeks was compared.

Although the results in the PRP-only group were better than those of the microdermabrasion-only group, the best results were obtained in a shorter time with combination therapy (Ibrahim et al., 2015).

Lichen Planus and Subtypes

PRP has been tested in many dermatoses in recent years in order to benefit from its local anti-inflammatory effects. The efficacy of PRP has been demonstrated in a case of resistant oral lichen planus (Merigo et al., 2018).

Again, in case reports of lichen planopilaris, PRP has been shown to be effective and reliable (Bolanča et al., 2016).

However, no study has been found on these subjects, only case reports are available. In addition to case reports on lichen sclerosus, a study was conducted in 2019. In this study, the effectiveness of PRP was mentioned (Goldstein et al., 2019).

Conclusion

Platelet-rich plasma applications are increasingly being used in skin diseases and cosmetic dermatology. Although the results obtained in the studies are promising, controlled studies in large patient populations are needed in order to obtain definitive data on the standardization of applications and efficacy.

References

Abuaf, O. K., Yildiz, H., Baloglu, H., Bilgili, M. E., Simsek, H. A., & Dogan, B. (2016). Histologic evidence of new collagen formulation using platelet rich plasma in skin rejuvenation: A prospective controlled clinical study. *Annals of Dermatology, 28*(6), 718. https://doi.org/10.5021/ad.2016.28.6.718.

Alser, O. H., & Goutos, I. (2018). The evidence behind the use of platelet-rich plasma (PRP) in scar management: A literature review. *Scars, Burns & Healing, 4*, 205951311880877. https://doi.org/10.1177/2059513118808773.

Asif, M., Kanodia, S., & Singh, K. (2016). Combined autologous platelet-rich plasma with microneedling verses microneedling with distilled water in the treatment of atrophic acne scars: A concurrent split-face study. *Journal of Cosmetic Dermatology, 15*(4), 434-443. https://doi.org/10.1111/jocd.12207.

Bolanča, Ž., Goren, A., Getaldić-Švarc, B., Vučić, M., & Šitum, M. (2016). Platelet-rich plasma as a novel treatment for lichen planopillaris: PRP as a novel treatment for LPP. *Dermatologic Therapy, 29*(4), 233-235. https://doi.org/10.1111/dth.12343.

Chakravdhanula, U., Anbarasu, K., Verma, V. K., & Beevi, S. S. (2016). Clinical efficacy of platelet rich plasma in combination with methotrexate in chronic plaque psoriatic patients: PRP-based adjunct therapy for plaque psoriasis. *Dermatologic Therapy, 29*(6), 446-450. https://doi.org/10.1111/dth.12388.

Chatterjee, M., & Vasudevan, B. (2014). Recent advances in melasma. *Pigment International, 1*(2), 70. https://doi.org/10.4103/2349-5847.147044.

Dhillon, R. S., Schwarz, E. M., & Maloney, M. D. (2012). Platelet-rich plasma therapy—Future or trend? _Arthritis Research & Therapy, 14_(4), 219. https://doi.org/10.1186/
ar3914.

Dhurat, R., & Sukesh, M. (2014). Principles and methods of preparation of platelet-rich plasma: A review and author's perspective. *Journal of Cutaneous and Aesthetic Surgery, 7*(4), 189. https://doi.org/10.4103/0974-2077.150734.

Domaszewska-Szostek, A., Polak, A., Słupecka-Ziemilska, M., Krzyżanowska, M., & Puzianowska-Kuźnicka, M. (2023). Current status of cell-based therapies for vitiligo. *International Journal of Molecular Sciences, 24*(4), Art. 4. https://doi.org/10.3390/ijms24043357.

EL-Komy, M. H. M., Hassan, A. S., Raheem, H. M. A., Doss, S. S., EL-Kaliouby, M., Saleh, N. A., & Saleh, M. A. (2015). Platelet-rich plasma for resistant oral erosions of pemphigus vulgaris: A pilot study. *Wound Repair and Regeneration, 23*(6), 953-955. https://doi.org/10.1111/wrr.12363.

Foster, T. E., Puskas, B. L., Mandelbaum, B. R., Gerhardt, M. B., & Rodeo, S. A. (2009). Platelet-rich plasma: From basic science to clinical applications. *The American Journal of Sports Medicine, 37*(11), 2259-2272. https://doi.org/10.1177/036354650 9349921.

Gawdat, H. I., Hegazy, R. A., Fawzy, M. M., & Fathy, M. (2014). Autologous platelet-rich plasma: Topical versus intradermal after fractional ablative carbon dioxide laser treatment of atrophic acne scars. *Dermatologic Surgery, 40*(2), 152-161. https://doi.org/10.1111/dsu.12392.

Goldstein, A. T., Mitchell, L., Govind, V., & Heller, D. (2019). A randomized double-blind placebo-controlled trial of autologous platelet-rich plasma intradermal injections for the treatment of vulvar lichen sclerosus. *Journal of the American Academy of Dermatology, 80*(6), 1788-1789. https://doi.org/10.1016/j.jaad.2018.12.060.

Hofny, E. R. M., Abdel-Motaleb, A. A., Ghazally, A., Ahmed, A. M., & Hussein, M. R. A. (2019). Platelet-rich plasma is a useful therapeutic option in melasma. *Journal of Dermatological Treatment, 30*(4), 396-401. https://doi.org/10.1080/09546634.2018.1524821.

Ibrahim, Z. A. E.-S., El-Tatawy, R. A., El-Samongy, M. A., & Ali, D. A. M. (2015). Comparison between the efficacy and safety of platelet-rich plasma vs. microdermabrasion in the treatment of striae distensae: Clinical and histopathological study. *Journal of Cosmetic Dermatology, 14*(4), 336-346. https://doi.org/10.1111/ jocd.12160.

Ibrahim, Z. A., El-Ashmawy, A. A., El-Tatawy, R. A., & Sallam, F. A. (2016). The effect of platelet-rich plasma on the outcome of short-term narrowband-ultraviolet B phototherapy in the treatment of vitiligo: A pilot study. *Journal of Cosmetic Dermatology, 15*(2), 108-116. https://doi.org/10.1111/jocd.12194.

Kadry, M., Tawfik, A., Abdallah, N., Badawi, A., & Shokeir, H. (2018). Platelet-rich plasma versus combined fractional carbon dioxide laser with platelet-rich plasma in the treatment of vitiligo: A comparative study. *Clinical, Cosmetic and Investigational Dermatology, Volume 11*, 551-559. https://doi.org/10.2147/CCID.S178817.

Kang, B. K., Shin, M. K., Lee, J. H., & Kim, N. I. (2014). Effects of platelet-rich plasma on wrinkles and skin tone in Asian lower eyelid skin: Preliminary results from a prospective, randomised, split-face trial. *European Journal of Dermatology, 24*(1), 100-101. https://doi.org/10.1684/ejd.2014.2267.

Kaur, I., & Jakhar, D. (2019). Intramatricial platelet-rich plasma therapy: A novel treatment modality in refractory nail disorders. *Dermatologic Therapy, 32*(2), e12831. https://doi.org/10.1111/dth.12831.

Kim, D.-S., Park, S.-H., & Park, K.-C. (2004). Transforming growth factor-β1 decreases melanin synthesis via delayed extracellular signal-regulated kinase activation. *The International Journal of Biochemistry & Cell Biology, 36*(8), 1482-1491. https://doi.org/10.1016/j.biocel.2003.10.023.

Kim, I. S., Park, K. Y., Kim, B. J., Kim, M. N., Kim, C. W., & Kim, S. E. (2012). Efficacy of intradermal radiofrequency combined with autologous platelet-rich plasma in striae distensae: A pilot study: Combination treatment in striae distensae. *International Journal of Dermatology, 51*(10), 1253-1258. https://doi.org/10.1111/j.1365-4632.2012.05530.x.

Lee, J. W., Kim, B. J., Kim, M. N., & Mun, S. K. (2011). The efficacy of autologous platelet rich plasma combined with ablative carbon dioxide fractional resurfacing for acne scars: A simultaneous split-face trial. *Dermatologic Surgery, 37*(7), 931-938. https://doi.org/10.1111/j.1524-4725.2011.01999.x.

Leo, M. S., Kumar, A. S., Kirit, R., Konathan, R., & Sivamani, R. K. (2015). Systematic review of the use of platelet-rich plasma in aesthetic dermatology. *Journal of Cosmetic Dermatology, 14*(4), 315-323. https://doi.org/10.1111/jocd.12167.

Mehryan, P., Zartab, H., Rajabi, A., Pazhoohi, N., & Firooz, A. (2014). Assessment of efficacy of platelet-rich plasma (PRP) on infraorbital dark circles and crow's feet wrinkles. *Journal of Cosmetic Dermatology, 13*(1), 72-78. https://doi.org/10.1111/ jocd.12072.

Mercuri, S. R., Vollono, L., & Paolino, G. (2020). The usefulness of platelet-rich plasma (PRP) for the treatment of vitiligo: State of the art and review. *Drug Design,*

Development and Therapy, Volume 14, 1749-1755. https://doi.org/10.2147/DDDT.S239912.

Merigo, E., Oppici, A., Parlatore, A., Cella, L., Clini, F., Fontana, M., & Fornaini, C. (2018). Platelet-rich plasma (PRP) rinses for the treatment of non-responding oral lichen planus: A case report. *Biomedicines, 6*(1), 15. https://doi.org/10.3390/biomedicines6010015.

Park, K. Y., Kim, I. S., Kim, B. J., & Kim, M. N. (2012). Letter: Autologous fat grafting and platelet-rich plasma for treatment of facial contour defects. *Dermatologic Surgery, 38*(9), 1572. https://doi.org/10.1111/j.1524-4725.2012.02515.x.

Pixley, J. N., Cook, M. K., Singh, R., Larrondo, J., & McMichael, A. J. (2023). A comprehensive review of platelet-rich plasma for the treatment of dermatologic disorders. *Journal of Dermatological Treatment, 34*(1), 2142035. https://doi.org/10.1080/09546634.2022.2142035.

Psoriasis: Epidemiology, clinical features, and quality of life. (n.d.). Retrieved March 11, 2023, from https://ard.bmj.com/content/64/suppl_2/ii18.short.

Redaelli, A., Romano, D., & Marciano, A. (2010). Face and neck revitalization with platelet-rich plasma (PRP): Clinical outcome in a series of 23 consecutively treated patients. *Journal of Drugs in Dermatology: JDD, 9*(5), 446-472.

Shin, M.-K., Lee, J.-H., Lee, S.-J., & Kim, N.-I. (2012). Platelet-rich plasma combined with fractional laser therapy for skin rejuvenation. *Dermatologic Surgery, 38*(4), 623-630. https://doi.org/10.1111/j.1524-4725.2011.02280.x.

Suh, D.-H., Lee, S.-J., Lee, J.-H., Kim, H.-J., Shin, M.-K., & Song, K.-Y. (2012). Treatment of striae distensae combined enhanced penetration platelet-rich plasma and ultrasound after plasma fractional radiofrequency. *Journal of Cosmetic and Laser Therapy, 14*(6), 272-276. https://doi.org/10.3109/14764172.2012.738916.

Treatment of inflammatory nail disorders—Dehesa—2012—Dermatologic Therapy—Wiley Online Library. (n.d.). Retrieved March 11, 2023, from https://onlinelibrary.wiley.com/doi/abs/10.1111/j.1529-8019.2012.01516.

Willemsen, J. C. N., Lindenblatt, N., & Stevens, H. P. J. D. (2013). Results and long-term patient satisfaction after gluteal augmentation with platelet-rich plasma-enriched autologous fat. *European Journal of Plastic Surgery, 36*(12), 777-782. https://doi.org/10.1007/s00238-013-0887-3.

Yuksel, E. P., Sahin, G., Aydin, F., Senturk, N., & Turanli, A. Y. (2014). Evaluation of effects of platelet-rich plasma on human facial skin. *Journal of Cosmetic and Laser Therapy, 16*(5), 206-208. https://doi.org/10.3109/14764172.2014.949274.

Chapter 21

The Role of PRP in Reproductive Medicine

Savaş Karakuş*, **MD**
Department of Obstetrics and Gynecology, Cumhuriyet University School of Medicine, Sivas, Turkiye

Abstract

Although the etiology of in vitro fertilization (IVF) failures has not been fully elucidated, the quality of transferred embryos and endometrial receptivity are the main factors that determine the success of implantation. The condition of the uterine cavity is known to be effective in the implantation process. The quality and number of ovum also increase the number of pregnancies obtained. Various methods have been tried to increase endometrial thickness and impact the ovary. Platelet-rich plasma (PRP) is one of them.

The PRP method can be defined in detail as administering plasma rich in platelets and growth factors to organs and/or tissues for treatment purposes. It has been used for a long time to help tissue and organ repair in the treatment of various injuries, particularly in branches such as orthopedics, plastic reconstructive and aesthetic surgery, and medical aesthetics.

In the PRP method, plasma is acquired by separating the blood taken from the patient by a special procedure. The obtained plasma is rich in platelets, whose main function in the body is blood coagulation. This plasma is given back to the patient through injection. Platelets help cell regeneration with the growth factors in their content. Administering PRP in the case of a thin endometrium is still an experimental intervention, there is no convincing scientific evidence that PRP

---

* Corresponding Author's Email: karakussavas@yahoo.com.

In: Current Clinical Recommendations ...
Editors: Nazan Yurtcu and Emel Güler
ISBN: 979-8-89113-723-3

applications are beneficial due to early menopause and deficiency of the ovarian reserve, and it is an experimental practice.

As an experimental intervention, PRP can only be administered under controlled research conditions, with the approval of the ethical committee and the permission for the experimental intervention acquired from the relevant units of the Ministry of Health, by explaining the possible risks.

Keywords: PRP, ovarian reserve, endometrial thickness

Introduction

Infertility is the absence of pregnancy for one year or more despite regular unprotected sexual intercourse. Infertility is classified as primary and secondary infertility. Infertility is called "primary infertility" in couples who have never had children and "secondary infertility" in couples who have had children before or have a history of miscarriage or stillbirth.

The purpose of infertility treatment should first be to find the cause of infertility and correct it. Considering the main causes of infertility, it is defined as male infertility, tubal and pelvic pathologies, ovulatory disorder, and unexplained infertility (Speroff et al., 2005).

Advancements in infertility treatment have increased its success rates. Thus, the expectations of infertile couples and their search for help in this regard have increased. Therefore, an increasing number of couples apply for infertility treatment. In vitro fertilization (IVF) represents a method that starts with controlled ovarian hyperstimulation with gonadotropins and continues with the aspiration of oocytes from the ovaries under transvaginal ultrasound, fertilization performed in the laboratory, and transcervical transfer of embryos into the uterus and is carried out in coordination with each other (Zarinara et al., 2016).

Infertility is a health problem with significant developments in diagnosis and treatment. The widespread use of assisted reproductive techniques (ARTs), the change in the perception in society, couples who have children at a later age, and the increased awareness of individuals of infertility and technological treatments have been factors in the formation of advancements in infertility diagnosis and treatment. Thus, couples experiencing infertility problems have become more sensitive and prone to receiving medical support and treatment.

Causes of Female Infertility

1. Ovulation disorders (Polycystic ovary syndrome, etc.)
2. Congestion in the tubes
3. Antisperm antibodies
4. Endometriosis
5. Pathologies in the uterus
6. Thyroid hormone disorders
7. Past infections related to genital organs
8. Previous surgeries related to the uterus and ovary
9. High prolactin levels
10. Decreased ovarian reserve due to advanced age
11. Cervical factor
12. Smoking
13. Being overweight
14. Closed cervix
15. Not having regular sexual intercourse
16. Early menopause
17. Adhesion in the endometrium
18. Luteal phase failure
19. Having undergone chemotherapy and radiotherapy treatment
20. Vaginismus

The following treatment methods are usually applied in couples who have decided to undergo treatment;

1. Ovulation induction,
2. Insemination,
3. Treatment according to the causes of infertility,
4. IVF

Treatment of Infertility

Nowadays, the increase in the number of in vitro fertilization centers and developments in the health sector ensure that infertility is perceived as a treatable disease and the rates of presenting to the hospital with successful treatment have increased significantly. At this point, it is important for individuals to receive successful treatment. Hence, the treatment process should be patient-specific and modifiable because the medical history and evaluations of the couple, economic levels, ages, religious beliefs, and cultural values differ and are important.

Evaluating patients appropriately before the treatment, using the methods determined accordingly in the treatment, and ensuring the patient's compliance with the treatment are important for the success of the treatment.

The success of IVF cycles depends on the complex relationship between endometrial receptivity and embryo quality. During the implantation window, endometrial receptivity is characterized by some morphological and functional changes. Endometrial thickness (ET) is a parameter that can be easily measured by transvaginal ultrasonography. Therefore, EC is essential to evaluate the condition of the endometrium. Nevertheless, the impact of ART on endometrial tissue and its thickness is still controversial nowadays. Although some studies report that pregnancy rates improve with increasing ET, there are studies in which this relationship has not been determined (Liao et al., 2022). There is no generally accepted limit value for ET in the studies conducted. However, in the literature, during the administration of human chorionic gonadotropin, an ET value of less than 7 mm is considered thin, and a value greater than 14 mm is considered an increase in endometrial thickness (Cagli et al., 2022; Prevedourakis et al., 1994).

Age, Number, and Quality of Oocytes and Embryos

It is known that reproductive functions are adversely affected by age in females. Females over the age of 35 who undergo IVF are more likely to have aneuploidies and mosaicism involving sex chromosomes and autosomal chromosomes (Munné et al., 2007).

Some studies have shown that aneuploidy can be detected in approximately half of the embryos in recurrent implantation failure cases (Magli et al., 2007; Kuliev et al., 2007). These cases have a high rate of chromosomal abnormalities, even in the presence of good morphology and division. The incidence of chromosomal abnormalities in embryos increases more in cases of previously unsuccessful IVF (Kuliev et al., 2007).

The annual cycle numbers and birth rates increase each year with advancements in assisted reproductive techniques. Treatment modalities also change with the development of exogenous gonadotropins and other drugs used for controlled ovarian stimulation. With patient-friendly treatment protocols, it is aimed to use fewer medications and obtain the highest pregnancy rates. It has been demonstrated that pregnancy rates increase with the increase in the number of mature oocytes obtained while targeting the development of more than one oocyte (Cohlen et al., 2005; Siristatidis et al., 2022).

Pregnancy rates decrease when the number of oocytes is low, and the risk of OHSS complications increases when the number of oocytes is high (David et al., 2020).

Endometrial Receptivity

Significant changes in the expression of specific endometrial molecules suggest that not only morphological but also functional endometrial defects play a role in recurrent implantation failures. Endometrial receptivity depends on adequate stimulation of estrogen and progesterone in glandular and stromal cells. This occurs through steroid effects or direct effects onreceptors or through paracrine mediators. In addition to the Noyes criteria used in the evaluation of endometrial function, alternative methods such as Doppler imaging, molecular markers, and gene profiling have been developed.

However, it is noteworthy that human progesterone receptor gene polymorphisms have not been fully linked to implantation failure to date (Rahnama et al., 2019).

A method that can change various causal factors proposed in this field or increase the possibility of implantation through a direct molecular mechanism has not been determined.

The high number of eggs and endometrial thickness increase the success of the IVF treatment. Various methods have been tried to increase endometrial thickness and increase the quality and number of the ovum. Platelet-rich plasma (PRP) is one of them.

The PRP method can be defined as injecting plasma rich in platelets and growth factors into organs and/or tissues for treatment purposes. It has recently been used in the treatment of various conditions, from hair loss to sports injuries. The purpose of PRP injections is to use the patient's blood cells to accelerate healing in a specific area. Owing to the PRP procedure, a natural rejuvenation is achieved without administering foreign substances and medications to the body. Recently, it has been suggested that it can be used in the treatment of females with infertility problems due to ovarian failure and thin endometrium.

Platelet-rich plasma is composed of two components: plasma and platelets. Platelets are blood cells that have an important role during wound healing. Platelets contain growth factors that, in addition to ensuring coagulation, can also trigger cell proliferation and stimulate tissue regeneration or healing in the treated area. To prepare PRP, which has a high platelet count, a blood sample is taken from the patient and centrifuged. The plasma obtained when the dense part is separated from the platelets accumulated in the upper part of the blood sample is the ready-made PRP.

The PRP acquired from the patient's blood sample is injected into the ovary or endometrium wall. The purpose here is to increase the density of growth factors in a certain area. These growth factors are used to accelerate the wound-healing process. Nevertheless, it should be known that PRP applied to the ovary affects the growth and maturation process of the ovum differently from wound healing. The biological mechanism behind PRP injections has not been fully clarified yet. Furthermore, another issue that should be kept in mind is that the possible activity durations of the growth factors contained in PRP are very short after injection.

The Site of PRP Injection into the Ovary in a Low Ovarian Reserve

The number of eggs and the egg quality of the woman are among the most important parameters that increase the chance of conception in IVF treatment. Age is one of the most significant factors affecting egg reserves. The number of eggs decreases rapidly when the woman's age is over 37. Some women younger than 40 may also experience a rapid decrease in the number of eggs due to early menopause. FSH (Follicle-stimulating hormone), AMH (Anti-müllerian hormone) tests, and ultrasonography are used to determine the egg reserve in the ovaries. Pregnancy can be achieved with in vitro fertilization treatment in women with reduced egg count.

PRP started to gain popularity with the claims that ovarian functions would start again with the injection of PRP into the ovaries of eight non-menstruating women in the menopause phase (aged between 45-50 years) in a publication from Greece. In later periods, under the influence of the press, case series presenting the results of PRP application in women with premature ovarian failure or decreased ovarian reserve were published in scientific journals. Furthermore, several reviews on the subject were extensively published by some clinics (Atkinson et al., 2021; Petryk et al., 2020).

A review by Atkinson et al. (2021) examined patients with inadequate response to IVF treatment, patients with premature ovarian failure, patients around menopause, and patients in menopause. As a result, it was claimed that "patients' hormonal status and ovarian reserve improve" (Petryk et al., 2020).

In case of series, studies of the hormone values of patients receiving PRP injection before and after PRP application may yield results showing the benefits of PRP. However, the values "before–after" fluctuate naturally anyway. Initially, low values may appear to be increasing, while initially, high values may appear to be decreasing. This is called the "return toward the mean law," which can make a treatment examined in "before-after" studies appear more beneficial than it actually is. In other words, observations such as decreased FSH, increased AMH, or increased number of follicles and eggs after PRP injection may actually depend on this simple law, not on PRP.

When assessing the benefits of PRP, the result should be an increase in the couple's chances of returning home with an infant, not an increase in the hormone level or the number of follicles. It can be argued that this procedure is successful if the difference in the rates of live birth is in favor of patients who have undergone PRP injection compared to a control group that has not undergone PRP injection.

Important shortcomings are that the studies include only selected patient series, a control group is absent, and details of the mechanism of how PRP might work on the ovaries are unknown.

As a result, there is no convincing scientific evidence that PRP application is beneficial due to early menopause and ovarian reserve deficiency, and it is an experimental practice. In light of the available information, it is not yet accepted practice to present PRP injection as an effective treatment to increase ovarian reserves and to perform it outside of research conditions.

The Site of PRP Injection due to a Thin Endometrium Thin Endometrium

It is still a controversial issue whether a thin endometrium has an adverse effect on pregnancy outcomes in IVF treatments. Studies have shown that significant negative impacts of a thin endometrium on pregnancy outcomes may occur in the presence of a thinner endometrium, perhaps 5 mm, rather than the generally accepted 7 mm limit (Shakerian et al., 2021).

Most of the existing studies reporting the results of PRP injection in order to thicken the endometrium and improve pregnancy outcomes in the case of a thin endometrium by making use of the growth factors it contains are selected case series, and there are no studies with a control group to show whether the applied treatment is really effective (El-Toukhy et al., 2021).

PRP "before–after" studies that evaluate endometrial thickness may be affected by the "return toward the mean law" mentioned above.

Most studies claiming the benefits of PRP applications are in the form of uncontrolled case series.

Although Eftekhar et al. (2018) reported that endometrial thickness increased more in the group administered with PRP injection in a randomized controlled trial they conducted with 43 patients administered with PRP injection and 40 patients in the control group, no statistically significant increase was found in the ongoing pregnancy rates. However, the success of a procedure is the number of children taken home.

In the case of a thin endometrium, the application of PRP is still an experimental intervention, and there is a need for studies involving large numbers of patients to perform PRP injection outside the research conditions for the treatment of a thin endometrium and present it as an effective treatment.

Conclusion

Before increasing the ovarian reserve, PRP has been widely used for tissue healing and repair in sports injuries, rheumatic disease treatment, hair loss, and skin cosmetic applications. However, as a result of controlled trials, it has been understood that PRP applications are not beneficial in the field of orthopedics and physical therapy (Dietrich et al., 2017).

Experts also warn that the irregularity in the development of embryos that may occur with PRP application may cause significant changes in growing infants and possibly lead to an increased risk of disease in children.

Hence, it is not approved by the American Food and Drug Administration and is accepted as an experimental practice. As an experimental intervention, PRP can only be applied under controlled research conditions, with ethical committee approval and permission for experimental intervention obtained from the relevant units of the Ministry of Health, by explaining the possible risks.

References

Atkinson, L., Martin, F., & Sturmey, R. G. (2021). Intraovarian injection of platelet-rich plasma in assisted reproduction: too much too soon? *Human Reproduction, 36*, 1737–1750. https://doi.org/10.1093/humrep/deab106.

Cagli, F., Dolanbay, M., Gülseren, V., Gurler, A. D., & Aygen, E. M. (2022). Does endometrial thickness affect pregnancy outcomes in isolated male infertility IVF cycles? A retrospective cohort study. *Journal of Obstetrics and Gynaecology, 42*(7), 3199–3203. https://doi.org/10.1080/01443615.2022.2109141.

Cohlen, B., Cantineau, A., D'Hooghe, T., & te Velde, E. (2005). Multiple pregnancy after assisted reproduction. *The Lancet, 366*(9484), 452–453. https://doi.org/10.1016/s0140-6736(05)67055-9.

Dietrich, F., Hammerman, M., & Blomgran, P. (2017). Effect of platelet-rich plasma on rat Achilles tendon healing is related to microbiota. *Acta Orthopaedica, 88*, 416–421. https://doi.org/10.1080/17453674.2017.1293447.

Eftekhar, M., Neghab, N., Naghshineh, E., & Khani, P. (2018). Can autologous platelet-rich plasma expand endometrial thickness and improve pregnancy rate during frozen-thawed embryo transfer cycle? A randomized clinical trial. *Taiwanese Journal of Obstetrics and Gynecology, 57*, 810–813. https://doi.org/10.1016/j.tjog.2018.10.007.

El-Toukhy, T., Coomarasamy, A., Khairy, M., Sunkara, K., Seed, P., Khalaf, Y., & Braude, P. (2008). The relationship between endometrial thickness and the outcome of medicated frozen embryo replacement cycles. *Fertility and Sterility, 89*, 832–839. https://doi.org/10.1016/j.fertnstert.2007.04.031.

Kuliev, A., & Verlinsky, Y. (2003). The role of preimplantation genetic diagnosis in women of advanced reproductive age. *Current Opinion in Obstetrics and Gynecology, 15*(3), 233–238. https://doi.org/10.1097/00001703-200306000-00004.

Liao, Z., Liu, C., Cai, L., Shen, L., Sui, C., Zhang, H., & Qian, K. (2022). The effect of endometrial thickness on pregnancy, maternal, and perinatal outcomes of women in fresh cycles after IVF/ICSI: A systematic review and meta-analysis. *Frontiers in Endocrinology, 12*, 814648. https://doi.org/10.3389/fendo.2021.814648.

Magli, M. C., Gianaroli, L., Ferraretti, A. P., Lappi, M., Ruberti, A., & Farfalli, V. (2007). Embryo morphology and development are dependent on the chromosomal complement. *Fertility and Sterility, 87*(3), 534–541. https://doi.org/10.1016/j.fertnstert.2006.07.1512.

Munné, S., Chen, S., Colls, P., Garrisi, J., Zheng, X., Cekleniak, N., Lenzi, M., Hughes, P., Fischer, J., Garrisi, M., Cohen, J., & Tomkin, G. (2007). Maternal age, morphology, development, and chromosome abnormalities in over 6000 cleavage-stage embryos. *Reproductive Biomedicine Online, 14*(5), 628–634. https://doi.org/10.1016/s1472-6483(10)61057-7.

Petryk, N., & Petryk, M. (2020). Ovarian rejuvenation through platelet-rich autologous plasma (PRP) – A chance to have a baby without donor eggs, improving the life quality of women suffering from early menopause without synthetic hormonal treatment. *Reproductive Sciences, 27*, 1975–1982. https://doi.org/10.1007/s43032-020-00266-8.

Prevedourakis, C., Loutradis, D., Kalianidis, C., Markis, N., & Asavantinos, D. (1994). Hysterosalpingography and hysteroscopy in female infertility. *Human Reproduction, 9*, 2353–2355. https://doi.org/10.1093/oxfordjournals.humrep.a138451.

Rahnama, R., Rafiee, M., Fouladi, S., Akbari-Fakhrabadi, M., Mehrabian, F., & Rezaei, A. (2019). Gene expression analysis of membrane progesterone receptors in women with recurrent spontaneous abortion: A case-control study. *BMC Research Notes, 12*(1), 790. https://doi.org/10.1186/s13104-019-4787-x.

Shakerian, B., Turkgeldi, E., Yildiz, S., Keles, I., & Ata, B. (2021). Endometrial thickness is not predictive for live birth after embryo transfer, even without a cutoff. *Fertility and Sterility, 116*, 130–137. https://doi.org/10.1016/j.fertnstert.2021.02.041.

Siristatidis, C., Stavros,S., Dafopoulos, K., Sergentanis, T., Domali, E., Drakakis, P., & Loutradis, D. (2022). A randomized controlled trial on the efficacy and safety of low-dose hCG in a short protocol with GnRH agonist and ovarian stimulation with recombinant FSH (rFSH) during the follicular phase in infertile women undergoing ART. *Reproductive Sciences, 29*(2), 497–505. https://doi.org/10.1007/s43032-021-00683-3.

Speroff, L., & Fritz, M. A. (2005). *Clinical Gynaecologic Endocrinology and Infertility* (7th ed., pp.1013-1067). Lippincott Williams & Wilkins.

Zarinara, A., Zeraati, H., Kamali, K., Mohammad, K., Shahnazari, P., & Akhondi, M. M. (2016). Models predicting success of infertility treatment: A systematic review. *Journal of Reproduction and Infertility, 17*(2), 68–81.

Chapter 22

PRP Treatment for Tendon Healing

Yücel Bilgin*, **MD**
and Saltuk Buğra Güler, MD
Department of Orthopedics and Traumatology, Bursa Uludag University, Bursa, Turkiye

Abstract

The use of Platelet-Rich Plasma (PRP) in the treatment of tendon injuries has gained significant attention. Tendons, which connect muscles to bones, frequently experience injuries. PRP is a plasma solution derived from the patient's own blood and contains a high concentration of platelets. Platelets release growth factors that are essential for blood clotting and initiate the healing process. PRP is used to expedite the natural healing of tendon injuries. Research studies have demonstrated that PRP promotes tendon healing and reduces pain. It is believed that PRP stimulates tendon cells, increases collagen production, and facilitates tissue remodeling. However, debates regarding the efficacy of PRP persist, necessitating further research. In summary, PRP is considered a potential treatment option for tendon injuries due to its potential to accelerate the healing process. Nonetheless, additional studies are required to evaluate its full effectiveness and long-term outcomes.

Keywords: platelet-rich plasma, tendon, injury, healing, blood

---

* Corresponding Author's Email: dryucelbilgin@gmail.com.

In: Current Clinical Recommendations ...
Editors: Nazan Yurtcu and Emel Güler
ISBN: 979-8-89113-723-3

Introduction

Tendon injuries are common and can result in pain, functional limitations, and prolonged recovery. Tendon injuries are injuries that occur as a result of the tendon tissue being subjected to sudden force or trauma. Injuries usually occur during sports activities and sudden movements. Consequently, researchers and medical professionals have been actively exploring new treatment modalities to enhance the healing process and improve outcomes. PRP has received significant attention in recent years for its potential in tendon healing.

Tendons are vital connective tissue structures that transmit forces from muscles to bones. However, its limited blood supply contributes to a slower healing process compared to other tissues. This delayed healing response often leads to compromised function and an increased risk of re-injury.

PRP is a regenerative medicine technique that involves the extraction and concentration of platelets from the patient's own blood. Platelets contain numerous growth factors and bioactive proteins that play a fundamental role in tissue repair and regeneration (Beitia et al., 2023). When applied to tendon injuries, PRP is believed to accelerate healing by stimulating cellular responses, promoting collagen synthesis, and facilitating tissue remodeling (Chalidis et al., 2023).

The objective of this chapter is to explore the effect of PRP on tendon healing. We will conduct a review of the existing literature, including research studies and clinical trials, to assess the efficacy and potential benefits of PRP as a treatment modality for tendon injuries.

In Vivo and In Vitro Effects of PRP on Tendon Healing

A considerable number of in vitro and in vivo studies have investigated the effects of PRP on tendon healing. In vitro studies can be divided into those conducted on animals in experimental settings and those performed on humans.

In a 2007 study by Schnabel et al. (Schnabel et al., 2007), the impact of platelet-rich plasma (PRP) on tendon cells derived from the flexor digitorum superficialis of horses was explored. The results demonstrated that PRP increased the levels of collagen type I (COL1A1) and collagen type III (COL3A1), while simultaneously reducing the levels of matrix metalloproteinase-13 (MMP-13). Similarly, a separate study conducted in 2015 by Zhou et al. (Zhou et al., 2015) investigated the effects of PRP on patellar tendon cells obtained from rabbits. Their findings indicated that PRP enhanced the expression of anabolic genes such as alpha-smooth muscle actin (α-SMA), collagen type I, and collagen type III.

In terms of in vivo studies, Anitua et al. (Anitua et al., 2006) conducted research in 2006 where they applied PRP to intact sheep Achilles tendons, resulting in increased cell density and vascularity. Lyras et al. (Lyras et al., 2011) investigated the effects of PRP on a model of full-thickness Achilles tendon rupture in a 2011 study. They demonstrated that PRP accelerated tendon healing by increasing levels of IGF-1 in the epi-tendon. Bosch et al. (Bosch et al., 2011) revealed in a 2011 study that PRP enhanced collagen organization during tendon healing. Additionally, Xu et al. (Xu et al., 2017) determined in a 2017 study using a rat model of full-thickness Achilles tendon rupture that PRP promoted cell maturation and collagen organization. Han et al. (Han et al., 2019) found in their 2019 study on a full-thickness rotator cuff rupture model that PRP increased the levels of VEGF, PDGF, EGF, and TGF-β. Moreover, in a 2020 study (Kobayashi et al., 2020) using a rat patellar tendon rupture model, PRP expedited tendon recovery time, increased tendon thickness, and improved vascularity. Furthermore, Yu et al. (Yu et al., 2021) reported in their investigation of a partial Achilles tendon rupture model in rats that PRP enhanced fibroblast orientation and collagen matrix on the 5th day while reducing cell apoptosis. They also observed an increase in new collagen fibers on the 10th day.

An experimental study conducted by Gürger et al. (Gurger et al., 2021) established a rat model of rotator cuff tendon rupture to explore the histological and biomechanical effects of combining ozone with PRP on the healing process. The study included a total of 28 rats divided into four groups. The findings revealed an increase in collagen fiber continuity and orientation in the groups where ozone was added. Additionally, the group that received a combination of PRP and ozone demonstrated the highest level of biomechanical strength among all the groups.

In the literature, there are many in vivo and in vitro studies examining the effect of PRP on tendon healing. These studies have generally shown that PRP has positive contributions to tendon healing at the molecular level. This effect has been experimentally demonstrated in many tendons, such as the rotator cuff, flexor tendons, and Achilles tendon.

Use of PRP in the Treatment of Acute Tendon Injuries

In this section, the effect of PRP on the healing of acute tendon injuries will be discussed. Its effect on chronic tendinopathies is described in other parts of the book. The effectiveness of PRP has been studied in the treatment of acute tendon injuries, particularly Achilles tendon rupture. Here are the findings from selected studies:

A randomized controlled clinical trial by Schepull et al. (2011) included 30 patients with surgically treated Achilles tendon rupture. PRP was administered to 14 patients in addition to surgical treatment. No significant differences were found between the PRP group and the control group in terms of elastic modulus, heel raise index, and clinical outcomes.

De Carli et al. (2016) studied 30 patients with Achilles tendon rupture who underwent surgical treatment, with half receiving PRP. No significant differences were observed in clinical results, jumping ability, or tendon morphology between the PRP group and the non-PRP group.

Zou et al. (2016) conducted a prospective study on acute Achilles tendon injury treated surgically with the injection of PRP into the paratenon. The PRP group showed better ankle joint range of motion, higher SF-36 scores, and improved calf circumference compared to the control group.

Other studies, such as those by Boesen et al. (2020), Boksh et al. (2022), and Keene et al. (2019), also reported no significant differences in clinical and functional outcomes between the PRP and control groups in conservative or non-operative treatment of Achilles tendon rupture.

The data in the literature listed above are controversial in terms of showing the effect of PRP in the treatment of acute Achilles tendon rupture. Although most literature does not show anyadditional benefit, there is also data showing that it is beneficial. There is still a need for studies involving larger case series on this subject.

Conclusion

Acute tendon injuries are common problems faced by athletes and active individuals. Appropriate treatment methods and strategies are important for the effective healing of such injuries.

Platelet-Rich Plasma (PRP) is a product obtained by concentrating platelets in the blood. Platelets are important cells that contain factors that promote healing, such as growth factors, cytokines, and other biological substances. Therefore, it makes sense to consider PRP as a potential treatment option to promote tendon healing.

Studies on the effects of PRP on acute tendon healing have yielded conflicting results. Some studies have suggested that PRP accelerates tendon healing and reduces pain. In these studies, it was observed that PRP increased the blood supply of the tendon, promoted cell proliferation, and collagen synthesis. However, other studies have had fewer positive results on the effectiveness of PRP.

In conclusion, in vivo and in vitro studies on tendon healing using PRP have shown promising effects based on molecular data. Numerous studies have demonstrated its potential to improve the healing process, increase tendon strength, and accelerate healing in a variety of tendon pathologies. Research findings indicate that PRP therapy can lead to increased collagen production, enhanced cell proliferation, and enhanced vascularization, all of which contribute to improved tendon healing. However, despite the positive results, the results of clinical studies are controversial. Despite the studies showing that it is beneficial, there are also publications showing that it does not provide additional benefits. There is still a need for studies involving larger case series on this subject. In addition, clinical studies are needed on other tendons in the human body other than the Achilles tendon. It is important to note that the therapeutic benefits of PRP may vary depending on several factors such as the severity of tendon injury, patient characteristics, and the specific PRP preparation protocols used.

References

Anitua, E., Sanchez, M., Nurden, A. T., Zalduendo, M., De La Fuente, M., Orive, G., Azofra, J., & Andia, I. (2006). Autologous fibrin matrices: A potential source of biological mediators that modulate tendon cell activities. *Journal of Biomedical Materials Research. Part A,* 77(2), 285–293. https://doi.org/10.1002/JBM.A.30585.

Beitia, M., Delgado, D., Mercader, J., Gimeno, I., Espregueira-Mendes, J., Aizpurua, B., & Sánchez, M. (2023). The effect of short-term cryopreservation on the properties and functionality of platelet-rich plasma. *Platelets,* 34(1), 2210243. https://doi.org/10.1080/09537104.2023.2210243.

Boesen, A. P., Boesen, M. I., Hansen, R., Barfod, K. W., Lenskjold, A., Malliaras, P., & Langberg, H. (2020). Effect of Platelet-Rich Plasma on Nonsurgically Treated Acute Achilles Tendon Ruptures: A Randomized, Double-Blinded Prospective Study. *The American Journal of Sports Medicine,* 48(9), 2268–2276. https://doi.org/

10.1177/0363546520922541.

Boksh, K., Elbashir, M., Thomas, O., Divall, P., & Mangwani, J. (2022). Platelet-Rich Plasma in acute Achilles tendon ruptures: A systematic review and meta-analysis. *Foot* (Edinburgh, Scotland), 53. https://doi.org/10.1016/J.FOOT.2022.101923.

Bosch, G., René van Weeren, P., Barneveld, A., & van Schie, H. T. M. (2011). Computerised analysis of standardised ultrasonographic images to monitor the repair of surgically created core lesions in equine superficial digital flexor tendons following treatment with intratendinous platelet rich plasma or placebo. *The Veterinary Journal,* 187(1), 92–98. https://doi.org/10.1016/J.TVJL.2009.10.014.

Chalidis, B., Givissis, P., Papadopoulos, P., & Pitsilos, C. (2023). Molecular and Biologic Effects of Platelet-Rich Plasma (PRP) in Ligament and Tendon Healing and Regeneration: A Systematic Review. *International Journal of Molecular Sciences,* 24(3). https://doi.org/10.3390/IJMS24032744.

De Carli, A., Lanzetti, R. M., Ciompi, A., Lupariello, D., Vadalà, A., Argento, G., Ferretti, A., Vulpiani, M. C., & Vetrano, M. (2016). Can platelet-rich plasma have a role in Achilles tendon surgical repair? *Knee Surgery, Sports Traumatology, Arthroscopy: Official Journal of the ESSKA,* 24(7), 2231–2237. https://doi.org/10.1007/S00167-015-3580-1.

Gurger, M., Once, G., Yilmaz, E., Demir, S., Calik, I., Say, Y., Kavakli, A., Key, S., Gurbuz, M. U., & Bingollu, O. (2021). The effect of the platelet-rich plasma and ozone therapy on tendon-to-bone healing in the rabbit rotator cuff repair model. *Journal of Orthopaedic Surgery and Research,* 16(1). https://doi.org/10.1186/S13018-021-02320-W.

Han, L., Fang, W. L., Jin, B., Xu, S. C., Zheng, X., & Hu, Y. G. (2019). Enhancement of tendon-bone healing after rotator cuff injuries using combined therapy with mesenchymal stem cells and platelet rich plasma. *European Review for Medical and Pharmacological Sciences,* 23(20), 9075–9084. https://doi.org/10.26355/EURREV_201910_19310.

Keene, D. J., Alsousou, J., Harrison, P., Hulley, P., Wagland, S., Parsons, S. R., Thompson, J. Y., O'Connor, H. M., Schlüssel, M. M., Dutton, S. J., Lamb, S. E., & Willett, K. (2019). Platelet rich plasma injection for acute Achilles tendon rupture: PATH-2 randomised, placebo controlled, superiority trial. *BMJ* (Clinical Research Ed.), 367. https://doi.org/10.1136/BMJ.L6132.

Kobayashi, Y., Saita, Y., Takaku, T., Yokomizo, T., Nishio, H., Ikeda, H., Takazawa, Y., Nagao, M., Kaneko, K., & Komatsu, N. (2020). Platelet-rich plasma (PRP) accelerates murine patellar tendon healing through enhancement of angiogenesis and collagen synthesis. *Journal of Experimental Orthopaedics,* 7(1), 1–10. https://doi.org/10.1186/S40634-020-00267-1/FIGURES/6.

Lyras, D. N., Kazakos, K., Georgiadis, G., Mazis, G., Middleton, R., Richards, S., O'Connor, D., & Agrogiannis, G. (2011). Does a single application of PRP alter the expression of IGF-I in the early phase of tendon healing? *The Journal of Foot and Ankle Surgery: Official Publication of the American College of Foot and Ankle Surgeons,* 50(3), 276–282. https://doi.org/10.1053/J.JFAS.2011.02.010.

Schepull, T., Kvist, J., Norrman, H., Trinks, M., Berlin, G., & Aspenberg, P. (2011). Autologous platelets have no effect on the healing of human achilles tendon ruptures: a randomized single-blind study. *The American Journal of Sports Medicine,* 39(1), 38–47. https://doi.org/10.1177/0363546510383515.

Schnabel, L. V., Mohammed, H. O., Miller, B. J., McDermott, W. G., Jacobson, M. S., Santangelo, K. S., & Fortier, L. A. (2007). Platelet rich plasma (PRP) enhances anabolic gene expression patterns in flexor digitorum superficialis tendons. *Journal of Orthopaedic Research: Official Publication of the Orthopaedic Research Society,* 25(2), 230–240. https://doi.org/10.1002/jor.20278.

Xu, K., Al-ani, M. K., Sun, Y., Xu, W., Pan, L., Song, Y., Xu, Z. L., Pan, X., & Yang, L. (2017). Platelet-rich plasma activates tendon-derived stem cells to promote regeneration of Achilles tendon rupture in rats. *Journal of Tissue Engineering and Regenerative Medicine,* 11(4), 1173–1184. https://doi.org/10.1002/term.2020.

Yu, T. Y., Pang, J. H. S., Lin, L. P., Cheng, J. W., Liu, S. J., & Tsai, W. C. (2021). Platelet-Rich Plasma Releasate Promotes Early Healing in Tendon After Acute Injury. *Orthopaedic Journal of Sports Medicine,* 9(4). https://doi.org/10.1177/2325967121990377.

Zhou, Y., Zhang, J., Wu, H., Hogan, M. C. V., & Wang, J. H. C. (2015). The differential effects of leukocyte-containing and pure platelet-rich plasma (PRP) on tendon stem/progenitor cells - implications of PRP application for the clinical treatment of tendon injuries. *Stem Cell Research & Therapy,* 6(1). https://doi.org/10.1186/s13287-015-0172-4.

Zou, J., Mo, X., Shi, Z., Li, T., Xue, J., Mei, G., & Li, X. (2016). A Prospective Study of Platelet-Rich Plasma as Biological Augmentation for Acute Achilles Tendon Rupture Repair. *BioMed Research International,* 2016(Special Issue), 1-8. https://doi.org/10.1155/2016/9364170.

Chapter 23

Efficacy of PRP Injection in Plantar Fasciitis

Abdülhalim Akar[*], MD
Department of Orthopedics and Traumatology, Private Emsey Hospital, Istanbul, Turkiye

Abstract

Plantar fasciitis (PF) is very common in the community and is one of the most common causes of heel pain. It is especially seen in those with foot anomalies, those who stand for a long time, runners, and obese people. PF is a degenerative disease that occurs in the calcaneal tubercle, which is the origin of the plantar fascia. Platelet-rich plasma (PRP) therapy is used as a safe treatment option for tendon, muscle, bone, and cartilage injuries. PRP therapy can be a good alternative, especially in resistant cases, due to the high amount of growth factors and cytokines it contains. With PRP treatment, both good functional and pain-reducing results can be obtained.

Keywords: plantar fasciitis, platelet-rich plasma, injection

Introduction

The plantar fascia is a thin fibrous connective tissue located on the sole of the foot between the calcaneus and the toes. It supports the medial longitudinal arch of the foot, absorbs the load on the foot, and supports the stability of the foot during walking (Bolgla & Malone, 2004; Kane et al., 2001).

[*] Corresponding Author's Email: ahalimakar@gmail.com.

In: Current Clinical Recommendations ...
Editors: Nazan Yurtcu and Emel Güler
ISBN: 979-8-89113-723-3

Plantar fasciitis (PF) is one of the most common causes of heel pain. It occurs in approximately 11% to 15% of the adult population (Cole et al., 2005; Schwartz & Su, 2014). Although PF can be seen at all ages, it most commonly occurs between the ages of 40 and 60. There is no difference between the male and female genders (Martin et al., 1998; Taunton, 2002). The diagnosis can be made by anamnesis and clinical examination. Rarely, further investigations may be required. Patients with plantar fasciitis mostly consult the physician with heel pain that occurs when first walking on the ground in the morning. Pain typically occurs in the medial calcaneal tubercle and is exacerbated by pressure on this area when the toes are in dorsiflexion. Many treatment methods are used in the treatment of plantar fasciitis. Non-steroidal anti-inflammatory agents and steroid injections, cold application, plantar fasciitis insoles, and plantar fascia stretching exercises are recommended as medical treatment. Even surgical treatments are applied in patients with very resistant PF (Johnson et al., 2014; Salvi, 2015).

Platelet-rich plasma (PRP) injections have been used quite frequently in ligament and tendon pathologies in recent years. Due to its high cytokine and cell content, it increases tendon regeneration in local applications. Compared to whole blood, PRP contains approximately 25 times more platelets and has been shown to accelerate recovery in muscle and tendon diseases with the growth factors it contains (Anitua et al., 2005; Cole et al., 2005; Hall et al., 2009; McCarrel & Fortier, 2009).

Anatomy

Plantar fascia starts from the periosteum of the medial calcaneal tubercle and extends to the metatarsal heads. The plantar fascia is a fibrous connective tissue located along the longitudinal axis of the foot. Although the heel part is in the form of a thin layer, the middle part of the fascia is quite thick and progresses towards all metatarsal heads by wrapping the flexor tendons. It is supported by an elastic multilobular fat pad in the heel area. This adipose tissue absorbs up to 110% of body weight during walking and 250% during running (Gefen et al., 2001).

Etiology

PF is a degenerative disease usually caused by microtears due to overuse. Pes planus, pes cavus, and decreased ankle movements have been shown to be predisposing factors. In the pes cavus anomaly, excessive stress occurs in the heel because the foot does not distribute the load equally. In most patients, tension may develop in the posterior leg muscles such as the soleus and gastrocnemius. About half of patients develop a calcaneal spur, which causes very sharp pain in the center of the heel. PF is frequently seen in long-distance runners and older adults. Other risk factors have been shown to be obesity, long-term periods, and aging.

Treatment Methods

Conservative treatments are mostly preferred for the treatment of PF. The symptoms of the patients regress after 12-18 months of conservative treatment. The most commonly used treatment methods are plantar fascia stretching exercises, ice compress applications, silicone insoles, pain relievers, corticosteroid corticosteroids and PRP injections, iontophoresis, and extracorporeal shock wave therapy.

Plantar Fascia Stretching Exercises and Ice Compress Applications

It is usually the first method to start treatment and is frequently preferred by physicians because it is both inexpensive and easy to use. The ice compress is applied for 10 minutes at the end of each day and immediately after getting out of bed in the morning. It has been shown in the literature that plantar fascia-specific stretching exercises are quite effective (Digiovanni et al., 2006). While the patient is in a sitting position, the patient forces their toes to dorsiflexion with one hand and feels the tension here applying pressure to the medial calcaneal tubercle with the other hand (Figure 1). The patient is asked to do this exercise at least 3 times and for 30 seconds. It is recommended to do exercises, especially before walking on the ground first thing in the morning.

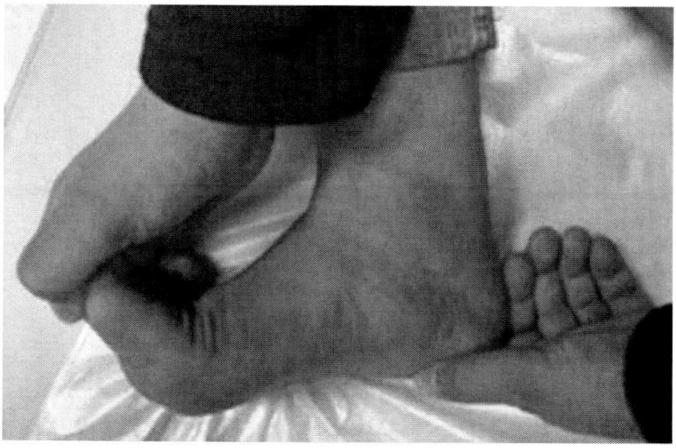

Figure 1. While the fingers are forced into dorsiflexion, the tension in the plantar fascia is felt with the other hand (Author's own archive).

NSAID

The use of anti-inflammatory agents is controversial in the treatment of plantar fasciitis. Various rates have been reported on the treatment success of NSAI drugs in studies (Wolgin et al., 1994). The most important advantage of NSAI drugs is that these drugs are easy and inexpensive to obtain. GIS and renal side effects are among the most important disadvantages (McCarthy, 1998).

Corticosteroid Injections

A steroid injection may be a good option for patients with PF who are resistant to other treatments. In patients who will be injected with steroids, it should be ensured that there is no tumor or infection in that area. More than 70% success rates have been reported in studies (Kane et al., 2001). However, single steroid injections are often insufficient and repeated injections are required. This may cause complications in patients such as fat pad atrophy and plantar fascia ruptures (Acevedo & Beskin, 1998; Neufeld & Cerrato, 2008; Ogden et al., 2002).

Focal Extracorporeal Shock Wave Therapy

It has been shown in the literature that focal extracorporeal shock wave therapy (ESWT) is effective in cases of persistent PF. Its effectiveness has been shown especially in cases that do not respond to other conservative treatments. ESWT is a non-invasive treatment that takes 10 to 15 minutes (Ibrahim et al., 2010; Malay et al., 2006).

Surgical Treatment

Failure rates of approximately 10% have been reported for all conservative treatments. In these patients, surgery is performed to release the plantar fascia from the calcaneal tubercle. However, complications such as nerve damage, infection, and tarsal instability may occur after surgery (Kinley et al., 1993; Tomczak & Haverstock, 1995).

PRP

Local PRP injection therapy is a relatively new treatment for chronic ligament and tendon diseases. PRP is obtained by centrifugation of platelet-rich plasma from the patient's whole blood. When approximately 25 cc of whole blood venous is taken from the patient, 3-4 cc of PRP is obtained after centrifugation. A straight line is drawn from the posterior border of the medial malleolus from the injection entry point to the sole of the foot. It is determined as 1 finger or 1.5 cm proximal to the sole of the foot (Figure 2). After the injection site is sterilized, the injection is made into the most tense and sensitive area of the plantar fascia. Intermittent ice compresses are recommended for 2 days after the injection. Putting a full load on it for 3 days is not allowed. The patient is recommended to wear for 2 weeks and not to do strenuous exercises such as jogging. After the patient is checked in the outpatient clinic for control in the first month after the injection, they are allowed to play sports as they can tolerate.

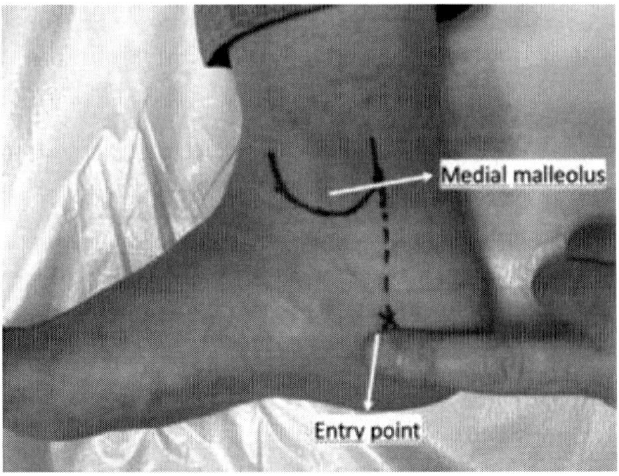

Figure 2. Injection entry point (Author's own archive).

In many studies in the literature, it has been stated that PRP is effective, especially in chronic cases (Gonnade et al., 2018). In the study by Monto et al., it was shown that PRP gives better long-term results than steroid injection in persistent chronic cases (Monto, 2014). Mahindra et al., on the other hand, examined the results of the third month after PRP and steroid injection, and the PRP injection was found to be significantly superior at the end of the third month (Mahindra et al., 2016). In the Peerbooms study, the first year results of the patients who received corticosteroid injection with PRP were examined and it was shown that both the pain was less and functional results were better in the PRP group. No complications were observed in the PRP group during the 1-year follow-up period (Peerbooms et al., 2019). Especially considering the side effects of steroid injections, PRP may be a safer method.

Conclusion

PRP treatment is widely used in muscle and tendon disorders, and its effectiveness has been shown especially in the treatment of chronic and resistant plantar fasciitis. PRP is a good treatment option in refractory cases that do not respond to conservative treatment, thanks to its dense platelet and growth factors.

References

Acevedo, J. I., & Beskin, J. L. (1998). Complications of plantar fascia rupture associated with corticosteroid injection. *Foot & Ankle International,* 19(2), 91–97. https://doi.org/10.1177/107110079801900207.

Anitua, E., Andí, I., Sanchez, M., Azofra, J., del Mar Zalduendo, M., de la Fuente, M., Nurden, P., & Nurden, A. T. (2005). Autologous preparations rich in growth factors promote proliferation and induce VEGF and HGF production by human tendon cells in culture. *Journal of Orthopaedic Research,* 23(2), 281–286. https://doi.org/10.1016/ j.orthres.2004.08.015.

Bolgla, L. A., & Malone, T. R. (2004). Plantar fasciitis and the windlass mechanism: a biomechanical link to clinical practice. *Journal of Athletic Training,* 39(1), 77–82. https://www.journalofathletictraining.org.

Cole, C., Seto, C., & Gazewood, J. (2005). Plantar fasciitis: Evidence-based review of diagnosis and therapy. *Am Fam Physician,* 72(11), 2237-2242. PMID: 16342847.

Digiovanni, B. F., Nawoczenski, D. A., Malay, D. P., Graci, P. A., Williams, T. T., Wilding, G. E., & Baumhauer, J. F. (2006). Plantar fascia-specific stretching exercise improves outcomes in patients with chronic plantar fasciitis. *The Journal of Bone & Joint Surgery,* 88(8), 1775–1781. https://doi.org/10.2106/JBJS.E.01281.

Gefen, A., Megido-Ravid, M., & Itzchak, Y. (2001). In vivo biomechanical behavior of the human heel pad during the stance phase of gait. *Journal of Biomechanics*, 34(12), 1661–1665. https://doi.org/10.1016/S0021-9290(01)00143-9.

Gonnade, N., Bajpayee, A., Elhence, A., Lokhande, V., Mehta, N., Mishra, M., & Kaur, A. (2018). Regenerative efficacy of therapeutic quality platelet-rich plasma injections versus phonophoresis with kinesiotaping for the treatment of chronic plantar fasciitis: A prospective randomized pilot study. *Asian Journal of Transfusion Science,* 12(2), 105. https://doi.org/10.4103/ajts.AJTS_48_17.

Hall, M. P., Band, P. A., Meislin, R. J., Jazrawi, L. M., & Cardone, D. A. (2009). Platelet-rich plasma: Current concepts and application in sports medicine. *Journal of the American Academy of Orthopaedic Surgeons, 17*(10), 602–608. https://doi.org/10.5435/00124635-200910000-00002.

Ibrahim, M. I., Donatelli, R. A., Schmitz, C., Hellman, M. A., & Buxbaum, F. (2010). Chronic plantar fasciitis treated with two sessions of radial extracorporeal shock wave therapy. *Foot & Ankle International, 31*(5), 391–397. https://doi.org/10.3113/FAI.2010.0391.

Johnson, R. E., Haas, K., Lindow, K., & Shields, R. (2014). Plantar fasciitis. *Orthopaedic Nursing, 33*(4), 198–204. https://doi.org/10.1097/NOR.0000000000000063.

Kane, D., Greaney, T., Shanahan, M., Duffy, G., Bresnihan, B., Gibney, R., & FitzGerald, O. (2001). The role of ultrasonography in the diagnosis and management of idiopathic plantar fasciitis. *Rheumatology, 40*(9), 1002–1008. https://doi.org/10.1093/rheumatology/40.9.1002.

Kinley, S., Frascone, S., Calderone, D., Wertheimer, S. J., Squire, M. A., & Wiseman, F. A. (1993). Endoscopic plantar fasciotomy versus traditional heel spur surgery: a prospective study. *The Journal of Foot and Ankle Surgery: Official Publication of the American College of Foot and Ankle Surgeons, 32*(6), 595–603.

Mahindra, P., Yamin, M., Selhi, H. S., Singla, S., & Soni, A. (2016). Chronic plantar fasciitis: Effect of platelet-rich plasma, corticosteroid, and placebo. *Orthopedics, 39*(2), e285-9. https://doi.org/10.3928/01477447-20160222-01.

Malay, D. S., Pressman, M. M., Assili, A., Kline, J. T., York, S., Buren, B., Heyman, E. R., Borowsky, P., & LeMay, C. (2006). Extracorporeal shockwave therapy versus placebo for the treatment of chronic proximal plantar fasciitis: Results of a randomized, placebo-controlled, double-blinded, multicenter intervention trial. *The Journal of Foot and Ankle Surgery, 45*(4), 196–210. https://doi.org/10.1053/j.jfas.2006.04.007.

Martin, R. L., Irrgang, J. J., & Conti, S. F. (1998). Outcome study of subjects with insertional plantar fasciitis. *Foot & Ankle International, 19*(12), 803–811. https://doi.org/10.1177/107110079801901203.

McCarrel, T., & Fortier, L. (2009). Temporal growth factor release from platelet-rich plasma, trehalose lyophilized platelets, and bone marrow aspirate and their effect on tendon and ligament gene expression. *Journal of Orthopaedic Research, 27*(8), 1033–1042. https://doi.org/10.1002/jor.20853.

McCarthy, D. (1998). Nonsteroidal anti-inflammatory drug-related gastrointestinal toxicity: definitions and epidemiology. *The American Journal of Medicine, 105*(5), 3S-9S. https://doi.org/10.1016/S0002-9343(98)00274-5.

Monto, R. R. (2014). Platelet-rich plasma efficacy versus corticosteroid injection treatment for chronic severe plantar fasciitis. *Foot & Ankle International, 35*(4), 313–318. https://doi.org/10.1177/1071100713519778.

Neufeld, S. K., & Cerrato, R. (2008). Plantar fasciitis: Evaluation and treatment. *Journal of the American Academy of Orthopaedic Surgeons, 16*(6), 338–346. https://doi.org/10.5435/00124635-200806000-00006.

Ogden, J. A., Alvarez, R. G., & Marlow, M. (2002). Shockwave therapy for chronic proximal plantar fasciitis: A meta-analysis. *Foot & Ankle International, 23*(4), 301–308. https://doi.org/10.1177/107110070202300402.

Peerbooms, J. C., Lodder, P., den Oudsten, B. L., Doorgeest, K., Schuller, H. M., & Gosens, T. (2019). Positive effect of platelet-rich plasma on pain in plantar fasciitis: A double-blind multicenter randomized controlled trial. *The American Journal of Sports Medicine, 47*(13), 3238–3246. https://doi.org/10.1177/0363546519877181.

Salvi, A. E. (2015). Targeting the plantar fascia for corticosteroid injection. *The Journal of Foot and Ankle Surgery, 54*(4), 683–685. https://doi.org/10.1053/j.jfas.2014.10.011.

Schwartz, E. N., & Su, J. (2014). Plantar fasciitis: a concise review. *Perm J., 18*(1), e105-7. https://doi.org/10.7812/TPP/13-113.

Taunton, J. E. (2002). A retrospective case-control analysis of 2002 running injuries. *British Journal of Sports Medicine, 36*(2), 95–101. https://doi.org/10.1136/bjsm.36.2.95.

Tomczak, R. L., & Haverstock, B. D. (1995). A retrospective comparison of endoscopic plantar fasciotomy to open plantar fasciotomy with heel spur resection for chronic plantar fasciitis/heel spur syndrome. *The Journal of Foot and Ankle Surgery, 34*(3), 305–311. https://doi.org/10.1016/S1067-2516(09)80065-3.

Wolgin, M., Cook, C., Graham, C., & Mauldin, D. (1994). Conservative treatment of plantar heel pain: Long-term follow-up. *Foot & Ankle International, 15*(3), 97–102. https://doi.org/10.1177/107110079401500303.

Index

P

R

S

T

V

W